WORLD HEALTH ORGANIZATION

INTERNATIONAL AGENCY FOR RESEARCH ON CANCER

IARC MONOGRAPHS
ON THE
EVALUATION OF THE
CARCINOGENIC RISK
OF CHEMICALS TO HUMANS

Some Metals and Metallic Compounds

VOLUME 23

This publication represents the views and expert opinions
of an IARC Working Group on the
Evaluation of the Carcinogenic Risk of Chemicals to Humans
which met in Lyon,
23-30 October 1979

Juillet 1980

INTERNATIONAL AGENCY FOR RESEARCH ON CANCER

IARC MONOGRAPHS

In 1971, the International Agency for Research on Cancer (IARC) initiated a programme on the evaluation of the carcinogenic risk of chemicals to humans involving the production of critically evaluated monographs on individual chemicals.

The objective of the programme is to elaborate and publish in the form of monographs critical reviews of data on carcinogenicity for groups of chemicals to which humans are known to be exposed, to evaluate these data in terms of human risk with the help of international working groups of experts in chemical carcinogenesis and related fields, and to indicate where additional research efforts are needed.

International Agency for Research on Cancer 1980

ISBN 92 832 1223 1

PRINTED IN SWITZERLAND

CONTENTS

IARC WORKING GROUP ON THE EVALUATION OF THE CARCINOGENIC

RISK OF CHEMICALS TO HUMANS:

SOME METALS AND METALLIC COMPOUNDS

Lyon, 23-30 October 1979

Members[1]

F.K. Dzhioev, Laboratory of Chemical Carcinogenesis, N.N. Petrov Research Institute of Oncology, 68 Leningradskaya Street, Pesochny-2, Leningrad 188646, USSR

B.A. Fowler, Research Biologist, Laboratory of Organ Function and Toxicology, National Institute of Environmental Health Sciences, PO Box 12233, Research Triangle Park, NC 27709, USA

A. Furst, Director, Institute of Chemical Biology, University of San Francisco, Harney Science Center, San Francisco, CA 94117, USA

J.M. Harrington, London School of Hygiene and Tropical Medicine, Keppel Street (Gower Street), London WC1E 7HT, UK

P.F. Infante, Director, Office of Carcinogen Identification and Classification, Occupational Safety and Health Administration, US Department of Labor, 200 Constitution Avenue, NW, Washington DC 20210, USA

M. Kuratsune, Department of Public Health, Kyushu University, Faculty of Medicine, Fukuoka 812, Japan

A. G. Levis, Institute of Animal Biology, University of Padua, Via Loredan 10, 35100 Padua, Italy

G. Matanoski, Department of Epidemiology, School of Hygiene and Public Health, Johns Hopkins University, 615 N. Wolfe, Baltimore, MD 21218, USA *(Co-rapporteur section 3.3)*

[1] Unable to attend: J. Hasa, Czechoslovak Centre for the Environment, Tr. L. Novomeského 2, 816 43 Bratislava, Czechoslovakia; R. Ahlberg, Health and Safety Department, International Metalworkers' Federation, route des Acacias 54 bis, 1227 Geneva, Switzerland

N. Nelson, Professor and Chairman, Institute of Environmental Medicine, New York University Medical Center, 550 First Avenue, New York, NY 10016, USA *(Chairman)*

D. Neubert, Institut für Toxikologie und Embryonal-Pharmakologie der Freien Universität Berlin, Garystrasse 9, 1000 Berlin 33, Federal Republic of Germany *(Vice-chairman ; co-rapporteur section 3.2)*

G. Nordberg, Department of Community Health and Environmental Medicine, School of Medicine, Odense University, J.B. Winsløwsvej 19, 5000 Odense C, Denmark

R.M. Stern, Danish Welding Industry, Park Allé 345, 2600 Glostrup, Denmark

F.W. Sunderman, Jr, Professor of Laboratory Medicine and Pharmacology, University of Connecticut School of Medicine, 263 Farmington Avenue, Farmington, CT 06032, USA *(Co-rapporteur section 3.1)*

B. Teichmann, Department of Chemical Carcinogenesis, Zentralinstitut für Krebsforschung, Akademie der Wissenschaften der DDR, Lindenberger Weg 80, 1115 Berlin-Buch, German Democratic Republic

S. Venitt, Chemical Carcinogenesis Division, Institute of Cancer Research, Pollards Wood Research Station, Nightingales Lane, Chalfont St Giles, Bucks HP8 4SP, UK

Representative from the National Cancer Institute

J.I. Munn, National Cancer Institute, Landow Building - Room 8C25, 7910 Woodmont Avenue, Bethesda, MD 20014, USA

Representative from SRI International

O.H. Johnson, Senior Industrial Economist, Chemical-Environmental Program, SRI International, 333 Ravenswood Avenue, Menlo Park, CA 94025, USA *(Rapporteur sections 2.1 and 2.2)*

Representative from the Commission of the European Communities

A. Berlin, Commission of the European Communities, Health and Safety Directorate, Batiment Jean Monnet, Plateau du Kirchberg, Luxembourg, Grand Duchy of Luxembourg

Representative from the European Council of Chemical Manufacturers' Federation

E. Loser, Bayer AG, Institut für Toxikologie, Friedrich-Ebert-Strasse 217-319, 5600 Wuppertal 1, Federal Republic of Germany

Representative from the US Manufacturing Chemists' Association

R.L. O'Connell, Director, Corporate Health Affairs, Olin Corporation, 120 Long Ridge Road, Stamford, CT 06904, USA

Secretariat

C. Agthe, Division of Human Cancer and Field Programmes

H. Bartsch, Division of Chemical and Biological Carcinogenesis *(Co-rapporteur section 3.2)*

J.R.P. Cabral, Division of Chemical and Biological Carcinogenesis

M. Friesen, Division of Chemical and Biological Carcinogenesis

L. Griciute[1], Division of Chemical and Biological Carcinogenesis

V. Khudoley, Division of Chemical and Biological Carcinogenesis

D. Mietton, Division of Chemical and Biological Carcinogenesis *(Library assistant)*

R. Montesano, Division of Chemical and Biological Carcinogenesis *(Co-rapporteur section 3.1)*

C. Partensky, Division of Chemical and Biological Carcinogenesis *(Technical editor)*

I. Peterschmitt, Division of Chemical and Biological Carcinogenesis, WHO, Geneva *(Bibliographic researcher)*

R. Saracci, Division of Human Cancer and Field Programmes *(Co-rapporteur section 3.3)*

L. Tomatis, Director, Division of Chemical and Biological Carcinogenesis *(Head of the Programme)*

V.B. Vouk, Division of Environmental Health, WHO, Geneva

E.A. Walker, Division of Chemical and Biological Carcinogenesis *(Rapporteur sections 1 and 2.3)*

E. Ward, Montignac, France *(Editor)*

---

[1] Present address: The Oncological Institute of the Lithuanian SSR, 2 Polocko Street, 232007 Vilnius, Lithuanian SSR

J.D. Wilbourn, Division of Chemical and Biological Carcinogenesis *(Secretary)*

H. Yamasaki, Division of Chemical and Biological Carcinogenesis

Secretarial assistance

A. Beevers

M.-J. Ghess

A. Personnaz

J. Smith

NOTE TO THE READER

The term 'carcinogenic risk' in the *IARC Monograph* series is taken to mean the probability that exposure to the chemical will lead to cancer in humans.

Inclusion of a chemical in the monographs does not imply that it is a carcinogen, only that the published data have been examined. Equally, the fact that a chemical has not yet been evaluated in a monograph does not mean that it is not carcinogenic.

Anyone who is aware of published data that may alter the evaluation of the carcinogenic risk of a chemical for humans is encouraged to make this information available to the Division of Chemical and Biological Carcinogenesis, International Agency for Research on Cancer, Lyon, France, in order that the chemical may be considered for re-evaluation by a future Working Group.

Although every effort is made to prepare the monographs as accurately as possible, mistakes may occur. Readers are requested to communicate any errors to the Division of Chemical and Biological Carcinogenesis, so that corrections can be reported in future volumes.

IARC MONOGRAPH PROGRAMME ON THE EVALUATION OF THE CARCINOGENIC RISK OF CHEMICALS TO HUMANS

PREAMBLE

BACKGROUND

In 1971, the International Agency for Research on Cancer (IARC) initiated a programme on the evaluation of the carcinogenic risk of chemicals to humans with the object of producing monographs on individual chemicals[1]. The criteria established at that time to evaluate carcinogenic risk to humans were adopted by all the working groups whose deliberations resulted in the first 16 volumes of the *IARC Monograph* series. In October 1977, a joint IARC/WHO *ad hoc* Working Group met to re-evaluate these guiding criteria; this preamble reflects the results of their deliberations(1) and those of a subsequent IARC *ad hoc* Working Group which met in April 1978(2).

OBJECTIVE AND SCOPE

The objective of the programme is to elaborate and publish in the form of monographs critical reviews of data on carcinogenicity for groups of chemicals to which humans are known to be exposed, to evaluate these data in terms of human risk with the help of international working groups of experts in chemical carcinogenesis and related fields, and to indicate where additional research efforts are needed.

The monographs summarize the evidence for the carcinogenicity of individual chemicals and other relevant information. The critical analyses of the data are intended to assist national and international authorities in formulating decisions concerning preventive measures. No recommendations are given concerning legislation, since this depends on risk-benefit evaluations, which seem best made by individual governments and/or other International agencies. In this connection, WHO recommendations on food additives(3), drugs(4), pesticides and contaminants(5) and occupational carcinogens(6) are particularly informative.

---

[1] Since 1972, the programme has undergone considerable expansion, primarily with the scientific collaboration and financial support of the US National Cancer Institute, Bethesda, MD

The *IARC Monographs* are recognized as an authoritative source of information on the carcinogenicity of environmental chemicals. The first users' survey, made in 1976, indicates that the monographs are consulted routinely by various agencies in 24 countries.

Since the programme began in 1971, 23 volumes have been published[7] in the *IARC Monograph* series, and 515 separate chemical substances have been evaluated (see also cumulative index to the monographs, p. 419   ). Each volume is printed in 4000 copies and distributed *via* the WHO publications service (see inside covers for a listing of IARC publications and back outside cover for distribution and sales services).

SELECTION OF CHEMICALS FOR MONOGRAPHS

The chemicals (natural and synthetic, including those which occur as mixtures and in manufacturing processes) are selected for evaluation on the basis of two main criteria: (a) there is evidence of human exposure, and (b) there is some experimental evidence of carcinogenicity and/or there is some evidence or suspicion of a risk to humans. In certain instances, chemical analogues were also considered. The scientific literature is surveyed for published data relevant to the monograph programme. In addition, the IARC *Survey of Chemicals Being Tested for Carcinogenicity*[8] often indicates those chemicals that are to be scheduled for future meetings.

Inclusion of a chemical in a volume does not imply that it is carcinogenic, only that the published data have been examined. The evaluations must be consulted to ascertain the conclusions of the Working Group. Equally, the fact that a chemical has not appeared in a monograph does not mean that it is without carcinogenic hazard.

As new data on chemicals for which monographs have already been prepared and new principles for evaluating carcinogenic risk receive acceptance, re-evaluations will be made at subsequent meetings, and revised monographs will be published as necessary.

WORKING PROCEDURES

Approximately one year in advance of a meeting of a working group, a list of the substances to be considered is prepared by IARC staff in consultation with other experts. Subsequently, all relevant biological data are collected by IARC; in addition to the published literature, US Public Health Service Publication No. 149[9] has been particularly valuable and has been used in conjunction with other recognized sources of information on chemical carcinogenesis and systems such as CANCERLINE, MEDLINE and TOXLINE. The major collection of data and the preparation of first drafts for the sections on chemical and physical properties, on production, use, occurrence and on analysis are carried out by SRI International, Stanford, CA, USA under a separate contract with the US National Cancer

Institute. Most of the data so obtained on production, use and occurrence refer to the United States and Japan; SRI International and IARC supplement this information with that from other sources in Europe. Bibliographical sources for data on mutagenicity and teratogenicity are the Environmental Mutagen Information Center and the Environmental Teratology Information Center, both located at the Oak Ridge National Laboratory, TN, USA.

Six to nine months before the meeting, reprints of articles containing relevant biological data are sent to an expert(s), or are used by the IARC staff, for the preparation of first draft monographs. These drafts are edited by IARC staff and are sent prior to the meeting to all participants of the Working Group for their comments. The Working Group then meets in Lyon for seven to eight days to discuss and finalize the texts of the monographs and to formulate the evaluations. After the meeting, the master copy of each monograph is verified by consulting the original literature, then edited and prepared for reproduction. The monographs are usually published within six months after the Working Group meeting.

DATA FOR EVALUATIONS

With regard to biological data, only reports that have been published or accepted for publication are reviewed by the working groups, although a few exceptions have been made. The monographs do not cite all of the literature on a particular chemical: only those data considered by the Working Group to be relevant to the evaluation of the carcinogenic risk of the chemical to humans are included.

Anyone who is aware of data that have been published or are in press which are relevant to the evaluations of the carcinogenic risk to humans of chemicals for which monographs have appeared is urged to make them available to the Division of Chemical and Biological Carcinogenesis, International Agency for Research on Cancer, Lyon, France.

THE WORKING GROUP

The tasks of the Working Group are five-fold: (a) to ascertain that all data have been collected; (b) to select the data relevant for the evaluation; (c) to ensure that the summaries of the data enable the reader to follow the reasoning of the committee; (d) to judge the significance of the results of experimental and epidemiological studies; and (e) to make an evaluation of the carcinogenic risk of the chemical.

Working Group participants who contributed to the consideration and evaluation of chemicals within a particular volume are listed, with their addresses, at the beginning of each publication (see p. 5   ). Each member serves as an individual scientist and not as a representative of any organization or government. In addition, observers are often invited from national and international agencies, organizations and industries.

GENERAL PRINCIPLES FOR EVALUATING THE CARCINOGENIC RISK OF CHEMICALS

The widely accepted meaning of the term 'chemical carcinogenesis', and that used in these monographs, is the induction by chemicals of neoplasms that are not usually observed, the earlier induction by chemicals of neoplasms that are usually observed, and/or the induction by chemicals of more neoplasms than are usually found - although fundamentally different mechanisms may be involved in these three situations. Etymologically, the term 'carcinogenesis' means the induction of cancer, that is, of malignant neoplasms ; however, the commonly accepted meaning is the induction of various types of neoplasms or of a combination of malignant and benign tumours. In the monographs, the words 'tumour' and 'neoplasm' are used interchangeably (In scientific literature the terms 'tumourigen', 'oncogen', and 'blastomogen', have all been used synonymously with 'carcinogen', although occasionally 'tumourigen' has been used specifically to denote a substance that induces benign tumours).

Experimental Evidence

Qualitative aspects

Both the interpretation and evaluation of a particular study as well as the overall assessment of the carcinogenic activity of a chemical involve several qualitatively important considerations, including: (a) the experimental parameters under which the chemical was tested, including route of administration and exposure, species, strain, sex, age, etc.; (b) the consistency with which the chemical has been shown to be carcinogenic, e.g., in how many species and at which target organ(s); (c) the spectrum of neoplastic response, from benign neoplasia to multiple malignant tumours; (d) the stage of tumour formation in which a chemical may be involved: some chemicals act as complete carcinogens and have initiating and promoting activity, while others are promoters only; and (e) the possible role of modifying factors.

There are problems not only of differential survival but of differential toxicity, which may be manifested by unequal growth and weight gain in treated and control animals. These complexities should also be considered in the interpretation of data, or, better, in the experimental design.

Many chemicals induce both benign and malignant tumours ; few instances are recorded in which only benign neoplasms are induced by chemicals that have been studied extensively. Benign tumours may represent a stage in the evolution of a malignant neoplasm or they may be 'end-points' that do not readily undergo transition to malignancy. If a substance is found to induce only benign tumours in experimental animals, the chemical should be suspected of being a carcinogen and requires further investigation.

Hormonal carcinogenesis

Hormonal carcinogenesis presents certain distinctive features: the chemicals involved occur both endogenously and exogenously; in many instances, long exposure is required; tumours occur in the target tissue in association with a stimulation of non-neoplastic growth, but in some cases, hormones promote the proliferation of tumour cells in a target organ. Hormones that occur in excessive amounts, hormone-mimetic agents and agents that cause hyperactivity or imbalance in the endocrine system may require evaluative methods comparable with those used to identify chemical carcinogens; particular emphasis must be laid on quantitative aspects and duration of exposure. Some chemical carcinogens have significant side effects on the endocrine system, which may also result in hormonal carcinogenesis. Synthetic hormones and anti-hormones can be expected to possess other pharmacological and toxicological actions in addition to those on the endocrine system, and in this respect they must be treated like any other chemical with regard to intrinsic carcinogenic potential.

Quantitative aspects

Dose-response studies are important in the evaluation of carcinogenesis: the confidence with which a carcinogenic effect can be established is strengthened by the observation of an increasing incidence of neoplasms with increasing exposure.

The assessment of carcinogenicity in animals is frequently complicated by recognized differences among the test animals (species, strain, sex, age), route(s) of administration and in dose/duration of exposure; often, target organs at which a cancer occurs and its histological type may vary with these parameters. Nevertheless, indices of carcinogenic potency in particular experimental systems [for instance, the dose-rate required under continuous exposure to halve the probability of the animals remaining tumourless(10)] have been formulated in the hope that, at least among categories of fairly similar agents, such indices may be of some predictive value in other systems, including humans.

Chemical carcinogens differ widely in the dose required to produce a given level of tumour induction, although many of them share common biological properties, which include metabolism to reactive [electrophilic(11-13)] intermediates capable of interacting with DNA. The reason for this variation in dose-response is not understood, but it may be due either to differences within a common metabolic process or to the operation of qualitatively distinct mechanisms.

Statistical analysis of animal studies

Tumours which would have arisen had an animal lived longer may not be observed because of the death of the animal from unrelated causes, and this possibility must be allowed for. Various analytical techniques have been developed which use the assumption of independence of competing risks to allow for the effects of intercurrent mortality on the final numbers of tumour-bearing animals in particular treatment groups.

For externally visible tumours and for neoplasms that cause death, methods such as Kaplan-Meier (i.e., 'life-table', 'product-limit', or 'actuarial') estimates(10), with associated significance tests(14,15), are recommended.

For internal neoplasms which are discovered 'incidentally'(14) at autopsy but which did not cause the death of the host, different estimates(16) and significance tests(14,15) may be necessary for the unbiased study of the numbers of tumour-bearing animals.

All of these methods(10,14-16) can be used to analyse the numbers of animals bearing particular tumour types, but they do not distinguish between animals with one or many such tumours. In experiments which end at a particular fixed time, with the simultaneous sacrifice of many animals, analysis of the total numbers of internal neoplasms per animal found at autopsy at the end of the experiment is straightforward. However, there are no adequate statistical methods for analysing the numbers of particular neoplasms that kill an animal.

Evidence of Carcinogenicity in Humans

Evidence of carcinogenicity in humans can be derived from three types of study, the first two of which usually provide only suggestive evidence: (1) reports concerning individual cancer patients (case reports), including a history of exposure to the supposed carcinogenic agent; (2) descriptive epidemiological studies in which the incidence of cancer in human populations is found to vary (spatially or temporally) with exposure to the agent; and (3) analytical epidemiological studies (e.g., case-control or cohort studies) in which individual exposure to the agent is found to be associated with an increased risk of cancer.

An analytical study that shows a positive association between an agent and a cancer may be interpreted as implying causality to a greater or lesser extent, if the following criteria are met: (a) there is no identifiable positive bias (By 'positive bias' is meant the operation of factors in study design or execution which lead erroneously to a more strongly positive association between an agent and disease than in fact exists. Examples of positive bias include, in case-control studies, better documentation of exposure to the agent for cases than for controls, and, in cohort studies, the use of better means of detecting cancer in individuals exposed to the agent than in individuals not exposed); (b) the possibility of positive confounding has been considered (By 'positive confounding' is meant a situation in which the relationship between an agent and a disease is rendered more strongly positive than it truly is as a result of an association between that agent and another agent which either causes or prevents the disease. An example of positive confounding is the association between coffee consumption and lung cancer, which results from their joint association with cigarette smoking); (c) the association is unlikely to be due to chance alone; (d) the association is strong; and (e) there is a dose-response relationship.

In some instances, a single epidemiological study may be strongly indicative of a cause-effect relationship; however, the most convincing evidence of causality comes when several independent studies done under different circumstances result in 'positive' findings.

Analytical epidemiological studies that show no association between an agent and a cancer ('negative' studies) should be interpreted according to criteria analogous to those listed above: (a) there is no identifiable negative bias; (b) the possibility of negative confounding has been considered; and (c) the possible effects of misclassification of exposure or outcome have been weighed.

In addition, it must be recognized that in any study there are confidence limits around the estimate of association or relative risk. In a study regarded as 'negative', the upper confidence limit may indicate a relative risk substantially greater than unity; in that case, the study excludes only relative risks that are above this upper limit. This usually means that a 'negative' study must be large to be convincing. Confidence in a 'negative' result is increased when several independent studies carried out under different circumstances are in agreement.

Finally, a 'negative' study may be considered to be relevant only to dose levels within or below the range of those observed in the study and is pertinent only if sufficient time has elapsed since first human exposure to the agent. Experience with human cancers of known etiology suggests that the period from first exposure to a chemical carcinogen to development of clinically observed cancer is usually measured in decades and may be in excess of 30 years.

Experimental Data Relevant to the Evaluation of Carcinogenic Risk to Humans

No adequate criteria are presently available to interpret experimental carcinogenicity data directly in terms of carcinogenic potential for humans. Nonetheless, utilizing data collected from appropriate tests in animals, positive extrapolations to possible human risk can be approximated.

Information compiled from the first 23 volumes of the *IARC Monographs*(17-19) shows that of the 37 chemicals, groups of chemicals or manufacturing processes now generally accepted to cause or probably to cause cancer in humans, all but possibly two (arsenic and benzene) of those which have been tested appropriately produce cancer in at least one animal species. For several of the chemicals that are carcinogenic for humans (aflatoxins, 4-aminobiphenyl, diethylstilboestrol, melphalan, mustard gas and vinyl chloride), evidence of carcinogenicity in experimental animals preceded evidence obtained from epidemiological studies or case reports.

In general, the evidence that a chemical produces tumours in experimental animals is of two degrees: (a) *sufficient evidence* of carcinogenicity is provided by the production of malignant tumours; and (b) *limited evidence* of carcinogenicity reflects qualitative and/or quantitative limitations of the experimental results.

For many of the chemicals evaluated in the first 23 volumes of the *IARC Monographs* for which there is *sufficient evidence* of carcinogenicity in animals, data relating to carcinogenicity for humans are either insufficient or nonexistent. In the absence of adequate data on humans, it is reasonable, for practical purposes, to regard such chemicals as if they presented a carcinogenic risk to humans.

Sufficient evidence of carcinogenicity is provided by experimental studies that show an increased incidence of malignant tumours: (i) in multiple species or strains, and/or (ii) in multiple experiments (routes and/or doses), and/or (iii) to an unusual degree (with regard to incidence, site, type and/or precocity of onset). Additional evidence may be provided by data concerning dose-response, mutagenicity or structure.

In the present state of knowledge, it would be difficult to define a predictable relationship between the dose (mg/kg bw/day) of a particular chemical required to produce cancer in test animals and the dose which would produce a similar incidence of cancer in humans. The available data suggest, however, that such a relationship may exist(20,21), at least for certain classes of carcinogenic chemicals. Data that provide *sufficient evidence* of carcinogenicity in test animals may therefore be used in an approximate quantitative evaluation of the human risk at some given exposure level, provided that the nature of the chemical concerned and the physiological, pharmacological and toxicological differences between the test animals and humans are taken into account. However, no acceptable methods are currently available for quantifying the possible errors in such a procedure, whether it is used to generalize between species or to extrapolate from high to low doses. The methodology for such quantitative extrapolation to humans requires further development.

Evidence for the carcinogenicity of some chemicals in experimental animals may be *limited* for two reasons. Firstly, experimental data may be restricted to such a point that it is not possible to determine a causal relationship between administration of a chemical and the development of a particular lesion in the animals. Secondly, there are certain neoplasms, including lung tumours and hepatomas in mice, which have been considered of lesser significance than neoplasms occurring at other sites for the purpose of evaluating the carcinogenicity of chemicals. Such tumours occur spontaneously in high incidence in these animals, and their malignancy is often difficult to establish. An evaluation of the significance of these tumours following administration of a chemical is the responsibility of particular Working Groups preparing individual monographs, and it has not been possible to set down rigid guidelines; the relevance of these tumours must be determined by considerations which include experimental design and completeness of reporting.

Some chemicals for which there is *limited evidence* of carcinogenicity in animals have also been studied in humans with, in general, inconclusive results. While such chemicals may indeed be carcinogenic to humans, more experimental and epidemiological investigation is required.

Hence *'sufficient evidence'* of carcinogenicity and *'limited evidence'* of carcinogenicity do not indicate categories of chemicals: the inherent definitions of those terms indicate varying degrees of experimental evidence, which may change if and when new data on the chemicals become available. The main drawback to any rigid classification of chemicals with regard to their carcinogenic capacity is the as yet incomplete knowledge of the mechanism(s) of carcinogenesis.

In recent years, several short-term tests for the detection of potential carcinogens have been developed. When only inadequate experimental data are available, positive results in validated short-term tests (see p. 23) are an indication that the compound is a potential carcinogen and that it should be tested in animals for an assessment of its carcinogenicity. Negative results from short-term tests cannot be considered sufficient evidence to rule out carcinogenicity. Whether short-term tests will eventually be as reliable as long-term tests in predicting carcinogenicity in humans will depend on further demonstrations of consistency with long-term experiments and with data from humans.

EXPLANATORY NOTES ON THE MONOGRAPH CONTENTS

Chemical and Physical Data (Section 1)

The Chemical Abstracts Service Registry Number, the latest Chemical Abstracts Primary Name (9th Collective Index)(22) and the IUPAC Systematic Name(23) are recorded in section 1. Other synonyms and trade names are given, but no comprehensive list is provided. Further, some of the trade names are those of mixtures in which the compound being evaluated is only one of the ingredients.

The structural and molecular formulae, molecular weight and chemical and physical properties are given. The properties listed refer to the pure substance, unless otherwise specified, and include, in particular, data that might be relevant to carcinogenicity (e.g., lipid solubility) and those that concern identification. In this volume, ultra-violet spectrometric data are expressed in a new symbol devised by the International Union of Spectroscopists, A (1%, 1 cm), i.e., absorbance of a 1% solution examined as a 1-cm layer.

A separate description of the composition of technical products includes available information on impurities and formulated products.

Production, Use, Occurrence and Analysis (Section 2)

The purpose of section 2 is to provide indications of the extent of past and present human exposure to this chemical.

Synthesis

Since cancer is a delayed toxic effect, the dates of first synthesis and of first commercial production of the chemical are provided. In addition, methods of synthesis used in past and present commercial production are described. This information allows a reasonable estimate to be made of the date before which no human exposure could have occurred.

Production

Since Europe, Japan and the United States are reasonably representative industrialized areas of the world, most data on production, foreign trade and uses are obtained from those countries. It should not, however, be inferred that those nations are the sole or even the major sources or users of any individual chemical.

Production and foreign trade data are obtained from both governmental and trade publications by chemical economists in the three geographical areas. In some cases, separate production data on organic chemicals manufactured in the United States are not available because their publication could disclose confidential information. In such cases, an indication of the minimum quantity produced can be inferred from the number of companies reporting commercial production. Each company is required to report on individual chemicals if the sales value or the weight of the annual production exceeds a specified minimum level. These levels vary for chemicals classified for different uses, e.g., medicinals and plastics; in fact, the minimal annual sales value is between $1000 and $50,000 and the minimal annual weight of production is between 450 and 22, 700 kg. Data on production in some

European countries are obtained by means of general questionnaires sent to companies thought to produce the compounds being evaluated. Information from the completed questionnaires is compiled by country, and the resulting estimates of production are included in the individual monographs.

Use

Information on uses is meant to serve as a guide only and is not complete. It is usually obtained from published data but is often complemented by direct contact with manufacturers of the chemical. In the case of drugs, mention of their therapeutic uses does not necessarily represent current practice nor does it imply judgement as to their clinical efficacy.

Statements concerning regulations and standards (e.g., pesticide registrations, maximum levels permitted in foods, occupational standards and allowable limits) in specific countries are mentioned as examples only. They may not reflect the most recent situation, since such legislation is in a constant state of change; nor should it be taken to imply that other countries do not have similar regulations.

Occurrence

Information on the occurrence of a chemical in the environment is obtained from published data including that derived from the monitoring and surveillance of levels of the chemical in occupational environments, air, water, soil, foods and tissues of animals and humans. When available, data on the generation, persistence and bioaccumulation of a chemical are also included.

Analysis

The purpose of the section on analysis is to give the reader an indication, rather than a complete review, of methods cited in the literature. No attempt is made to evaluate critically or to recommend any of the methods.

Biological Data Relevant to the Evaluation of Carcinogenic Risk to Humans (Section 3)

In general, the data recorded in section 3 are summarized as given by the author; however, comments made by the Working Group on certain shortcomings of reporting, of statistical analysis or of experimental design are given in square brackets. The nature and extent of impurities/contaminants in the chemicals being tested are given when available.

Carcinogenicity studies in animals

The monographs are not intended to cover all reported studies. Some studies are purposely omitted (a) because they are inadequate, as judged from previously described criteria(24-27) (e.g., too short a duration, too few animals, poor survival); (b) because they only confirm findings that have already been fully described; or (c) because they are judged irrelevant for the purpose of the evaluation. In certain cases, however, such studies are mentioned briefly, particularly when the information is considered to be a useful supplement to other reports or when it is the only data available. Their inclusion does not, however, imply acceptance of the adequacy of their experimental design and/or of the analysis and interpretation of their results.

Mention is made of all routes of administration by which the compound has been adequately tested and of all species in which relevant tests have been done(5, 26). In most cases, animal strains are given [General characteristics of mouse strains have been reviewed (28)]. Quantitative data are given to indicate the order of magnitude of the effective carcinogenic doses. In general, the doses and schedules are indicated as they appear in the paper; sometimes units have been converted for easier comparison. Experiments in which the compound was administered in conjunction with known carcinogens and experiments on factors that modify the carcinogenic effect are also reported. Experiments on the carcinogenicity of known metabolites, chemical precursors, analogues and derivatives are also included.

Other relevant biological data

Lethality data are given when available, and other data on toxicity are included when considered relevant. The metabolic data are restricted to studies that show the metabolic fate of the chemical in animals and humans, and comparisons of data from animals and humans are made when possible. Information is also given on absorption, distribution, excretion and placental transfer.

Effects on reproduction and prenatal toxicity

Data on effects on reproduction, teratogenicity, feto- and embryotoxicity from studies in experimental animals and from observations in humans are also included. There appears to be no causal relationship between teratogenicity (29) and carcinogenicity, but chemicals often have both properties. Evidence of prenatal toxicity suggests transplacental transfer, which is a prerequisite for transplacental carcinogenesis.

Indirect tests (mutagenicity and other short-term tests)

Data from indirect tests are also included. Since most of these tests have the advantage of taking less time and being less expensive than mammalian carcinogenicity studies, they are generally known as 'short-term' tests. They comprise assay procedures which rely on the induction of biological and biochemical effects in *in vivo* and/or *in vitro* systems. The end-point of the majority of these tests is the production not of neoplasms in animals but of changes at the molecular, cellular or multicellular level: these include the induction of DNA damage and repair, mutagenesis in bacteria and other organisms, transformation of mammalian cells in culture, and other systems.

The short-term tests are proposed for use (a) in predicting potential carcinogenicity in the absence of carcinogenicity data in animals, (b) as a contribution in deciding which chemicals should be tested in animals, (c) in identifying active fractions of complex mixtures containing carcinogens, (d) for recognizing active metabolites of known carcinogens in human and/or animal body fluids and (e) to help elucidate mechanisms of carcinogenesis.

Although the theory that cancer is induced as a result of somatic mutation suggests that agents which damage DNA *in vivo* may be carcinogens, the precise relevance of short-term tests to the mechanism by which cancer is induced is not known. Predictions of potential carcinogenicity are currently based on correlations between responses in short-term tests and data from animal carcinogenicity and/or human epidemiological studies. This approach is limited because the number of chemicals known to be carcinogenic in humans is insufficient to provide a basis for validation, and most validation studies involve chemicals that have been evaluated for carcinogenicity only in animals. The selection of chemicals is in turn limited to those classes for which data on carcinogenicity are available. The results of validation studies could be strongly influenced by such selection of chemicals and by the proportion of carcinogens in the series of chemicals tested; this should be kept in mind when evaluating the predictivity of a particular test. The usefulness of any test is reflected by its ability to classify carcinogens and noncarcinogens, using the animal data as a standard; however, animal tests may not always provide a perfect standard. The attainable level of correlation between short-term tests and animal bioassays is still under investigation.

Since many chemicals require metabolism to an active form, tests that do not take this into account may fail to detect certain potential carcinogens. The metabolic activation systems used in short-term tests (e.g., the cell-free systems used in bacterial tests) are meant to approximate the metabolic capacity of the whole organism. Each test has its advantages and limitations; thus, more confidence can be placed in the conclusions when negative or positive results for a chemical are confirmed in several such test systems. Deficiencies in metabolic competence may lead to misclassification of chemicals, which means that not all tests are suitable for assessing the potential carcinogenicity of all classes of compounds.

The present state of knowledge does not permit the selection of a specific test(s) as the most appropriate for identifying potential carcinogenicity. Before the results of a particular test can be considered to be fully acceptable for predicting potential carcino- genicity, certain criteria should be met: (a) the test should have been validated with respect to known animal carcinogens and found to have a high capacity for discriminating between carcinogens and noncarcinogens, and (b), when possible, a structurally related carcinogen(s) and noncarcinogen(s) should have been tested simultaneously with the chemical in question. The results should have been reproduced in different laboratories, and a prediction of car- cinogenicity should have been confirmed in additional test systems. Confidence in positive results is increased if a mechanism of action can be deduced and if appropriate dose-response data are available. For optimum usefulness, data on purity must be given.

The short-term tests in current use that have been the most extensively validated are the *Salmonella typhimurium* plate-incorporation assay(30-34), the X-linked recessive lethal test in *Drosophila melanogaster*(35), unscheduled DNA synthesis(36) and *in vitro* transform- ation(34,37). Each is compatible with current concepts of the possible mechanism(s) of car- cinogenesis.

An adequate assessment of the genetic activity of a chemical depends on data from a wide range of test systems. The monographs include, therefore, data not only from those already mentioned, but also on the induction of point mutations in other systems(38-43), on structural(44) and numerical chromosome aberrations, including dominant lethal effects (45), on mitotic recombination in fungi(38) and on sister chromatid exchanges(46-48).

The existence of a correlation between quantitative aspects of mutagenic and carcino- genic activity has been suggested (5,45-51) , but it is not sufficiently well established to allow general use.

Further information about mutagenicity and other short-term tests is given in references 46-54.

Case reports and epidemiological studies

Observations in humans are summarized in this section.

Summary of Data Reported and Evaluation (Section 4)

Section 4 summarizes the relevant data from animals and humans and gives the critical views of the Working Group on those data.

Experimental data

Data relevant to the evaluation of the carcinogenicity of the chemical in animals are summarized in this section. The animal species mentioned are those in which the carcinogenicity of the substance was clearly demonstrated. Tumour sites are also indicated. If the substance has produced tumours after prenatal exposure or in single-dose experiments, this is indicated. Dose-response data are given when available.

Results from validated mutagenicity and other short-term tests and from tests for prenatal toxicity are reported if the Working Group considered the data to be relevant.

Human data

Case reports and epidemiological studies that are considered to be pertinent to an assessment of human carcinogenicity are described. Human exposure to the chemical is summarized on the basis of data on production, use and occurrence. Other biological data which are considered to be relevant are also mentioned.

Evaluation

This section comprises the overall evaluation by the Working Group of the carcinogenic risk of the chemical to humans. All of the data in the monograph, and particularly the summarized information on experimental and human data, are considered in order to make this evaluation.

References

1. IARC (1977)   IARC Monograph Programme on the Evaluation of the Carcinogenic Risk of Chemicals to Humans.   Preamble.   *IARC intern. tech. Rep. No. 77/002*

2. IARC (1978)   Chemicals with *sufficient evidence* of carcinogenicity in experimental animals - *IARC Monographs* volumes 1-17.   *IARC intern. tech. Rep. No. 78/003*

3. WHO (1961) Fifth Report of the Joint FAO/WHO Expert Committee on Food Additives. Evaluation of carcinogenic hazard of food additives. *WHO tech. Rep. Ser., No. 220*, pp. 5, 18, 19

4. WHO (1969) Report of a WHO Scientific Group. Principles for the testing and evaluation of drugs for carcinogenicity. *WHO tech. Rep. Ser. , No. 426*, pp. 19, 21, 22

5. WHO (1974)   Report of a WHO Scientific Group.   Assessment of the carcinogenicity and mutagenicity of chemicals. *WHO tech. Rep. Ser., No. 546*

6. WHO (1964) Report of a WHO Expert Committee. Prevention of cancer. *WHO tech. Rep. Ser., No. 276*, pp. 29, 30

7. IARC (1972-1980)   *IARC Monographs on the Evaluation of the Carcinogenic Risk of Chemicals to Humans*, Volumes 1-23, Lyon, France

    Volume 1 (1972) Some Inorganic Substances, Chlorinated Hydrocarbons, Aromatic Amines, *N*-Nitroso Compounds and Natural Products (19 monographs), 184 pages

    Volume 2 (1973) Some Inorganic and Organometallic Compounds (7 monographs), 181 pages

    Volume 3 (1973) Certain Polycyclic Aromatic Hydrocarbons and Heterocyclic Compounds (17 monographs), 271 pages

    Volume 4 (1974) Some Aromatic Amines, Hydrazine and Related Substances, *N*-Nitroso Compounds and Miscellaneous Alkylating Agents (28 monographs), 286 pages

    Volume 5 (1974) Some Organochlorine Pesticides (12 monographs), 241 pages

    Volume 6 (1974) Sex Hormones (15 monographs), 243 pages

Volume 7 (1974) Some Anti-thyroid and Related Substances, Nitrofurans and Industrial Chemicals (23 monographs), 326 pages

Volume 8 (1975) Some Aromatic Azo Compounds (32 monographs), 357 pages

Volume 9 (1975) Some Aziridines, *N*-, *S*- and *O*-Mustards and Selenium (24 monographs), 268 pages

Volume 10 (1976) Some Naturally Occurring Substances (32 monographs), 353 pages

Volume 11 (1976) Cadmium, Nickel, Some Epoxides, Miscellaneous Industrial Chemicals and General Considerations on Volatile Anaesthetics (24 monographs), 306 pages

Volume 12 (1976) Some Carbamates, Thiocarbamates and Carbazides (24 monographs), 282 pages

Volume 13 (1977) Some Miscellaneous Pharmaceutical Substances (17 monographs), 255 pages

Volume 14 (1977) Asbestos (1 monograph), 106 pages

Volume 15 (1977) Some Fumigants, the Herbicides 2,4-D and 2,4,5-T, Chlorinated Dibenzodioxins and Miscellaneous Industrial Chemicals (18 monographs), 354 pages

Volume 16 (1978) Some Aromatic Amines and Related Nitro Compounds - Hair Dyes, Colouring Agents, and Miscellaneous Industrial Chemicals (32 monographs), 400 pages

Volume 17 (1978) Some *N*-Nitroso Compounds (17 monographs), 365 pages

Volume 18 (1978) Polychlorinated Biphenyls and Polybrominated Biphenyls (2 monographs), 140 pages

Volume 19 (1979) Some Monomers, Plastics and Synthetic Elastomers, and Acrolein (17 monographs), 513 pages

Volume 20 (1979) Some Halogenated Hydrocarbons (25 monographs), 609 pages

Volume 21 (1979) Sex Hormones (II) (22 monographs), 583 pages

Volume 22 (1980) Some Non-Nutritive Sweetening Agents (2 monographs), 208 pages

Volume 23 (1980) Some Metals and Metallic Compounds (4 monographs), 438 pages

8.   IARC (1973-1979) *Information Bulletin on the Survey of Chemicals Being Tested for Carcinogenicity*, Numbers 1-8, Lyon, France

Number 1 (1973) 52 pages
Number 2 (1973) 77 pages
Number 3 (1974) 67 pages
Number 4 (1974) 97 pages
Number 5 (1975) 88 pages
Number 6 (1976) 360 pages
Number 7 (1978) 460 pages
Number 8 (1979) 604 pages

9.   PHS 149 (1951-1976) Public Health Service Publication No. 149, *Survey of Compounds which have been Tested for Carcinogenic Activity*, Washington DC, US Government Printing Office

1951   Hartwell, J.L., 2nd ed., Literature up to 1947 on 1329 compounds, 583 pages

1957   Shubik, P. & Hartwell, J.L., Supplement 1, Literature for the years 1948-1953 on 981 compounds, 388 pages

1969   Shubik, P. & Hartwell, J.L., edited by Peters, J.A., Supplement 2, Literature for the years 1954-1960 on 1048 compounds, 655 pages

1971   National Cancer Institute, Literature for the years 1968-1969 on 882 compounds, 653 pages

1973   National Cancer Institute, Literature for the years 1961-1967 on 1632 compounds, 2343 pages

1974   National Cancer Institute, Literature for the years 1970-1971 on 750 compounds, 1667 pages

1976   National Cancer Institute, Literature for the years 1972-1973 on 966 compounds, 1638 pages

10. Pike, M.C. & Roe, F.J.C. (1963) An actuarial method of analysis of an experiment in two-stage carcinogenesis. *Br. J. Cancer, 17*, 605-610

11. Miller, E.C. & Miller, J.A. (1966) Mechanisms of chemical carcinogenesis: nature of proximate carcinogens and interactions with macromolecules. *Pharmacol. Rev., 18*, 805-838

12. Miller, J.A. (1970) Carcinogenesis by chemicals: an overview - G.H.A. Clowes Memorial Lecture. *Cancer Res., 30*, 559-576

13. Miller, J.A. & Miller, E.C. (1976) *The metabolic activation of chemical carcinogens to reactive electrophiles.* In: Yuhas, J.M., Tennant, R.W. & Reagon, J.D., eds, *Biology of Radiation Carcinogenesis*, New York, Raven Press

14. Peto, R. (1974) Guidelines on the analysis of tumours rates and death rates in experimental animals. *Br. J. Cancer, 29*, 101-105

15. Peto, R. (1975) Letter to the editor. *Br. J. Cancer, 31*, 697-699

16. Hoel, D.G. & Walburg, H.E., Jr (1972) Statistical analysis of survival experiments. *J. natl Cancer Inst., 49*, 361-372

17. IARC Working Group (1980) An evaluation of chemicals and industrial processes associated with cancer in humans based on human and animal data : *IARC Monographs* Volumes 1 to 20. *Cancer Res., 40*, 1-12

18. IARC (1979) *IARC Monographs on the Evaluation of the Carcinogenic Risk of Chemicals to Humans, Supplement 1, Chemicals and Industrial Processes Associated with Cancer in Humans*, Lyon, France

19. IARC (1979) *Annual Report 1979*, Lyon, International Agency for Research on Cancer, pp. 89-99

20. Rall, D.P. (1977) *Species differences in carcinogenesis testing.* In: Hiatt, H.H., Watson, J.D. & Winsten, J.A., eds, *Origins of Human Cancer*, Book C, Cold Spring Harbor, NY, Cold Spring Harbor Laboratory, pp. 1383-1390

21. National Academy of Sciences (NAS) (1975) *Contemporary Pest Control Practices and Prospects: the Report of the Executive Committee*, Washington DC

22. Chemical Abstracts Service (1978) *Chemical Abstracts Ninth Collective Index (9CI), 1972-1976*, Vols 76-85, Columbus, Ohio

23. International Union of Pure & Applied Chemistry (1965) *Nomenclature of Organic Chemistry*, Section C, London, Butterworths

24. WHO (1958) Second Report of the Joint FAO/WHO Expert Committee on Food Additives. Procedures for the testing of intentional food additives to establish their safety and use. *WHO tech. Rep. Ser., No. 144*

25. WHO (1967) Scientific Group. Procedures for investigating intentional and unintentional food additives. *WHO tech. Rep. Ser., No. 348*

26. Berenblum, I., ed. (1969) Carcinogenicity testing. *UICC tech. Rep. Ser., 2*

27. Sontag, J.M., Page, N.P. & Saffiotti, U. (1976) Guidelines for carcinogen bioassay in small rodents. *Natl Cancer Inst. Carcinog. tech. Rep. Ser., No. 1*

28. Committee on Standardized Genetic Nomenclature for Mice (1972) Standardized nomenclature for inbred strains of mice. Fifth listing. *Cancer Res., 32*, 1609-1646

29. Wilson, J.G. & Fraser, F.C. (1977) *Handbook of Teratology*, New York, Plenum Press

30. Ames, B.N., Durston, W.E., Yamasaki, E. & Lee, F.D. (1973) Carcinogens are mutagens: a simple test system combining liver homogenates for activation and bacteria for detection. *Proc. natl Acad. Sci. USA, 70*, 2281-2285

31. McCann, J., Choi, E., Yamasaki, E. & Ames, B.N. (1975) Detection of carcinogens as mutagens in the *Salmonella*/microsome test: assay of 300 chemicals. *Proc. natl Acad. Sci. USA, 72*, 5135-5139

32. McCann, J. & Ames, B.N. (1976) Detection of carcinogens as mutagens in the *Salmonella*/microsome test: assay of 300 chemicals: discussion. *Proc. natl Acad. Sci. USA, 73*, 950-954

33. Sugimura, T., Sato, S., Nagao, M., Yahagi, T., Matsushima, T., Seino, Y., Takeuchi, M. & Kawachi, T. (1977) *Overlapping of carcinogens and mutagens.* In: Magee, P.N., Takayama, S., Sugimura, T. & Matsushima, T., eds, *Fundamentals in Cancer Prevention*, Baltimore, University Park Press, pp. 191-215

34. Purchase, I.F.M., Longstaff, E., Ashby, J., Styles, J.A., Anderson, D., Lefevre, P.A. & Westwood, F.R. (1976) Evaluation of six short term tests for detecting organic chemical carcinogens and recommendations for their use. *Nature, 264*, 624-627

35. Vogel, E. & Sobels, F.H. (1976) *The function of* Drosophila *in genetic toxicology testing.* In: Hollaender, A., ed., *Chemical Mutagens: Principles and Methods for Their Detection*, Vol. 4, New York, Plenum Press, pp. 93-142

36. San, R.H.C. & Stich, H.F. (1975) DNA repair synthesis of cultured human cells as a rapid bioassay for chemical carcinogens. *Int. J. Cancer, 16*, 284-291

37. Pienta, R.J., Poiley, J.A. & Lebherz, W.B. (1977) Morphological transformation of early passage golden Syrian hamster embryo cells derived from cryopreserved primary cultures as a reliable *in vitro* bioassay for identifying diverse carcinogens. *Int. J. Cancer, 19*, 642-655

38. Zimmermann, F.K. (1975) Procedures used in the induction of mitotic recombination and mutation in the yeast *Saccharomyces cerevisiae*. *Mutat. Res., 31*, 71-86

39. Ong, T.-M. & de Serres, F.J. (1972) Mutagenicity of chemical carcinogens in *Neurospora crassa*. *Cancer Res., 32*, 1890-1893

40. Huberman, E. & Sachs, L. (1976) Mutability of different genetic loci in mammalian cells by metabolically activated carcinogenic polycyclic hydrocarbons. *Proc. natl Acad. Sci. USA, 73*, 188-192

41. Krahn, D.F. & Heidelburger, C. (1977) Liver homogenate-mediated mutagenesis in Chinese hamster V79 cells by polycyclic aromatic hydrocarbons and aflatoxins. *Mutat. Res., 46*, 27-44

42. Kuroki, T., Drevon, C. & Montesano, R. (1977) Microsome-mediated mutagenesis in V79 Chinese hamster cells by various nitrosamines. *Cancer Res., 37*, 1044-1050

43. Searle, A.G. (1975) The specific locus test in the mouse. *Mutat. Res., 31*, 277-290

44. Evans, H.J. & O'Riordan, M.L. (1975) Human peripheral blood lymphocytes for the analysis of chromosome aberrations in mutagen tests. *Mutat. Res., 31*, 135-148

45. Epstein, S.S., Arnold, E., Andrea, J., Bass, W. & Bishop, Y. (1972) Detection of chemical mutagens by the dominant lethal assay in the mouse. *Toxicol. appl. Pharmacol., 23*, 288-325

46. Perry, P. & Evans, H.J. (1975) Cytological detection of mutagen-carcinogen exposure by sister chromatid exchanges. *Nature, 258*, 121-125

47. Stetka, D.G. & Wolff, S. (1976) Sister chromatid exchanges as an assay for genetic
    damage induced by mutagen-carcinogens. I. *In vivo* test for compounds requiring
    metabolic activation. *Mutat. Res., 41*, 333-342

48. Bartsch, H. & Grover, P.L. (1976) *Chemical carcinogenesis and mutagenesis.* In:
    Symington, T. & Carter, R.L. eds, *Scientific Foundations of Oncology*, Vol. IX,
    Chemical Carcinogenesis, London, Heinemann Medical Books Ltd, pp. 334-342

49. Hollaender, A., ed (1971a,b, 1973, 1976) *Chemical Mutagens: Principles and Methods
    for Their Detection,* Vols 1-4, New York, Plenum Press

50. Montesano, R. & Tomatis, L., eds (1974) *Chemical Carcinogenesis Essays
    (IARC Scientific Publications No. 10),* Lyon, International Agency for Research
    on Cancer

51. Ramel, C., ed. (1973) Evaluation of genetic risk of environmental chemicals: report of
    a symposium held at Skokloster, Sweden, 1972. *Ambio Spec. Rep., No. 3*

52. Stoltz, D.R., Poirier, L.A., Irving, C.C., Stich, H.F., Weisburger, J.H. & Grice, H.C.
    (1974) Evaluation of short-term tests for carcinogenicity. *Toxicol. appl.
    Pharmacol., 29*, 157-180

53. Montesano, R., Bartsch, H. & Tomatis, L., eds (1976) *Screening Tests in Chemical
    Carcinogenesis (IARC Scientific Publications No. 12),* Lyon, International Agency
    for Research on Cancer

54. Committee 17 (1976) Environmental mutagenic hazards. *Science, 187*, 503-514

GENERAL REMARKS ON THE SUBSTANCES CONSIDERED

This twenty-third volume of the *IARC Monographs* contains evaluations of the carcinogenicity of arsenic, beryllium, chromium and lead and their compounds. Many new data have become available since these substances were originally reviewed (beryllium and lead: IARC, 1972; arsenic, chromium and organic lead compounds: IARC, 1973). The availability of some data on carcinogenicity or mutagenicity was a prerequisite in the selection of the metallic compounds for review in these monographs.

Exceptionally, chemical data have been included for a few widely used compounds for which there were no biological data: lead tetroxide is the most important compound in this respect.

Regulatory status

In the statements concerning regulation in each of the monographs, the contents of the regulations and standards cited are more complex and detailed than is indicated by the brief descriptions given in the text. Reference to the bibliography and to the original texts is therefore essential for an appreciation of the meaning of these summaries. Additionally, as indicated in the preamble (p. 21), such legislation changes rapidly, and that cited in the monographs may not represent the current situation.

Problems in evaluating carcinogenic risk of metals and their compounds

At least two of the metals evaluated are essential trace elements; however, since they occur in various oxidation states and in compounds which have various solubilities, single metals may display a wide variety of biological activities.

Metals in the elemental form have the property of retaining their fundamental identity; accordingly, although they may be altered by natural or technological means, they may reappear in the biosphere at any time, in biologically important forms.

Metals, and especially those considered in this document, present special problems with respect to their description and to the extent of human exposure, for a number of reasons. These metals occur as ores of complex composition, frequently with significant contamination from other metallic substances, and are often byproducts of the refining process of related and/or unrelated materials. Production of metals therefore involves exposure of workers to mixtures of substances, the composition of which depends on the process used and the composition of the raw materials, both of which may change significantly over the years as new techniques are introduced and world markets vary.

Metallic materials occur most frequently industrially as binary (or more complex) alloys, the biological activity of which may depend on surface properties, morphology, etc. and which becomes significantly different from that of the pure metal. Since frequently a number of diverse operations take place in a single factory, individual workers are exposed to material from a wide variety of sources, not only during a single working day but also over a working lifetime. This situation is, of course, similar in most factories. Another complicating factor in metal industries is that there is often concomitant exposure to asbestos.

Many operations within the metal-working industry are dusty, and an extremely wide range of concentrations is encountered. In secondary processes (such as welding), the exact nature of the airborne material is frequently unknown, since it is an accidental byproduct of a particular technological process. Similar remarks are appropriate for industries producing or using metallic compounds; here the active material may either be in the form of metallic ions, or in the form of inorganic or organometallic complexes.

Although duration of exposure is frequently short, the possibility of permanent incorporation in the lung of material of low solubility may produce a hazard of unknown magnitude, especially in view of the high persistence of some of these materials (e.g., calcium chromate). Slow release of some metals may provide a chronic exposure that could be more carcinogenic than acute extremely high levels. Organic chemicals are often metabolized by the human system and may become indistinguishable from other organic compounds; thus, metals are often isolated from organs that may not have been associated with the original site of entry. It is important to investigate further how these metals may be incorporated into the human structure and how they may alter enzyme systems and become part of the living organism. Changes made by the human system to the original form of the metal may produce new materials that are potentially carcinogenic.

Since deposition, retention (i.e., effectual dose) and biological activity are related to particle size, type of compound, etc., a correlation of specific carcinogenic effects with specific exposures may be impossible, in spite of the experimental evidence of carcinogenic activity. The failure of most epidemiological studies to specify the form (oxidation state, solubility) of the metal compound under investigation can lead to serious difficulties in the interpretation of data from humans. Studies on arsenic and chromium exemplify this problem well. Clarification of this issue is of major importance in public health.

Short-term tests

Short-term tests for the detection of potential carcinogens that are based on mutagenicity in bacteria are conspicuously unsuccessful in detecting biological activity of metals, with the exception of hexavalent chromium compounds but including most of the other substances considered in this volume. Salts of arsenic, beryllium and lead, and chromium [III] compounds at very high doses, cause chromosomal aberrations and morphological transformation in cultured mammalian cells.

The absence of mutagenicity of arsenic, beryllium, lead and chromium [III] compounds may reflect either technical deficiencies in the bacterial tests or fundamental differences in the mechanism of metal carcinogenesis.

References

IARC (1972) *IARC Monographs on the Evaluation of Carcinogenic Risk of Chemicals to Man,* Vol. 1, Lyon, pp. 17-28, 40-50

IARC (1973) *IARC Monographs on the Evaluation of Carcinogenic Risk of Chemicals to Man,* Vol. 2, *Some Inorganic and Organometallic Compounds,* Lyon, pp. 48-73, 100-125, 150-160

THE MONOGRAPHS

ARSENIC and ARSENIC COMPOUNDS

Arsenic and inorganic arsenic compounds were first considered by an IARC Working Group in October 1972 (IARC, 1973). Since that time new data have become available, and these are included in the present monograph and have been taken into consideration in the evaluation.

A number of reviews on arsenic and its compounds are available, e.g., those by Fowler (1977), the National Academy of Sciences (1977) and Woolson (1975a). In addition, the UNEP/WHO (1980) have completed an Environmental Health Criteria Series draft report on arsenic.

1. Chemical and Physical Data

1.1 Synonyms, trade names and molecular formulae

Table 1. Synonyms (Chemical Abstracts Services names are given in bold), trade names and atomic or molecular formulae of arsenic and arsenic compounds

Chemical name	Chem. Abstr. Reg. Serial No.	Synonyms and trade names	Formula
Arsanilic acid	98-50-0	4-Aminobenzenearsonic acid; *para*-aminophenylarsenic acid; amino-phenylarsine acid; *para*-aminophenyl-arsine acid; *para*-aminophenylarsinic acid; 4-aminophenylarsonic acid; *para*-anilinearsonic acid; *para*-arsanilic acid; 4-arsanilic acid; **arsonic acid, (4-aminophenyl)-;** atoxylic acid Arsanilic acid-100; Premix; Pro Gen; Pro Gen 227; Progen 90	$C_6H_4NH_2 \cdot AsO(OH)_2$
Arsenic[a]	7440-38-2	Arsen; arsenic black; grey arsenic; metallic arsenic	As
Arsenic pentoxide[b]	1303-28-2	Arsenic acid; arsenic acid anhydride; arsenic anhydride; arsenic oxide; **arsenic oxide [As$_2$O$_5$];** arsenic [V] oxide; diarsenic pentoxide	As_2O_5

Table 1 (contd)

Chemical name	Chem. Abstr. Reg. Serial No.	Synonyms and trade names	Formula
Arsenic sulphide	1303-33-9	Arsenic sesquisulphide; **arsenic sulfide** $[As_2S_3]$; arsenic tersulphide; arsenic trisulphide; arsenic yellow; arsenious sulphide; arsenous sulphide; auripigment; C.I. 77086; C.I. pigment yellow 39; diarsenic trisulphide; orpiment King's Yellow (obsolete, now used for CdS-ZnO mixture)	As_2S_3
Arsenic trioxide[a,c]	1327-53-3	**Arsenic oxide $[As_2O_3]$**; arsenic [III] oxide; arsenic sesquioxide; arsenicum album; arsenious acid; arsenious oxide; arsenious trioxide; arsenite; arsenous acid; arsenous acid anhydride; arsenous anhydride; arsenous oxide; arsenous oxide anhydride; crude arsenic; diarsenic trioxide; white arsenic Arsenolite; Arsodent; Claudelite	As_2O_3
Arsine	7784-42-1	Arsenic hydrid $[AsH_3]$; arsenic hydride; arsenic trihydride; arseniuretted hydrogen; arsenous hydride; hydrogen arsenide	AsH_3
Calcium arsenate	7778-44-1	**Arsenic acid $[H_3AsO_4]$, calcium salt (2:3)**; calcium *ortho*arsenate; tricalcium arsenate Chip-cal; Pencal; Spra-cal	$Ca_3(AsO_4)_2$
Dimethylarsinic acid	75-60-5	Arsine oxide, hydroxydimethyl-; **arsinic acid, dimethyl-**; cacodylic acid; hydroxydimethylarsine oxide Agent Blue; Ansar 138; Arsan; Dilic; Phytar 138; Phytar 560; Rad-E-Cate 25; Silvisar 510	$(CH_3)_2AsO(OH)$
Lead arsenate	7784-40-9	**Arsenic acid $[H_3AsO_4]$, lead (2+) salt (1:1)**; acid lead arsenate; acid lead *ortho*arsenate; arsenate of lead; arsinette; lead acid arsenate; plumbous arsenate; schultenite; standard lead arsenate Gypsine; Soprabel; Talbot	$PbHAsO_4$

Table 1 (contd)

Chemical name	Chem. Abstr. Reg. Serial No.	Synonyms and trade names	Formula
Methanearsonic acid, disodium salt	144-21-8	Arrhenal; arsinyl; **arsonic acid, methyl-, disodium salt**; disodium methanearsenate; disodium methanearsonate; disodium methylarsonate	$CH_3AsO(ONa)_2$
		Ansar 184; Ansar 8100; Ansar DSMA Liquid; Arsynal; Cacodyl New; Chipco Crab Kleen; Cralo-E-Rad; Dal-E-Rad 100; Diarsen; Disomear; Di-Tac; DMA; DMA 100; DSMA; DSMA Liquid; Methar; Metharsan; Metharsinat; Namate; Neo-Asycodile; Sodar; Somar; Stenosine; Tonarsen; Tonarsin; Weed Broom; Weed-E-Rad; Weed-E-Rad DMA Powder; Weed-E-Rad 360; Weed-Hoe	
Methanearsonic acid, monosodium salt	2163-80-6	**Arsonic acid, methyl-, monosodium salt**; monosodium acid methanearsonate; monosodium acid metharsonate; monosodium methanearsonate; monosodium methylarsonate; monosodium methyl arsonate; MSMA; sodium acid methanearsonate	$CH_3AsO(OH)ONa$
		Ansar 170 H.C.; Ansar 170 L; Ansar 529 H.C.; Arsonate Liquid; Bueno 6; Daconate 6; Dal-E-Rad; Herb-All; Merge 823; Mesamate; Mesamate H.C.; Mesamate Concentrate; Mesamate 400; Mesamate 600; Phyban H.C.; Silvisar 550; Target MSMA; Trans-Vert; Weed 108; Weed-E-Rad; Weed-Hoe	
Potassium arsenate[d]	7784-41-0	**Arsenic acid [H_3AsO_4], monopotassium salt**; arsenic acid, monopotassium salt; monopotassium arsenate; monopotassium dihydrogen arsenate; potassium acid arsenate; potassium arsenate, monobasic; potassium dihydrogen arsenate; potassium hydrogen arsenate	KH_2AsO_4
		Macquer's Salt	
Potassium arsenite	13464-35-2	**Arsenenous acid, potassium salt**; arsenious acid, potassium salt; arsenious acid [H_3AsO_3], potassium salt; arsonic acid, potassium salt; potassium *meta*arsenite	$KH(AsO_2)_2$
		Fowler's Solution	

Table 1 (contd)

Chemical name	Chem. Abstr. Reg. Serial No.	Synonyms and trade names	Formula
Sodium arsenate[e]	7631-89-2	Arsenic acid, sodium salt; **arsenic acid, [H_3AsO_4], sodium salt;** sodium *ortho*-arsenate	Na_3AsO_4
Sodium arsenite	7784-46-5	**Arsenenous acid, sodium salt;** arsenious acid, sodium salt; sodium *meta*-arsenite; sodium *meta*arsenite Atlas 'A'; Chem Pels C; Chem-Sen 56; Kill-All; Penite; Prodalumnol	$NaAsO_2$
Sodium cacodylate	124-65-2	Arsine oxide, hydroxydimethyl-, sodium salt; **arsinic acid, dimethyl-, sodium salt;** cacodylic acid, sodium salt; [(dimethyl-arsino)oxy] sodium-As-oxide; hydroxydi-methylarsine oxide, sodium salt; sodium dimethylarsinate; sodium dimethylarsonate Alkarsodyl; Arsecodile; Arsicodile; Arsy-codile; Boll's Eye; Phytar 560; Rad-E-Cate 25; Silvisar	$(CH_3)_2AsO(ONa)$

[a] As_2O_3 is sometimes erroneously called 'arsenic'.

[b] The name 'arsenic acid' is commonly used for As_2O_5 as well as for the various hydrated products (H_3AsO_4, H_3AsO_3, $H_4As_2O_7$).

[c] As_2O_3 is sometimes called 'arsenic oxide', but this name is more properly used for As_2O_5.

[d] The other salts, K_3AsO_4 and K_2HAsO_4, do not appear to be produced commercially.

[e] The name 'sodium arsenate' is applied to both the disodium and the trisodium salts; it is therefore not always possible to determine which substance is under discussion.

1.2 Chemical and physical properties of the pure substances

Physical properties of the arsenic compounds considered in this monograph are given, when available, in Table 2 (from Weast (1977) unless otherwise specified). Information on solubility is given below.

Arsanilic acid - soluble in hot water, hot ethanol, amyl alcohol and aqueous alkaline carbon-ates; slightly soluble in acetic acid; insoluble in acetone, benzene, chloroform, diethyl ether and moderately dilute mineral acids (Windholz, 1976)

Arsenic - insoluble in water; soluble in nitric acid

Arsenic pentoxide - soluble in water (1500 g/l at 16°C), acids, alkali and ethanol

Arsenic sulphide - soluble in ethanol and alkali; slightly soluble in hot water; insoluble in cold water (5×10^{-4} g/l at 18°C); slowly soluble in hot hydrochloric acid (Windholz, 1976)

Arsenic trioxide - soluble in water (37 g/l at 20°C; 101.4 g/l at 100°C), alkali and hydrochloric acid

Arsine - soluble in chloroform, benzene and water (200 ml/l); slightly soluble in ethanol and alkali (Hawley, 1977)

Calcium arsenate - practically insoluble in water (0.13 g/l at 25°C)

Dimethylarsinic acid - soluble in water (829 g/l at 22°C) and ethanol; insoluble in diethyl ether

Lead arsenate - very slightly soluble in water; soluble in nitric acid

Methanearsonic acid, disodium salt - soluble in water (300 g/l at 25°C) and methanol; practically insoluble in organic solvents (Spencer, 1973)

Methanearsonic acid, monosodium salt - soluble in water (570 g/l at 25°C) and methanol; insoluble in organic solvents (Spencer, 1973)

Potassium arsenate - soluble in water (190 g/l at 6°C), glycerine (525 g/l), acids and ammonia; insoluble in ethanol

Potassium arsenite - soluble in water; slightly soluble in ethanol

Sodium arsenate - the dodecahydrate is soluble in water (389 g/l at 15.5°C), ethanol (16.7 g/l) and glycerine (500 g/l at 15°C)

Sodium arsenite - very soluble in water; slightly soluble in ethanol

Sodium cacodylate - very soluble in water (200 g/l at 15-20°C); soluble in ethanol (400 g/l at 25°C) and 90% ethanol (1000 g/l at 15-20°C)

Table 2. Physical properties of arsenic and arsenic compounds[a]

Chemical name	Atomic/molecular weight	Melting-point (°C)	Boiling-point (°C)	Density (g/cm³)	Crystal system
Arsanilic acid	217.07	232	–	1.957[20]	monoclinic needles from water or ethanol
Arsenic	74.92	817 (28 atm.) (triple-point)	613 (sublimes)	5.727[14]	hexagonal, rhombic
Arsenic pentoxide	229.84	315 (dec.)	–	4.32	amorphous
Arsenic sulphide	246.04	300	707	3.43	yellow or red monoclinic needles (change from yellow to red at ~170°C)
Arsenic trioxide[b]	197.84	312.3	465[c]	3.738	amorphous or vitreous
Arsine	77.95	-113.5[f]	-55 (dec. 230)[f]	2.695 (gas)[g] 1.689[8.4.9] (liq.)	colourless gas
Calcium arsenate	398.08	–	–	3.62	amorphic powder
Dimethylarsinic acid	138.00	200	–	–	prism
Lead arsenate	347.12	720 (dec.)	–	5.79	monoclinic leaves
Methanearsonic acid, disodium salt	183.9[d]	132-139[d]	–	–	crystalline[d]
Methanearsonic acid, monosodium salt	161.9[d]	115-119[d]	–	–	crystalline[d]

Table 2 (contd)

Chemical name	Atomic/molecular weight	Melting-point (°C)	Boiling-point (°C)	Density (g/cm³)	Crystal system
Potassium arsenate	180.04	288	–	2.867	tetrahedral
Potassium arsenite	254.8	–	–	–	powder
Sodium arsenate dodecahydrate	423.93	86.6	–	1.752-1.804	trigonal or hexagonal prism
Sodium arsenite	129.91	–	–	1.87	powder
Sodium cacodylate	159.98[e]	–	200[f]	–	crystalline[h]

[a]From Weast (1977), unless otherwise specified
[b]Vapour pressure 0.653 (200°C) (National Academy of Sciences, 1977)
[c]van Thoor (1968)
[d]Spencer (1973)
[e]Midwest Research Institute (1975)
[f]Hawley (1977)
[g]Specific gravity (air = 1)
[h]Berg (1979)

1.3 Technical products and impurities

Arsanilic acid is available in the US from one supplier, with a specification of 98% min. purity (Tridom/Fluka Company, 1979).

Commercial *arsenic* is available in the US as a technical grade, with a typical purity of 99%, and as a high purity grade for semiconductor use, with a purity of 99.999+% (Carapella, 1978). It is available in Japan in a grade of 98% purity.

Arsenic pentoxide has been available in the US as a technical grade. Aqueous solutions of various concentrations are sold for use as cotton defoliants and wood preservatives.

Arsenic sulphide is available in the US from one supplier in three grades: optical grade, 99.999% active; optical grade, glass, unspecified purity; and powder, 99% active (Atomergic Chemetals Company, undated).

Arsenic trioxide is available in the US as a 95% pure crude grade and as a 99% pure refined grade (Carapella, 1978). It is available as a 1% solution in about 5% hydrochloric acid and in 2 mg tablets (Modell, 1977). It was also available commercially as a paste (Wade, 1977).

Arsine is available in the US either alone or in a mixture with an inert carrier gas. Typical products are an electronic grade (liquid phase), 99.995% pure (hydrogen-free basis); a preparation in hydrogen, of light-emitting diode purity, containing <1 ppm each of nitrogen, oxygen, water and methane; and arsine in ultra-high purity background gases (Dopant Mixtures), containing concentrations of 5-1000 ppm, 1001-7500 ppm, 0.76-1.5% and 1.6-4.5% arsine, with argon, helium, hydrogen and nitrogen as background gases. The usual impurities in these products are hydrogen and, sometimes, air (Matheson Co., Inc., 1979). Arsine is also available in the US from another supplier in Grade 2.5 (chemically pure, 99.5%); Grade 4.5 (electronic), 99.995% min., containing <2 ppm phosphine; and Grade 2.5 or Grade 4.5 in mixtures with argon, helium, hydrogen and nitrogen, containing concentrations of 5-1000 ppm, 1001-5000 ppm, 1%, 5%, 10% and 15% arsine (Airco Industrial Gases, 1973).

Commercial *calcium arsenate* contains 61% calcium arsenate and 9% calcium arsenite (National Academy of Sciences, 1977) and an excess of lime and calcium carbonate (Metcalf, 1966).

Dimethylarsinic acid is available as a technical grade, containing 65% active ingredient and the following possible impurities: sodium chloride (Midwest Research Institute, 1975), sodium sulphate, methylarsonic acid and arsenic acid. Commercial formulations as concentrated water solutions may contain sodium cacodylate, the monosodium salt of methylarsonic acid and surfactants (Berg, 1979).

Lead arsenate is available as acid lead arsenate, which contains 33% arsenic pentoxide (van Thoor, 1968). It has been available in the US as a wettable powder (94-98% of the chemical), as a dust and as a paste. Lead arsenate available in Japan contains more than 32% arsenic pentoxide.

Methylarsonic acid, disodium salt is available for farm applications as a solution containing added surfactant (Berg, 1979).

Methylarsonic acid, monosodium salt is available for farm applications as a technical grade in combination with a surfactant, or in combination with sodium cacodylate, dimethylarsinic acid and a surfactant (Berg, 1979; Weed Science Society of America, 1979).

Potassium arsenate has been available in the US as a purified grade and a reagent grade.

Potassium arsenite is available from chemical reagent suppliers in a purified grade. It is also available in a 1% aqueous solution known as Fowler's solution (Modell, 1977).

Sodium arsenate has been available in the US as technical and chemically pure grades.

Sodium arsenite is available commercially in the US as a pure grade of 95-98% purity, and as a technical grade of 90-95% purity (Windholz, 1976). It was previously available in the US as an analytical grade powder, as powders containing 90 and 94% of the chemical and as solutions containing various levels (A 0.25% solution was available for use as a livestock dip, but most solutions contained 40-44% active ingredient).

Sodium cacodylate is available for farm applications as concentrated solutions, as a 25% solution with surfactant, in combination with dimethylarsinic acid or in combination with methanearsonic acid, monosodium salt and surfactant (Berg, 1979).

2. Production, Use, Occurrence and Analysis

2.1 Production and use

ARSANILIC ACID

(a) Production

Arsanilic acid was known as Bechamp's 'arsenic anilide' until 1907, when it was fully characterized (Ehrlich & Bertheim, 1907). It is produced commercially by the same process used prior to 1907, i.e., by heating aniline with arsenic pentoxide.

Currently, three companies in the US produce arsanilic acid; however, separate data on US production, imports and exports are not reported. It is also believed to be produced by one company in France and by one in the UK, although it may be produced elsewhere as well.

(b) Use

Arsanilic acid is used as an intermediate in the production of a variety of medicinal compounds, including *N*-carbamoylarsanilic acid (an antiprotozoan) and arsphenamine (used in the treatment of syphilis). It is used as an antiinfectant to treat: (1) haemorrhagic dysentery and vibrionic dysentery in swine, at levels of 230-360 g/ton of feed (Ladwig, 1978); and (2) protozoan coccidiosis in poultry, at a level of 0.04% in feed (Pomeroy, 1978). Arsanilic acid is also used as a growth promoter, at a level of approximately 90 g/ton of feed, for swine and poultry (Woolson, 1975b).

ARSENIC

(a) Production

The preparation of elemental arsenic by reduction of arsenic compounds was first described by Paracelsus in about 1520 A.D. (Windholz, 1976). Arsenic is prepared commercially either by reduction of arsenic trioxide with charcoal or by direct smelting of the minerals arsenopyrite (FeAsS) and loellingite ($FeAs_2$) (Carapella, 1978). In Japan, it is prepared commercially by sublimation and reduction of purified arsenic trioxide, although small amounts are made by chlorination of arsenic trioxide and reduction with hydrogen.

Arsenic was produced commercially in the US during the World Wars on a temporary basis and has been produced on a regular basis only since 1974 (Carapella, 1978); there is currently only one US producer and production data are not reported (see preamble, p. 20). Almost all of the 485 thousand kg of arsenic metal used in the US in 1971 was imported from Sweden. US imports of metallic arsenic in 1978 were 335 thousand kg; about 97% came from Sweden, and the remaining 3% from Canada, the Federal Republic of Germany, Japan and the UK. US imports of unspecified arsenic compounds in 1978 were 429 thousand kg: 61% came from France, 31% from the UK, 8% from the Federal Republic of Germany, and very small quantities from other countries (US Bureau of the Census, 1979a).

Japanese production of arsenic began prior to 1945. Approximately 7000 kg of a 99.999% pure grade were produced in 1978 and between 200-300 thousand kg of a 98% pure grade. Combined exports of arsenic and arsenic trioxide in 1978 were approximately 6000 kg.

Production of arsenic in Sweden in 1979 was 850 thousand kg. Available information indicated that arsenic is also produced by one company in France, two in the Federal Republic of Germany and two in the UK, although it may be produced elsewhere as well.

(b) Use

An approximate use pattern for arsenic in the US in 1971 has been reported as follows: alloying additive, 90%; electronic devices, 7%; and veterinary medicines, 3%. Metallic arsenic is currently used in alloys in combination with lead and copper, in semiconductor devices and in low-melting glasses (Carapella, 1978).

In Japan, arsenic is used as an alloying additive in the automotive industry and in semiconductors.

ARSENIC PENTOXIDE

(a) Production

Arsenic pentoxide was discovered in 1775 as a product of the reaction of arsenic trioxide with nitric acid (Mellor, 1947). It is manufactured commercially by the oxidation of arsenic trioxide with nitric acid followed by the dehydration of the intermediate crystalline *ortho*arsenic acid hydrate (Doak *et al.*, 1978).

There are believed to be 4 producers of arsenic pentoxide in the US. Separate data on US production, imports and exports are not reported, although total annual US production (exclusive of material used as a nonisolated intermediate) has probably not exceeded 681 thousand kg and imports are negligible.

Arsenic pentoxide, reported as arsenic acid (H_3AsO_4), was produced in Japan since before 1945. Production in 1973 was about one million kg but declined to between 400 and 500 thousand kg in 1978; 4000 kg of arsenic acid were imported in 1978, all from the Federal Republic of Germany, and 6000 kg of arsenic acid and arsenic trioxide were exported to Korea and Taiwan.

Production of arsenic pentoxide in Sweden in 1979 was 710 thousand kg. Available information indicated that arsenic pentoxide is also produced by one company in the Federal Republic of Germany and by three companies in the UK, although it may be produced elsewhere as well.

(b)   Use

Virtually all of the arsenic pentoxide or arsenic acid that is not used as an intermediate in the production of metal arsenates is reported to be used as a preharvest defoliant on cotton and as an ingredient in formulated wood preservatives. It can be used as an oxidizing agent (Doak *et al.*, 1978).

About 50% of the total arsenic pentoxide used in Japan before 1976 was as an intermediate in the production of lead arsenate. Of the 400-500 thousand kg of arsenic pentoxide (reported as arsenic acid) used in Japan in 1978, 90% was used for wood treatment and 10% as an intermediate in the production of sodium arsenate.

ARSENIC SULPHIDE

(a)   Production

Naturally-occurring arsenic sulphide, orpiment, was mentioned by Aristotle (van Thoor, 1968). It is not known when commercial production of arsenic sulphide began; current methods include either heating a mixture of arsenic trioxide and elemental sulphur or passing hydrogen sulphide through a solution of a trivalent arsenic compound in dilute hydrochloric acid (Doak *et al.*, 1978).

There is currently one producer of an undisclosed amount of high-purity arsenic sulphide in the US (see preamble, p. 20). Arsenic sulphide is also believed to be produced by one company in the Federal Republic of Germany, although it may be produced elsewhere as well.

(b)   Use

Arsenic sulphide is used: (1) for **dehairing** skins in tanning, (2) as a pigment, (3) in the manufacture of pyrotechnics and semiconductors, and (4) in the manufacture of infrared lenses and glass. Pigment applications are now almost negligible, since suitable synthetics of lower inherent toxicity have been developed. Recently, arsenic sulphide crystals have been evaluated for applications such as infra-red-transmitting glass, semiconductors and optical waveguides.

ARSENIC TRIOXIDE

(a)   Production

Arsenic trioxide was prepared in the first century A.D. by roasting arsenic sulphides (van Thoor, 1968). It is prepared commercially by recovery from copper or lead smelter flue dusts, which may contain as much as 30%. Condensation of the flue dust produces crude arsenic (90-95% arsenic trioxide), and resubliming produces white arsenic (99% arsenic tri-oxide). All arsenic trioxide in Japan, as well as minor quantities in the US is obtained from the roasting of arsenopyrite (FeAsS) (Carapella, 1978).

US production of arsenic trioxide in 1968 was estimated to be 3.5 million kg from domestic ores and 3.86 million kg from imported ores. Only one company currently produces arsenic trioxide, and separate production data are not reported (see preamble, p. 20). US imports of arsenic trioxide were 22.9 million kg in 1968, but dropped to 14.9 million kg in 1971 and to 9.35 million kg in 1978, when 49% came from France, 25% from Mexico, 22% from Sweden, and the remaining 4% from Belgium, Canada, the UK, the Federal Republic of Germany and Japan (US Bureau of the Census, 1979a). Separate US export data have not been available since 1947. In 1978, 4.1 million kg were produced in Mexico (US Bureau of Mines, 1979).

Japanese production of arsenic trioxide, which began before 1945, amounted to 50 thousand kg in 1978, down from 200 thousand kg in 1973. In 1978, imports (primarily from France, the People's Republic of China and Sweden) were 750 thousand kg, and combined exports of arsenic trioxide and arsenic were approximately 6000 kg.

Arsenic trioxide is produced by three companies in France, and one in each of the Federal Republic of Germany, Portugal, Spain, Sweden and the UK. In 1978, 6.9 million kg were produced in France and 6.8 million kg in Sweden; it was also produced in south-west Africa (7.3 million kg) and in other areas of the world (9.4 million kg), to give an estimated world production, excluding the US, of arsenic trioxide in 1978 of 34.5 million kg (US Bureau of Mines, 1979). In 1979, 8 million kg were produced in Sweden.

(b) Use

The use pattern for arsenic trioxide in the US in 1968 was estimated as follows: pesti-cides, 77%; glass, 18%; industrial inorganic chemicals, 4%; medicine, 1%. The use pattern in 1974 was: pesticides, 70%; glass and glassware, 20%; miscellaneous (including industrial chemicals, copper and lead alloys, and pharmaceuticals), 10% (Jiler, 1975). That in recent years (1975-1978) was: manufacture of agricultural chemicals (pesticides), 82%; glass and glassware, 8%; industrial chemicals, copper and lead alloys, and pharmaceuticals, 10% (US Bureau of Mines, 1979). Total annual US consumption of arsenic trioxide is an average of 27 million kg (US Occupational Safety & Health Administration, 1978).

The major use of arsenic trioxide in the US is as an intermediate in the synthesis of arsenical pesticides such as calcium, lead and sodium arsenates, sodium arsenite, and arsenic pentoxide. Arsenic trioxide compositions have been used as insecticides for dormant application on grapes, in insecticidal dips for goats and sheep, and, in combination with mercuric chloride, in fungicides for treating fenceposts. It was formerly used in baits for the control of grasshoppers and rodents (Berg, 1979).

The refined compound is used in the production of bottleglass and other types of glassware. It is used to prepare arsenic metal for use in copper and lead alloys (Carapella, 1978). Arsenic trioxide is also used in the purification of synthesis gas and in the manufacture of pigments.

In pharmaceutical applications (including veterinary use) it is used primarily for the manufacture of organic arsenical compounds, which are effective against sleeping sickness, and of arsanilic acid, which is used as a feed additive to promote the growth and health of chickens. Arsenic trioxide has been used in dental practice, as a paste with cocaine or morphine, for treatment of tooth cavities prior to filling (Wade, 1977). Solutions (e.g., Fowler's solution) and tablets containing arsenic trioxide are occasionally used in the treatment of leukaemia as a haematinic and in the treatment of some skin diseases (Modell,1977) (see also potassium arsenite). So-called 'asiatic pills' containing 0.08 g arsenic trioxide, were also used in the treatment of skin diseases (Neubauer, 1947).

In Japan, more than 794 thousand kg arsenic trioxide were used in 1978, primarily for intermediate uses.

ARSINE

(a)   Production

Arsine was discovered in 1775 by Scheele. Early preparation schemes included the reduction of arsenous or arsenic acid, the electrolysis of solutions of arsenous compounds and the action of water or dilute acids on metallic arsenides. It is now produced commercially either by the reaction of aluminium arsenide with water or hydrochloric acid or by the electrochemical reduction of arsenic compounds in acid solutions.

At present, two companies in the US produce an undisclosed amount of arsine (see preamble, p. 20). It is believed that there are also two producers of arsine in Belgium and one each in the Federal Republic of Germany and Italy, although it may be produced elsewhere as well.

(b) Use

Most arsine is used, either as a pure gas or in mixtures with an inert background gas, in the electronics industry in the manufacture of certain semiconductor components (e.g., gallium arsenide). It has also reportedly been used by the military as a poison gas (Hawley, 1977).

CALCIUM ARSENATE

(a) Production

Calcium arsenate was prepared in 1881 by heating a mixture of arsenic trioxide and lime (Mellor, 1947). It is prepared commercially by adding a solution of arsenic acid to milk of lime (van Thoor, 1968).

US production of calcium arsenate [70% $Ca_3(AsO_4)_2$] in 1942 was 38.1 million kg and in 1971, 409 thousand kg (US Bureau of the Census, 1976). No production data have been reported since 1971, although at least one US company produced calcium arsenate in 1978 (see preamble, p. 20). US imports in 1978 were 31.8 thousand kg, all of which came from Canada (US Bureau of the Census, 1979a). Separate US export data are not reported. Available information indicated that calcium arsenate is also produced by one company in each of France, Spain and the UK, although it may be produced elsewhere as well.

(b) Use

Calcium arsenate was first used as an insecticide in 1907 (Metcalf, 1966). Until 1960 it was used in the US on cotton for control of the boll weevil [where it is more effective than lead arsenate (National Academy of Sciences, 1977)] and of cotton-leaf worm (Carapella, 1978). It can be used for treatment of turf and lawns to control crabgrass, annual bluegrass, chickweed and certain soil insects, including Japanese beetle grubs (Berg, 1979). It has also been used as a pesticide on fruits, vegetables and potatoes (National Academy of Sciences, 1977).

Bordeaux mixture, a preparation containing 1-2% copper sulphate and calcium hydroxide and used since 1880 against fungal infections of vines, has been fortified with calcium arsenate (4 mg/ml) since 1917 (Ivankovic *et al.*, 1979) (see also lead arsenate).

DIMETHYLARSINIC ACID

(a)   Production

Dimethylarsinic acid was prepared in 1843 by the oxidation of cacodyl oxide using air or aqueous mercuric oxide (Prager *et al.*, 1922). It is prepared commercially by the alkylation of methanearsonic acid, disodium salt with methyl chloride, followed by addition of hydrochloric acid (Midwest Research Institute, 1975).

US production of dimethylarsinic acid was first reported in 1960 (US Tariff Commission, 1961), and one company currently produces an undisclosed amount (see preamble, p. 20). Separate data on imports and exports are not reported.

Available information indicated that dimethylarsenic acid is also produced by two companies in France, although it may be produced elsewhere as well.

(b)   Use

Dimethylarsinic acid was introduced as a herbicide in 1958 (Midwest Research Institute, 1975), and total US consumption in 1978 is estimated to have been 1.27 million kg. The use pattern in 1973 was as follows: nonselective weed control (including directed application in nonbearing citrus orchards), 52%; cotton defoliation, 42%; miscellaneous uses (including lawn renovation and unregistered uses), 5%; and forest management, 1% (Midwest Research Institute, 1975). Now dimethylarsinic acid is used as a silvicide, a nonselective herbicide and in cotton defoliation (Berg, 1979) and dessication. It was used as a crop destruction agent in Vietnam under the name Agent Blue (National Academy of Sciences, 1977).

LEAD ARSENATE

(a)   Production

Lead arsenate is prepared by reacting a suspension of lead oxide (litharge) with arsenic acid or reacting a solution of a lead salt (e.g., lead nitrate) with disodium arsenate (van Thoor, 1968).

Combined US production of acid and basic lead arsenate in 1944 was 41.2 million kg; by 1970 it had declined to 1.89 million kg; production of lead arsenate was 2.8 million kg in 1971 and 1.79 million kg in 1973 (US Bureau of the Census, 1978a). Two US companies currently produce an undisclosed amount (see preamble, p. 20). In 1977, 100 thousand kg were imported, all from the Republic of Korea (US Bureau of the Census, 1978b); exports in 1978 were 19.7 thousand kg (US Bureau of the Census, 1979b).

Available information indicated that lead arsenate is also produced by two companies in each of France and the UK and by one in each of the Federal Republic of Germany, Italy and Spain, although it may be produced elsewhere as well.

(b)   Use

Lead arsenate was first used in the US in 1892 for the control of the gypsy moth, *Porthetria dispar* (Metcalf, 1966). It was also used against the codling moth (e.g., in apple orchards) and other chewing insects (e.g., cotton boll weevil) and apparently found wide-spread use for insect control on tobacco. It was used extensively in the control of fruit insects, but it has been replaced in much of this use by synthetic organic chemicals (Berg, 1979). Current US consumption as an insecticide is negligible.

Lead arsenate is used in veterinary drugs for sheep and goats (National Academy of Sciences, 1977).

Outside the US, lead arsenate is used as an insecticide on fruit trees, vegetables, rubber, coffee, cocoa, grapefruit and as a herbicide in the treatment of turf (Berg, 1979). Bordeaux mixture originated in France as a spray to control the downy mildew disease, *Peronospora viticola*, of grapes, in about 1882, and was first used in the US in 1887. It is produced by mixing 9.5-12 g/l hydrated lime (calcium hydroxide) and 486.5 g/l copper sulphate in cold water to produce a colloid which remains in suspension for several hours and which when sprayed on foliage covers the leaves with a thin, tenacious film which gradually produces soluble copper. By the addition of lead arsenate or DDT, a mixture is made that is widely used to prevent and cure fungal and insect plant diseases on many crops (Metcalf, 1966).

In Japan, 530 kg of lead arsenate were used in 1971 and 300 thousand kg in 1976, all of which was imported.

METHANEARSONIC ACID, DISODIUM SALT

(a)   Production

Methanearsonic acid, disodium salt is prepared commercially by the reaction of sodium arsenite with methyl chloride.

US production was first reported in 1955 (US Tariff Commission, 1956). Although there are presently three US producers, separate production data are no longer reported (see preamble, p. 20). In 1978, US exports of methanearsonic acid and its salts (primarily to Venezuela and Argentina) amounted to 618 thousand kg; exports of herbicide preparations containing methanearsonic acid or its salts (primarily to Brazil) were 1.33 million kg (US Bureau of the Census, 1979b).

No information was available on whether methanearsonic acid and its salts are produced elsewhere.

(b)   Use

Methanearsonic acid, disodium salt is used as a selective postemergence herbicide; 679 thousand kg were used in the US in 1978. It was first used for cotton weed control in 1961. It can also be used for weed control on drainage ditch banks and in storage yards (Berg, 1979).

METHANEARSONIC ACID, MONOSODIUM SALT

(a)   Production

Methanearsonic acid, monosodium salt was prepared in 1883 by reacting sodium arsenite and methyl iodide in an aqueous alcohol solution (Prager *et al.*, 1922). It is prepared commercially from methanearsonic acid, disodium salt.

US production of methanearsonic acid, monosodium salt was first reported in 1967 (US Tariff Commission, 1969); there are currently two US producers, but production data are not reported (see preamble, p. 20). In 1978, US exports of methanearsonic acid and its salts (primarily to Venezuela and Argentina) amounted to 618 thousand kg; exports of herbicide preparations containing methanearsonic acid or its salts (primarily to Brazil) were 1.33 million kg (US Bureau of the Census, 1979b).

No information was available on whether methanearsonic acid and its salts are produced elsewhere.

(b) Use

In 1978, 4.85 million kg of methanearsonic acid, monosodium salt were used in the US. It is used as a herbicide for controlling weeds (Carapella, 1978) and can also be used for weed control on ditch banks, rights-of-way, storage yards and other non-crop areas as well as to control crabgrass and broadleaf in turf (Berg, 1979). Use of methanearsonic acid, monosodium salt in the US in 1975 is estimated to have been as follows: industrial and commercial herbicide uses, 64%; weed control in cotton fields, 26%; and lawns and turf, 10%.

POTASSIUM ARSENATE

(a) Production

Impure potassium arsenates were first prepared in 1589 by heating a mixture of arsenic trioxide and potassium nitrate (Mellor, 1947). Potassium arsenate has been prepared commercially by the reaction of arsenic acid with potassium hydroxide (van Thoor, 1968).

One US company reported production of an undisclosed amount (see preamble, p. 20) in 1979. Separate data on imports and exports are not reported. Available information indicated that potassium arsenate is also produced by one company in each of Italy and the UK, although it may be produced elsewhere as well.

(b) Use

Potassium arsenate is not believed to be used commercially in the US at present, although it has been reported to be useful in fly baits, for preserving hides, in textile printing and as a laboratory reagent.

POTASSIUM ARSENITE

(a) Production

Potassium arsenite was prepared in 1848 by boiling potassium hexaarsenite in a solution of potassium carbonate (Mellor, 1947). It is reportedly prepared for medicinal uses by the reaction of arsenic trioxide with potassium bicarbonate.

Production in the US is believed to be limited to a very small quantity produced by a few companies specializing in laboratory chemicals and analytical reagents (Pfaltz & Bauer, Inc., 1976). Separate data on production, imports and exports are not reported.

Available information indicated that potassium arsenite is produced by two companies in the UK and one in Italy, although it may be produced elsewhere as well.

(b) Use

Potassium arsenite (also known as Fowler's solution)[1] is a haematinic that has been used as a temporary medication for treatment of chronic myelogenous leukaemia. It is also used to treat certain skin lesions (Modell, 1977) and it was formerly used for the treatment of dermatitis herpetiformis and eczema (Wade, 1977). In veterinary medicine, it has reportedly been used in the treatment of pulmonary emphysema, chronic cough, anaemia, general debility and chronic skin disease in horses, cattle and dogs.

Although Fowler's solution is not generally deemed acceptable for widespread use, it should be noted that it is still listed in the *International Pharmacopoeia* (WHO, 1977).

SODIUM ARSENATE

(a) Production

Sodium arsenate was prepared in 1821 by crystallization of sodium hydroarsenate from a solution of arsenic acid and sodium carbonate and subsequent treatment with an excess of sodium carbonate (Mellor, 1947). It is probably prepared commercially by treating arsenic pentoxide or arsenic acid with sodium hydroxide.

US annual production of sodium arsenate in 1968 was estimated to have been slightly greater than the amount imported, which had averaged 138 thousand kg during the previous five years. Separate production data are not reported, however. In 1978, 300 kg were imported from the Federal Republic of Germany (US Bureau of the Census, 1979a).

---

[1] Fowler's solution may have various compositions. One typical preparation contains 1% arsenic trioxide, 1% potassium hydroxide solution, 2.8% dilute hydrochloric acid and chloroform in water (concentration unspecified) (Wade, 1977).

Japanese production of sodium arsenate in 1978 was approximately 60 thousand kg. Available information indicated that sodium arsenate is also produced by two companies in France, one in each of the Federal Republic of Germany and Italy and three in the UK, although it may be produced elsewhere as well.

(b)   Use

The major uses of sodium arsenate are believed to be in the formulation of wood preservatives known as Wolman salts and Boliden salts and as an insecticide in ant killers and animal dips.

SODIUM ARSENITE

(a)   Production

Sodium arsenite is produced commercially by the reaction of arsenic trioxide with sodium hydroxide. Four US companies currently produce it, but separate data on production, imports and exports are not reported. Available information indicated that it is also produced by one company in each of Belgium, Italy, Spain and the UK and by two in France, although it may be produced elsewhere as well.

(b)   Use

In 1954, about 2 million kg of sodium arsenite were used in the US; in 1975, 45.4 thousand kg were used in herbicides. It has been used as a herbicide since 1890 (National Academy of Sciences, 1977); however, in mid-1971 such use of sodium arsenite was drastically restricted in the US by government regulations. Preparations containing very low percentages of sodium arsenite are still permitted for ant control. The major application of sodium arsenite is still thought to be for herbicidal and pesticidal purposes, even though it has been gradually replaced in most of these areas by more efficient organic pesticides with lower mammalian toxicity. It is used mainly for weed control in industrial areas (Berg, 1979).

Sodium arsenite has been used in cattle and sheep dips, for debarking trees and for aquatic weed control (Carapella, 1978). It has also been used to destroy trees and stumps, in baits for grasshoppers, for armyworm and cutworm control and in soil treatment against termites (Berg, 1979).

Sodium arsenite has reportedly been used as an inhibitor of the corrosion caused in oil-well piping when oil wells are acidized with hydrochloric acid. In 1970, it was reported that 454 thousand kg were used for this purpose in the US, although organic inhibitors were said to be gradually replacing sodium arsenite.

It has reportedly been used as an intermediate in the production of arsenic-containing medicinals, arsenical soaps for taxidermists, copper acetoarsenite (Paris Green, a mosquito larvicide) and copper arsenite. Other applications are in wood preservation, pigments, hide preservation and textile dyeing. No information was available on the quantities used in these applications.

SODIUM CACODYLATE

(a) Production

Sodium cacodylate was obtained in 1842 by treatment of methylarsine oxide with methyl iodide and sodium hydroxide in methyl alcohol (Prager *et al.,* 1922). It is prepared commercially by the alkylation of methanearsonic acid, disodium salt with methyl chloride (Midwest Research Institute, 1975).

One US company reported production of an undisclosed amount (see preamble, p. 20) in 1979. Separate data on imports and exports are not reported. Available information indicated that sodium cacodylate is also produced by two companies in France, although it may be produced elsewhere as well.

(b) Use

Sodium cacodylate can be used as a herbicide in general weed control, for sod and turf renovation, for edging along pathways and on ornamental shrubs and nonbearing citrus trees (Berg, 1979).

2.2 Regulatory status (see also preamble, p. 21)

The WHO international standard (WHO, 1971), the WHO European standard (WHO, 1970), the European Community standard (EEC, 1975a), the US standard (US Environmental Protection Agency, 1976), as well as the Japanese standard (Ministry of Health & Welfare, 1978) for inorganic arsenic in drinking-water is 0.05 mg/l. In the European Community, a limit of 0.01, 0.05 or 0.1 mg/l is set for the characteristics of surface water intended for the abstraction of drinking-water, depending on the quality (physical, chemical or microbiological characteristics) of the surface water (EEC, 1975b). Effluent limitation guidelines for arsenic established in the US require that any process waste water discharged from copper smelting facilities and from primary copper refining facilities may not contain a concentration of arsenic exceeding the maximum daily limit of 20 mg/l or an average daily limit of 10 mg/l for 30 consecutive days. Process waste water from copper refining facilities discharged from a point source located in an area where the precipitation rate exceeds the evaporation rate during a one-year period may not contain a concentration of arsenic exceeding the maximum daily limit of 0.04 kg/kg of product or an average daily limit of 0.02 kg/kg of product for 30 consecutive days (US Environmental Protection Agency, 1975).

US effluent guidelines and standards for organometallic pesticide chemicals require that there should be no discharge of process waste water containing arsenic to navigable waters (US Environmental Protection Agency, 1978).

In the US, a permissible exposure limit at work of 10 $\mu g/m^3$ As, averaged over an 8-hour period, has been established for inorganic arsenic (all inorganic compounds containing arsenic except arsine, lead arsenate and calcium arsenate); the equivalent limit for calcium arsenate is 1 mg/m^3, that for arsine, 0.2 mg/m^3, and that for organic arsenic, measured as As, 0.5 mg/m^3 (US Occupational Safety & Health Administration, 1979). The TRK (Technical Guideline) limit for inorganic arsenic in the Federal Republic of Germany is 0.2 mg/m^3 As.

The maximum allowable workplace air concentrations for arsenic and its compounds (as As) are 0.3 mg/m^3 in the USSR, the German Democratic Republic and Czechoslovakia; and 0.05 mg/m^3 in Sweden (Winell, 1975). In Japan, the maximum allowable workplace air concentration for arsenic trioxide is 0.5 mg/m^3 and that for arsine 0.2 mg/m^3 (Japanese Society of Industrial Hygiene, 1978).

The US Food and Drug Administration regulates use of arsenic in veterinary medicine for nonfood animals and as a food additive in swine and poultry. Tolerances based on toxicity have been established for arsenic (measured as arsenic trioxide) in cotton hulls (0.9 mg/kg), in kidney and liver of horses and cattle (2.7 mg/kg), and in meat, fat and meat products of cattle and horses (0.7 mg/kg) (Interagency Regulatory Liaison Group, 1978). Maximum permitted levels of arsenic in feed stuffs are also set at the European Community level, 2 mg/kg, except for meal made from grass, dried lucerne, dried clover, dried sugar beet pulp and dried molasses sugar beet pulp (EEC, 1974, 1976).

The US Food and Drug Administration has also set tolerances for residues of arsenic-containing pesticides (Jelinek & Corneliussen, 1977); these are summarized in Table 3.

Lead arsenate has been prohibited from use as an insecticide in Japan since 1977.

Table 3. Tolerances for residues of arsenic-containing pesticides[a]

Code Fed. Regul., Title 40	Pesticide	Tolerance
Part 180.192	Calcium arsenate	3.5 mg/kg as As_2O_3; numerous fruits and vegetables
180.194	Lead arsenate	7 mg/kg as lead; numerous fruits and vegetables 1 mg/kg as lead; citrus fruits
180.196	Sodium arsenate	3.5 mg/kg as As_2O_3; grapes
180.289	Methanearsonic acid, monosodium salt	0.7 mg/kg as As_2O_3; cottonseed
	Methanearsonic acid, disodium salt	0.35 mg/kg as As_2O_3; citrus fruit
180.311	Dimethylarsinic acid	2.8 mg/kg as As_2O_3; cottonseed 1.4 mg/kg as As_2O_3; beef kidney and liver 0.7 mg/kg as As_2O_3; cattle meat, fat and by-products, other
180.335	Sodium arsenite	2.7 mg/kg as As_2O_3; beef and horse kidney and liver 0.7 mg/kg as As_2O_3; beef and horse meat, fat and by-products, other

[a]From Jelinek & Corneliussen (1977)

2.3 Occurrence

The occurence of arsenic and arsenic compounds in environmental samples was reviewed by the National Academy of Sciences (1977). The flow of arsenic in Sweden (Lindau,
1977) is presented schematically in Figure 1.

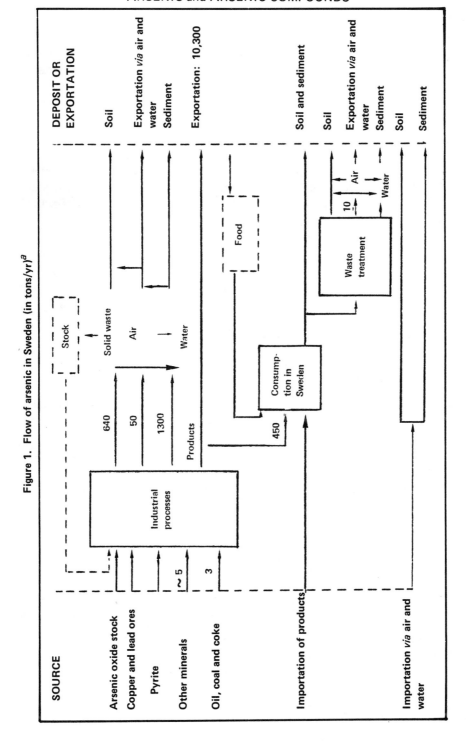

Figure 1. Flow of arsenic in Sweden (in tons/yr)[a]

[a]From Lindau, 1977

(a) Natural environment

Arsenic is widely distributed in the earth's crust, where it occurs in over 150 minerals. Its terrestrial abundance is approximately 5 mg/kg, although higher concentrations are associated with sulphide deposits: soils overlying sulphide ore deposits commonly contain several hundred mg/kg arsenic, and levels up to 8000 mg/kg have been reported. Sedimentary iron and manganese ores as well as phosphate rock deposits occasionally contain up to 2900 mg/kg arsenic (Carapella, 1978; National Academy of Sciences, 1977).

Arsenic constitutes 7-11% of the gold ores of Sweden and 2-3% of lead and copper ores (Carapella, 1978). It is also found in the ores used in tin smelting, zinc refining and cobalt smelting. The usual arsenic content of coal is about 25 mg/kg (Walsh & Keeney, 1975), an average of 14 mg/kg has been reported in US coal (Drever *et al.*, 1977)

Of the arsenic compounds included in this monograph, only three are known to occur in nature in mineral form: these are arsenic trioxide as arsenolite, lead arsenate as shultenite, and arsenic sulphide as orpiment. Although arsine does not occur naturally, it is formed when any inorganic arsenic-bearing material is brought into contact with zinc and sulphuric acid. It may, therefore, be formed accidentally by the reaction of arsenic impurities in commercial acids stored in metal tanks (Doak *et al.*, 1978).

(b) Air

Measurements made in 1950, 1953, 1961 and 1964 at 133 US stations showed average arsenic contents ranging from below the limit of detection to 750 ng/m^3; the average for all stations was about 30 ng/m^3. A level of 20 ng/m^3 was reported to be the average for US urban areas and the maximum in nonurban areas in 1968-1969, with most values <10 ng/m^3 (National Academy of Sciences, 1977). In 1974, annual average levels of <0.5-12 ppt (1.5-37 ng/m^3) were reported in air from 7 sites in the UK (Cawse, 1975). Air samples from an industrial area of Osaka, Japan in 1970 contained 25-90 ng/m^3 (National Academy of Sciences, 1977).

Arsenic trioxide and elemental arsenic are released into the atmosphere as by-products of the primary smelting of nonferrous ores, which contain up to 3% arsenic. In 1907, during an accident, the rate of emission of arsenic trioxide at a smelter in Anaconda, Montana, was 26,884 kg/day (National Academy of Sciences, 1977). During 1961 and 1962, the ambient air concentration of arsenic in Anaconda was 0-2500 ng/m^3 (Suta, 1978). In 1962, air samples from a US gold smelter were found to contain 0.06-13.0 mg/m^3 arsenic (Vallee, 1973). In Sweden, the air emission of arsenic from copper and lead smelters in 1979 was 40 thousand kg; due to the fact that previous production was higher, emissions in 1973 were 65 thousand kg.

During 1973 and 1974, atmospheric arsenic concentrations near 12 nonferrous smelters ranged from below detection to 0.854 $\mu g/m^3$. Those at secondary nonferrous smelters are insignificant (less than 0.003 $\mu g/m^3$). Large cities generally have a higher atmospheric arsenic concentration than do small cities because of emissions from coal-fired power plants; however, US power-plant emissions do not add appreciably to nominal urban background concentrations (Suta, 1978).

Arsenic emissions from pesticide manufacturing processes are 137-363 thousand kg/yr (depending upon the degree of control used by the industry); average ambient air concentrations at pesticide plants are between 0.003-0.8 $\mu g/m^3$ (Suta, 1978).

Because arsenic compounds are used for weed control and as dessicants for cotton, dust and gases emitted from cotton gins contain arsenic. At one US cotton gin in 1964, concentrations of airborne arsenic were 0.6-141 $\mu g/m^3$ 46-91 metres from the gin (National Academy of Sciences, 1977). In 1974, atmospheric concentrations of arsenic measured at sites 300 metres from several cotton gins producing 5 bales of cotton per day were estimated to be 0.25 $\mu g/m^3$ for gins with uncontrolled emissions and 0.037 $\mu g/m^3$ for gins with well-controlled emissions; at gins producing 20 bales per day, concentrations were 1 $\mu g/m^3$ for uncontrolled gins and 0.148 $\mu g/m^3$ for controlled gins. Atmospheric concentrations at sites 50 metres from cotton gins range from 1.804 $\mu g/m^3$ for well-controlled emissions (production of 5 bales per day) to 28.995 $\mu g/m^3$ for uncontrolled emissions (production of 20 bales per day) (Suta, 1978). The burning of cotton trash from cotton gins is another source of arsenic emissions, although the amounts released are not known (National Academy of Sciences, 1977).

Emissions of arsenic can result from the manufacture of glass, primarily from the glass-melting furnace: the arsenic volatilizes during glass melting and condenses on particulates. Uncontrolled arsenic emissions as high as 15 g/kg have been reported during the manufacture of lead glasses and 25 g/kg during the manufacture of borosilicate glasses (Suta, 1978).

(c) Cigarette smoke

Human exposure to arsenic occurs from tobacco smoke when the tobacco has been sprayed with arsenical pesticides. From 1932 to 1951, the arsenic content of US cigarettes had risen from 12.6 to 42 μg/cigarette. By 1969, levels in US cigarettes had declined to an average of 7.7 μg/g tobacco; however, as recently as 1966, Peruvian tobacco contained levels of arsenic as high as 22 μg/cigarette (Fishbein, 1976).

(d) Occupational exposure

The greatest worker exposure to arsenic occurs in the smelting of nonferrous metal in which arseniferous ores are commonly used (Utidjian, 1974). It has been estimated that 1.5 million workers are potentially exposed to inorganic arsenic compounds produced in this way (Fishbein, 1976; National Institute for Occupational Safety & Health, 1975). Gafafer (1964) listed 78 occupations in which there is potential exposure to arsenic; and 37 occupations in which there is potential exposure to arsine have been listed (US Department of Health, Education, & Welfare, 1964).

Birmingham *et al.* (1965), reporting an outbreak of arsenical dermatosis, estimated that 40 thousand kg of arsenic and 100 thousand kg of sulphur dioxide were burned off daily from a gold-smelting plant in which the dust collecting system failed to operate at the expected 90% efficiency. Average hourly exposure levels for 12 work areas within a copper smelter were reported to range from 0 in the engineering building and warehouse areas to 22.0 $\mu g/m^3$ in the reverberatory furnace areas. The overall average was 7.38 $\mu g/m^3$ (National Institute for Occupational Safety & Health, 1975).

A study of a large smelter population reported by Lee & Fraumeni (1969) classified work areas in terms of relative arsenic exposures. Exposure in the arsenic roaster areas was classified as 'heavy': levels ranged from 0.10-12.66 mg/m^3 As. Exposures in the reverberatory area, treater building and loading area were classified as 'medium', with levels ranging from 0.03-8.2 mg/m^3 As. Exposures in other areas of the plant that were classified as 'light' were to levels ranging from 0.001-1.2 mg/m^3 As.

In 1945, Watrous & McCaughey reported on conditions in a pharmaceutical factory manufacturing arsphenamine and related compounds from the basic intermediate arsanilic acid. In the manufacturing department, exposures varied from 0.002-0.60 mg/m^3 As_2O_3 (approximately 0.0015-0.456 mg/m^3 As), with an overall average of 0.17 mg/m^3 As_2O_3 (0.129 mg/m^3 As). In the packaging division, air concentrations ranged from 0.007-0.28 mg/m^3 As_2O_3 (0.005-0.213 mg/m^3 As), with a mean of 0.065 mg/m^3 As_2O_3 (0.049 mg/m^3 As).

Perry *et al.* (1948) conducted clinical and environmental investigations at a sheep-dip factory during 1945 and 1946. On 5 occasions over a 12-month period, general room samples were collected in the packing room, in the drying room, in the sieving room and near the kibbler operator; median concentrations were 0.071, 0.254, 0.373 and 0.696 mg/m^3 As, respectively. Combining all air samples (30 samples), the workers' exposure ranged from 0.058-4.038 mg/m^3 As, with a mean of 0.562 and a median of 0.379 mg/m^3 As. The level of 4.038 mg/m^3 was almost 4 times higher than the next highest level (1.051 mg/m^3 As).

Urinary arsenic levels were reported for exposed and nonexposed workers employed in a smelter (Pinto & McGill, 1953). In 147 samples from 124 nonexposed workers, the mean urinary arsenic level was 0.13 mg/l As, with 4 samples reported as containing 0.4 mg/l As or more; in 835 samples from 348 men exposed to arsenic trioxide dust, the average urinary level was 0.82 mg/l As, and 7 samples contained 4.0 mg/l As or more. The urinary level for the 'nonexposed' workers is consistent with that reported by Watrous & McCaughey (1945) for 13 persons with no known arsenic exposure, although other studies have shown considerably lower normal urinary arsenic levels [see section 2.3(i)].

Arsenic levels in the urine of smelter workers exposed to airborne arsenic trioxide (0.001-12.66 mg/m^3) ranged from 60-480 μg/l (National Institute for Occupational Safety & Health, 1975). Smith et al. (1977) reported urinary concentrations of total arsenic ranging from 24.7-66.1 μg/l in copper smelter workers exposed to airborne arsenic at levels of 8.3-52.7 μg/m^3. The urine contained four types of arsenic: arsenite, arsenate, methylarsonic acid and dimethylarsinic acid. The levels of these compounds were directly related to levels of arsenic exposure; dimethylarsinic acid in urine (17-64.I μg/l) showed the closest correlation with airborne arsenic levels.

Butzengeiger (1940) examined 180 vinedressers and cellarmen with symptoms of chronic arsenic intoxication. Arsenical insecticides were used in the vineyards, and workers reportedly were exposed not only when spraying but also by inhaling arsenic-containing dusts and plant debris when working in the vineyards. The homemade wine consumed by most of the workers was also believed to be contaminated with arsenic. Urinary arsenic levels, given in terms of arsenic trioxide per litre of urine, ranged from 0.1-0.8 mg/l; levels in hair ranged from 0.012-0.1 mg/g.

The effects of lead arsenate on orchard workers were studied from 1937 to 1940. Arsenic concentrations in the air were found to be highest when the workers were burning the pesticide containers (16.7 mg/m^3); next highest were during mixing of the pesticide (1.85 mg/m^3), then picking the fruit (0.88 mg/m^3), then spraying (0.14 mg/m^3) and then thinning the fruit (0.08 mg/m^3) (National Academy of Sciences, 1977). Tarrant & Allard (1972) found urinary arsenic levels of up to 0.93 mg/l in forestry workers using the monosodium salt of methanearsonic acid, compared with a level of up to 0.14 mg/l in the urine of nonexposed controls.

(e) Water and sediments

Arsenic occurs widely in natural waters. The arsenic contents of a variety of water bodies and several examples of unusually high arsenic levels are given in Table 4.

Table 4. Total arsenic content of water samples from various sources[a]

Water sample	Location	µg/l As
Rainwater	USA	0.82-17
	Japan	0.01-13.9
Lakes	Searles Lake, CA, USA	198,000-243,000
	California, USA	0-2000
	USA	0.1-117
	Japan	0.16-1.9
	Greece	1.1-54.5
Rivers	Fox, USA (polluted)	100-6000
	Sugar Creek, USA (polluted)	⟨ 10-1100
	USA	0.25-180
	Japan (40 rivers)	0.25-7.7
	Federal Republic of Germany	3.1-25
	Waikato, New Zealand	5-100
	Waiotapu Valley, New Zealand	trace-276,000
	Sweden	0.2-0.4
Canals	Florida, USA	⟨ 10-20
Wells	Minnesota, USA (contaminated)	11,800-21,000
	USA	0-2000
	Canada	0.5-7.5
	Taiwan	800
		10-1820[b]
Springs	Sebrenica, Yugoslavia	4607
	California, USA ⎫	
	Kamchatka, USSR ⎬	130-1000
	New Zealand ⎭	
	Algeria ⎫	
	Iceland ⎪	
	USSR ⎬	30-500
	Wyoming, USA ⎭	
Thermal springs	Alaska, California, Nevada & Wyoming, USA Iceland	20-3800
Drinking-water	Cordoba, Argentina	traces-1490
Groundwater	Modena Province, Italy	3.0-5.0
Subsurface	Modena Province, Italy	⟨ 0.4-2.1

Table 4 (contd)

Water sample	Location	µg/l As
Glacial ice	Sweden	2.0-3.8
	Antarctica	0.60-0.75
Unspecified	Chile	800
	Aomori Prefecture, Japan	30-3950

[a]From National Academy of Sciences (1977)

[b]From Tseng (1977); Tseng et al. (1968)

In spite of its ubiquitousness in nature, most arsenic in water is added through industrial discharges; the highest concentrations other than those occurring naturally in spring waters are usually in areas of high industrial activity. For example, in 1970, the arsenic content of 79% of 727 samples of US surface water was less than 10 µg/l. Only 2% of the samples contained more than 50 µg/l, and the highest concentration (1100 µg/l) was found downstream from a plant making arsenic compounds (Durum et al., 1971). Similarily, in 1974, levels of 1.5-2.0 µg/l arsenic were reported in the waters of Puget Sound, Washington, except for levels as high as 1000 µg/l within a few miles of a large copper smelter releasing about 272 thousand kg of arsenic into the atmosphere in stack dust and about the same amount in liquid effluent directly into Puget Sound (Safe Drinking Water Committee, 1977). Arsenic emissions to the Gulf of Bothnia off Sweden were 150 thousand kg in 1979; however, in 1973, when production levels were about twice the present ones, emissions to the Gulf amounted to 1.5 million kg.

Natural sources of arsenic in fresh waters include the erosion of surface rocks and volcanism. Although groundwater normally contains low levels of arsenic, averaging around 1 µg/l, waters of hot springs have been found to contain up to 13,700 µg/l and fumarolic gases up to 700 ppb (21.5 µg/m^3) (Safe Drinking Water Committee, 1977). For example, arsenic was discharged into a creek from certain California hot springs at levels up to 1000 µg/l (Eccles, 1976). The concentration was diluted, however, as the water flowed into the Los Angeles water supply, where concentrations were only about 30 µg/l.

Whanger et al. (1977) found that levels of up to 2000 µg/l in Oregon well-water were associated with volcanic rock deposits. Elevated levels of arsenic in groundwater have been attributed to its occurrence in bedrock, its dissolution in sulphide minerals upon oxidation and to the natural occurrence of arsenopyrite with gold, waste rock and tailings from gold mines (Grantham & Jones, 1977).

Arsenic can also be added to freshwater systems through waste waters containing detergent products, which may contain levels as high as 70 mg/l (Angino et al., 1970). Sandhu et al. (1978) suggested that leachings from septic tanks were responsible for arsenic contamination of well water.

Johnson & Pilson (1972) found average arsenic concentrations of 0.028 µg/l in the surface water and 0.044 µg/l in the deep water of the western North Atlantic Ocean. Studies of the vertical distribution of arsenate, which is 2-4 times more abundant that arsenite in seawater, in the Atlantic and Pacific Oceans show increased amounts with depth. It has been suggested that marine organisms, which take up arsenate, may be responsible for the downward transport of arsenic in the sea. Braman (1975) has reported arsenate levels of 1.45 µg/l in saline bay water and 1.29 µg/l in tidal flat water; arsenite levels were 0.12 µg/l in the bay water and 0.62 µg/l in the tidal flat.

Arsenate in both fresh and salt water is metabolized by bacteria and fungi to methylated compounds, predominantly dimethylarsinic acid (Woolson, 1977); and Braman & Foreback (1973) have reported arsenates, arsenites, methylarsonic acid and dimethylarsinic acid in natural waters to a total level as arsenic of 0.25-3.58 µg/l.

Arsenic levels in sediments from various locations ranged from 0.1-306 mg/kg As in the USA, 0-93.4 in Japan, 0-310 in the Rhine delta in The Netherlands and <2-5000 in the UK. Sediments from contaminated bodies of water contained up to 66,700 mg/kg As (National Academy of Sciences, 1977).

Kobayashi & Lee (1978) reported accumulations of up to 549 mg/kg arsenic in the sediment of lakes that had been treated with sodium arsenite as an aquatic herbicide.

(f) Soil and plants

Arsenic is found in detectable amounts in nearly all soils. In surveys of US soils, arsenic levels ranged from 0.2-40 mg/kg in uncontaminated soils (rarely more than 10 mg/kg) and up to 550 mg/kg in arsenic-treated soils (Walsh & Keeney, 1975).

Arsenic was reported to have accumulated to 2500 mg/kg in a fine soil containing high concentrations of hydrous iron and aluminium oxides or their cations. Little arsenic accumulates in sandy soils low in iron and aluminium compounds. It may be leached downward in sandy soils, although leaching is unlikely in heavier soils (National Academy of Sciences, 1977).

Soils are contaminated with arsenic by the use of pesticides, from smelting operations, from the burning of cotton wastes and from fallout from the burning of fuel. Concentrations of 194-389 mg/kg have been found in the top 15 cm of orchard soils that had been treated with lead arsenate pesticide from the early 1900s (National Academy of Sciences, 1977). Concentrations as high as 2553 mg/kg occur in the soil of orchards. The amount of arsenic that reaches the soil from inorganic arsenicals used as pesticides is decreasing, however, because the use of sodium arsenite as a defoliant has decreased in recent years, and lead arsenate has been replaced by carbamates and organophosphates (Walsh *et al.,* 1977).

Organoarsenicals, such as dimethylarsinic acid, methanearsonic acid, monosodium and disodium salts, and sodium cacodylate are adsorbed by clay soils. After rapid initial adsorption, changes occur which result in the redistribution of dimethylarsinic acid into a less soluble form associated with aluminium in the soil. Downward leaching of the methanearsonic acid salts has also been reported (Hiltbold, 1975). The methanearsonic acid salts and dimethylarsinic acid are fixed by iron and aluminium in the soil, although not as strongly as inorganic arsenate (National Academy of Sciences, 1977).

Arsenic accumulates in soil around smelters: soil samples within 1.6 km of a smelter stack contained 150 mg/kg arsenic, and the content decreased with distance from the stack. Levels as high as 380 mg/kg near smelters have also been reported (National Academy of Sciences, 1977).

The arsenic content of plants seldom exceeds a few mg/kg unless the plant or soil in which it grows has been treated with an arsenic compound. Highest levels in untreated and treated plants found in one survey were as follows (in mg/kg dry weight): cereals, 5 and 252; vegetables, 22.7 and 334; fruits, 2.4 and 1200; trees, 8000 and 1000; forage crops, 7.15 and 860; moss, 4 and 99; seaweed, 109 and 71.4; and aquatic plants (New Zealand), 13 and 1450. In grass treated with sodium arsenite, levels of 938-1462 mg/kg were found; and in grass treated with lead arsenate and arsenic trioxide, 15,000-60,000 mg/kg were observed (National Academy of Sciences, 1977).

There is wide variability in the relationship between the arsenic content of soil and that of plants. Alfalfa and grasses grown on a soil containing 2.5 mg/kg arsenic had 20-30 mg/kg on a dry weight basis. However, peas and beans grown in soil containing 126-157 mg/kg contained only 2.1 mg/kg in the vines and 0.88 mg/kg in the pods (National Academy of Sciences, 1977). In general, soil arsenic is well correlated with the arsenic concentration in the whole plant; but because plants tend to exclude arsenic from seeds and fruits, soil samples are not reliable predictors of concentrations likely to be found in edible plant tissue (Walsh *et al.,* 1977).

Tobacco leaves showed a decrease in arsenic content when arsenicals were removed from the list of recommended insecticides for use on tobacco. When no arsenic was applied to soil, tobacco generally contained less than 2 mg/kg. Vegetables grown in soils containing high concentrations of applied arsenic trioxide did not have a significant arsenic content; however, vegetables grown in lead arsenate-treated soils generally showed increased arsenic levels with increasing amounts of applied arsenic. No significant arsenic residues are found in cottonseed when the sodium and disodium salts of methanearsonic acid are applied after the cotton has reached a height of 7.6 cm and before early bloom (National Academy of Sciences, 1977).

Vegetation growing in soils near smelters which contained elevated levels of arsenic (due to air emissions) have elevated arsenic contents: e.g., 3.3 mg/kg in fresh sunflower leaves and 14.3 mg/kg in fresh barley straw (National Academy of Sciences, 1977).

When sodium arsenite was used as an aquatic herbicide in a Wisconsin lake, elevated arsenic concentrations were found in aquatic vegetation. A single sample of *Cladophora* contained 1258 mg/kg arsenic (dry weight), and fresh shoots of mature *Myriophyllum* stems contained between 228 and 261 mg/kg (dry weight).

(g)   Food

The World Health Organization calculated that the average total arsenic intake from diet in 1973 for Canada, the UK, the US and France varied from 25-33 μg/kg bw if all the dietary components contained acceptable amounts (WHO, 1973).

Other reports have suggested that arsenic is present in the US diet at levels of 0.05-0.16 mg/kg (wet weight). The daily dietary intakes of arsenic as arsenic trioxide in the US in 1967 and 1969 was calculated to have been 0.137 and 0.330 mg/person (Fishbein, 1976); by 1974, the average US daily intake of arsenic (as arsenic trioxide) had been reduced to 20 μg/day because of the decreased use of arsenical pesticides on food crops. The US Food and Drug Administration Total Diet Surveys from 1967 to 1974 reported that the highest levels of arsenic in the US food supply were in seafood, with a mean level of 1.4 mg/kg (as arsenic trioxide) in finfish (Jelinek & Corneliussen, 1977). Tinned seafood products have been found to have the following arsenic contents (in mg/kg): clams, 15.9; oysters, 16.0; smoked oysters, 45.8; lobsters, 22.1; and shrimp, 19.9 (National Academy of Sciences, 1977).

A survey in the UK indicated the following levels of arsenic in food (in mg/kg): cereals, 0.18; fats, 0.05; fruits and preserves, 0.07; root vegetables, 0.08; milk, 0.05; meat, 0.10; and fish, 2.0. In 1971, Canadian food products were reported to contain lower levels of arsenic, with only root vegetables and garden fruits having average arsenic levels greater than 0.01 mg/kg (National Academy of Sciences, 1977).

(h)   Animals

Although arsenic is present in all animals, domestic animals generally contain less than 0.3 mg/kg (wet weight basis), while wild animals have been reported to contain levels of up to 1 mg/kg. Animals that have been fed arsenic show higher concentrations in tissues: 0.29-0.92 mg/kg in pigs, 0.01-2.43 mg/kg in chickens and trace levels up to 3.0 mg/kg in rabbits. The hair of horses living close to a smelter exhaust stack and eating locally grown hay has been reported to contain up to 5.9 mg/kg (National Academy of Sciences, 1977).

(i)   Marine organisms

Marine organisms are exposed only to the low levels of arsenic found in the sea and bodies of freshwater; however, they contain the highest arsenic concentrations (0.01-198 mg/kg) of all animals. Crustaceae generally have the highest arsenic concentrations; the following levels have been reported (in mg/kg): shrimp, 0.95-41.6; clams, 0.36-18.0; prawns, 10.5-130.5; oysters, 0.3-52.5; lobsters, 0.02-54.5; scallops, 27.0-63.8; mussels, 0.01-89.2; and crawfish, 0.8-54.6. Fish oil contains more arsenic than most tissues, e.g., the arsenic content of the liver oil of black bass ranged from 7.37-77.31 mg/kg. Ocean fish generally have higher arsenic contents than freshwater fish, ranging up to 24.3 mg/kg for cod (National Academy of Sciences, 1977).

Lunde (1974) has reported arsenic levels in various fish species to range from 0.2-72.5 mg/kg. He also reported that marine organisms synthesize water- and lipid-soluble arseno-organic compounds from inorganic arsenic and that levels greater than 100 mg/kg of organic arsenic may be present, whereas inorganic arsenic levels rarely exceed 1 mg/kg.

(j)   Human tissues and secretions

Total human body arsenic content is between 3 and 4 mg and tends to increase with age. With the exception of hair, nails and teeth, most body tissues contain less than 0.3 mg/kg; the concentrations of arsenic found in normal human body tissues and in the tissues of persons exposed to a variety of arsenic sources are summarized in Table 5 (National Academy of Sciences, 1977).

The normal arsenic content of urine reportedly can vary from 0.1 to 1.0 mg/l (National Academy of Sciences, 1977). Schrenk & Schreibeis (1958) reported an average of 0.08 mg/l As based on 756 specimens from 29 persons with no known exposure; Perry *et al.* (1948) reported a mean of 0.085 mg/l for 54 controls; and Webster (1941) reported an average of 0.014 mg/l As based on samples from 43 adults and children. Whanger *et al.* (1977) reported levels of arsenic in the blood of Oregon residents ranging from 10-360 µg/l. The highest concentrations occurred in blood from people living in areas where there is arsenic-rich water.

High urinary arsenic levels have been found in people living downwind from a US smelter producing arsenic trioxide (Fishbein, 1976). Yoakum (1976) found that mean arsenic concentrations in the urine of children living near copper smelters ranged from 11.9-115.3 mg/l. Milham & Strong (1974) measured the urinary arsenic levels of children downwind from a smelter and found that arsenic levels decreased with distance from the smelter: levels were 0.3 mg/l at a distance of 0-0.4 miles, and 0.02 mg/l at a distance of 2.0-2.4 miles.

2.4 Analysis (see also preamble, p. 21)

Methods of analysis for arsenic and its compounds in environmental samples have been reviewed (Brown & Button, 1979; Henry *et al.,* 1979; Lauwerys *et al.,* 1979; Lewis, 1977; National Academy of Sciences, 1977; Talmi & Feldman, 1975).

Typical methods of analysis for determining levels of arsenic in environmental samples are summarized in Table 6. Abbreviations are: AAS, atomic absorption spectrometry; AES, atomic emission spectrometry; FAAS, flameless atomic absorption spectrometry; GC, gas chromatrography; ICP-AES, inductively coupled plasma-atomic emission spectroscopy; NAA, neutron activation analysis; SSMS, spark source mass spectrometry; UV, ultra-violet spectrometry; X-RF, X-ray fluorescence.

Table 5. Concentrations of arsenic in mg/kg
(fresh weight, unless otherwise specified) in normal tissues and in those from persons
exposed to arsenic

Tissue	Arsenic concentration (mg/kg)		
	Normal	Exposed	Exposure[a]
Hair	0.3-1.75	-	-
Distal	0.79	-	-
Proximal	0.03 [b]-1.92	-	-
	< 3.0	0.4-816	1
	0.997	3.58	2
Brain	0.001[b]-0.14	-	-
	-	1.0-1.4	3
	-	1.9	4
Teeth	0.003-0.635	-	-
Oesophagus	-	168	4
Thyroid	0.06-0.13	-	-
	0.001-0.314[b]	-	-
	0.003-0.332[b]	-	-
	-	0.002-0.093	2
Lung	0.08-0.17	-	-
	-	2.3-2.6	3
	-	20.0	4
	0.006-0.514[b]	-	-
	0.006-0.038	-	-
Heart	-	64.0	4
	0.002-0.078[b]	-	-
	0.001-0.016	-	-
Liver	0.09-0.30	-	-
	-	4.4-6.9	3
	-	12.8-143	4
	0.005-0.246[b]	-	-
Kidney	0.07-0.14	-	-
	-	0.4-1.3	3
	-	15.8-92	4
	-	81	4
	0.002-0.363[b]	-	-

Table 5 (contd)

| Tissue | Arsenic concentration (mg/kg) | | Exposure[a] |
	Normal	Exposed	
Pancreas	0.07	-	-
	-	94	4
	0.005-0.41[b]	-	-
Bladder	0.06	-	-
Gallbladder	-	41	4
Stomach	0.04	-	-
	-	0.1-0.3	3
Walls	-	5-246	4
Contents	-	5-8836	4
	0.003-0.104[b]	-	-
Intestine	0.07	-	-
Small	-	132	4
Large	-	259	4
Spleen	0.08-0.13	-	-
	-	0.5-2.2	3
	-	12.8	4
	0.001-0.132[b]	-	-
Bone	0.16-0.50	-	-
Calvarium	59-61 (in ash)	-	-
Rib	20-27 (in ash)	-	-
Nail	1.70	-	-
	0.04-0.11	7.1-17.8	5
	0.02-2.90[b]	-	-
	-	20-130	4
Blood	-	0.82-3.0	6
	0.01-0.59	-	-
	-	5.0	4
	0.001-0.920[b]	-	-
	0.01-0.13	0.03-0.27	7
Women, venous	0.06-1.44	-	-
Menstrual	0.18	-	-
Serum	0.000-0.0028	-	-
Skin	0.009-0.59[b]	-	-
Spinal cord	-	20.6	4

Table 5 (contd)

| | Arsenic concentration (mg/kg) | | |
Tissue	Normal	Exposed	Exposure[a]
Urine	0.01-0.22	0.04-0.9	1
	0.000-0.11	-	-
	-	27.2	4
Uterus	0.010-0.188[b]	-	-
Membrane	45.6	-	-
Aorta	0.003-0.570[b]	-	-
Adrenal	0.002-0.293[b]	-	-
Breast	0.030-0.221[b]	-	-
Muscle, pectoral	0.012-0.431[b]	-	-
Ovary	0.013-0.260[b]	-	-
Prostate	0.010-0.090[b]	-	-

[a]1, industrial; 2, pollution; 3, arsine; 4, poisoning; 5, arsenic polyneuritis ; 6, aerosol treatment; 7, feeding

[b]Dry weight

Table 6. Analytical methods for arsenic and arsenic compounds

Sample matrix	Sample preparation	Assay procedure	Sensitivity or limit of detection	Reference
Inorganic or total arsenic				
Air	Collect on filter; wet ash with nitric and perchloric acids; solubilize in nitric acid; pipette into graphite tube	FAAS	Working range: 0.1-1.3 mg/m³ air	SRI International (1976)
	Collect on filter; wet ash with nitric and sulphuric acids; convert to trivalent arsenic with potassium iodide and stannous chloride; reduce to arsine with zinc in an arsine generator	Visible spectro-photometry	0.0004 mg/m³	Kneip *et al.* (1976)
Arsenic trioxide	Sample at 3 l/min for 3 min; dissolve filter paper in sodium hydroxide	UV	>0.0006 mg/m³	Snyder & Isola (1979)
Water As(III)	Dilute; purge with nitrogen; treat with hydrochloric acid; add zinc; reduce to arsine	Visible spectro-photometry	0.001 mg/l	Clement & Faust (1973)
	Digest with nitric acid and hydrogen peroxide; stabilize with nickel nitrate	FAAS	0.078 mg/l	Fisher (1977)
	Use the enzyme glyceraldehyde-3-phosphate dehydrogenase	Fluorescence	0.02 mg/l	Goode & Matthews (1978)
	Adjust pH to 3; add sodium hydrogen sulphate; boil; neutralize and boil	Differential pulse polarography	0.007-0.02 µg/l	Henry *et al.* (1979)

Table 6 (contd)

Sample matrix	Sample preparation	Assay procedure	Sensitivity or limit of detection	Reference
Soils and plants	Homogenize; irradiate; dissolve in perchloric and nitric acids; add hydrogen fluoride; add perchloric acid; pass through stannous dioxide column	NAA		Gills (1977)
	Wet ash with nitric and perchloric acids; add hydrochloric acid, potassium iodide and stannous chloride; add pyridine solution of silver diethyldithiocarbamate; generate arsine	Spectrophotometry (535 nm)	0.01 mg/kg	Burke & Diamondstone (1977)
	Irradiate; wash with sulphuric, nitric, hydrochloric and hydrobromic acids; distill; precipitate arsenic sulphides with acetamide	NAA		Steinnes (1977)
Food and beverages				
Wines, fruit juices, raisins, rice, shellfish, beef liver	Dry ash with magnesium nitrate; rinse with hydrochloric acid; reduce to arsine with sodium borohydride in an arsine generator	AAS	0.02 mg/l (beverages) 0.02 mg/kg (foods)	Siemer et al. (1977)
Biological samples				
Beef extract	Irradiate; oxidize with nitric and sulphuric acids; through a series of reactions precipitate a $MgNH_4AsO_4$ complex	NAA	0.06 µg/kg	Korob et al. (1978)

Table 6 (contd)

Sample matrix	Sample preparation	Assay procedure	Sensitivity or limit of detection	Reference
Beef offal and fish	Digest with nitric, perchloric and sulphuric acids; dilute; generate arsine by reaction with sodium borohydride	AAS	6 ng	Flanjak (1978)
Fish (edible muscle)	Clean; irradiate; dissolve in nitric acid; separate arsenic on anion exchange column; wash with hydrochloric acid	NAA	1 ng	Anand (1978)
Blood	Freeze-dry; irradiate; dissolve in sodium hydroxide; mineralize with 96% sulphuric acid and 50% hydrogen peroxide; heat; cool; add 48% hydrobromic acid	NAA	0.005 mg/kg	Weers *et al.* (1978)
Whole blood, serum, urine	Digest with nitric acid and hydrogen peroxide; add perchloric and hydrobromic acids; distill off volatile bromides	ICP-AES	Amounts detected 0.016 mg/l (whole blood) 0.032 mg/l (serum) 0.036 mg/l (urine)	Nixon (1976)
Urine, hair, blood, dust	Wash with nitric, perchloric and sulphuric acids; heat with ammonium oxalate; generate arsine	AAS	<0.05 mg/kg (hair)	Yoakum (1976)
Liver	Dry; irradiate with 3MeV proton-induced X-rays	X-RF	0.2-2 mg/kg	Kemp *et al.* (1974)

Table 6 (contd)

Sample matrix	Sample preparation	Assay procedure	Sensitivity or limit of detection	Reference
Liver, leaves, coal	Irradiate; wash with nitric acid and water; cool in liquid nitrogen; dissolve in nitric acid, perchloric acid and hydrogen fluoride; separate arsenic with hydrated manganese dioxide	NAA		Gallorinl *et. al.* (1978)
Lung tissue	Homogenize; freeze-dry; irradiate; add sodium peroxide and potassium perchlorate; through a series of reactions precipitate a $MgNH_4AsO_4$ complex	NAA	0.01 mg/kg	Filby (1975)
Lung tissue and hilar node tissue	Homogenize; freeze-dry; ash; mix with ultra-pure graphite	SSMS	0.002 mg/kg	Brown & Taylor (1975)
Muscle	Freeze-dry; grind to powder; irradiate; wet-ash with perchloric and nitric acids; distill arsenic; separate by ion exchange	NAA		D'Hondt *et al.* (1977)
Hair	Wash; wet ash with sulphuric and nitric acids; add 30% hydrogen perioxide; add saturated ammonium oxalate; generate arsine by reaction with sodium borohydride	AAS	0.02 µg	Curatola *et al.* (1978)

Table 6 (contd)

Sample matrix	Sample preparation	Assay procedure	Sensitivity or limit of detection	Reference
Other				
Coal	Grind to powder; add nitric, perchloric and sulphuric acids; extract with toluene; pipette into graphite tube	FAAS	0.1 mg/kg	Aruscavage (1977)
Glacial ice	Irradiate; add concentrated sulphuric acid; evaporate; precipitate sulphides of arsenic by passing hydrogen sulphide through solution; treat with nitric and sulphuric acids; wash with hydrochloric acid	NAA	0.4 ng	Weiss & Bertine (1973)
Sewage sludge	Freeze- or oven-dry; irradiate	NAA	40 mg/kg	Egan & Spyrou (1977)
Organic arsenic				
Natural water (dimethylarsinic acid; monomethylarsine)	Strip out arsine with helium; form various arsine compounds as a function of pH	GC, AAS	0.05 ng	Andreae (1977)
Natural water, eggshells, seashells, urine (methylarsinic acid)	Reduce to arsines with sodium borohydride as a function of pH	AES	1 ng	Braman & Foreback (1973)

3. Biological Data Relevant to the Evaluation
of Carcinogenic Risk to Humans

A review is available (Leonard & Lauwerys, 1980).

3.1 Carcinogenicity studies in animals

(a) Oral administration

Mouse: Two groups of 50 C57Bl 6 mice received *arsenic trioxide* either in tap-water
or in 12% aqueous ethanol in the drinking-water.   The starting level of 4 mg/l was increased
monthly up to 34 mg/l and then held constant up to 24 months.   The same numbers of controls received water or 12% aqueous ethanol.   No mice that received arsenic trioxide in
aqueous ethanol lived longer than 9 months, and none of the corresponding controls survived
more than 12 months;   6 mice given arsenic trioxide in water and 2 of the corresponding
controls survived 18 months.   There was no excess of tumours in the treated groups (Hueper
& Payne, 1962).

Of 77 Swiss mice that received 0.01% *arsenic trioxide* in their drinking-water, 21 lived
up to 60 weeks; the tumour incidence was similar to that in controls (Baroni *et al.*, 1963;
Shubik *et al.*, 1962).

Treatment of Swiss mice with *sodium arsenite* in their drinking-water for lifespan at a
concentration equivalent to 5 μg/ml As, which represented an intake more than 10 times
greater than that of controls, was associated with a decreased incidence of spontaneous
tumours and with no evidence of the induction of other tumours; fewer treated males than
controls were alive at 18 months of age (Kanisawa & Schroeder, 1967) [The Working Group
noted the very low dose used in this experiment].

Groups of 30 NMRI mice of both sexes received one drop of a drug containing *arsenic
trioxide* (Psor-Intern) or of Fowler's solution orally once a week for 5 months (calculated
total dose, 7 mg arsenic trioxide per animal).   Higher incidences of ardenocarcinomas of the
skin, lung, peritoneum and lymph nodes were seen up to the end of the 14-month observation period (including time of treatment).   No tumours were seen in 15 control mice of
both sexes or their offspring observed up to 2 years.   Some treated animals produced offspring in which 'metastasizing tumours' were observed with no further treatment (Knoth,
1966/67) [The Working Group noted the very brief and incomplete description of the
study].

Groups of 18 male and 18 female (C57BL/6 x C3H/Anf)F_1 (B6C3F_1) mice and 18 male and 18 female (C57BL/6 x AKR)F_1 (B6AKF$_1$) mice were given daily doses (adjusted each day for body-weight change) of 46.4 mg/kg bw *dimethylarsinic acid* in the diet from 7 days of age until 28 days of age. Subsequently, the mice received a diet containing 121 mg/kg of diet of the compound for 18 months, at which time 11 male and 18 female B6C3F_1 mice and 17 male and 16 female B6AKF$_1$ mice were still alive. No increased incidence of tumours was observed compared with that in untreated and pooled controls (Innes *et al.*, 1969; National Technical Information Service, 1968).

In 30 female C3H/St mice given 10 mg/l *sodium arsenite* continuously in the drinking-water, the incidence of spontaneous mammary carcinomas was reduced, but the growth rate of tumours in those mice which developed them was increased markedly (Schrauzer & Ishmael, 1974).

Of 4 groups of 50 mice (strain unspecified), one was given 20 mg/l *arsenic trioxide* in drinking-water for life and was painted once 6 months after the beginning of the experiment with 7,12-dimethylbenz[a]anthracene (DMBA); the second was given arsenic trioxide and painted with croton oil 6 months after the experiment began; the third group was given arsenic trioxide alone; and the control group was given water only. One control mouse, 3 treated with arsenic alone, 8 treated with arsenic and croton oil and 6 treated with arsenic and DMBA developed skin papillomas. The author stated that the number of tumours produced was too small for statistical analysis (Sanderson, 1961) [The Working Group noted that no controls painted with DMBA or croton oil alone were used].

Arsenic trioxide was administered to Swiss mice as a 0.01% solution as drinking-water for 40-60 weeks in conjunction with twice weekly treatments with croton oil, single treatment with DMBA or two doses of urethane. Negative results were obtained in all 18/77, 37/50 and 28/50 mice that survived the three treatments, respectively (Baroni *et al.*, 1963).

Two groups of 30 female STS mice were fed 500 then 250 mg/kg of diet *arsanilic acid* or 338 then 169 mg/kg of diet *potassium arsenite* for 48 weeks 1 week after a single skin application of 5 μg DMBA; 2 weeks later, they were also given skin applications of 25 μl of a 0.5% solution of croton oil in benzene weekly throughout the experiment. The incidence of papillomas in the 2 groups treated with arsenic did not differ from that in a control group of 20 mice given DMBA and croton oil in benzene (Boutwell, 1963).

In a controlled study on 16 DBA, 20 BALB/c and 28 CxC3H mice, administration of 0.01% *arsenic trioxide* in the drinking-water for 4-13 weeks did not significantly enhance skin carcinogenesis by 3-methylcholanthrene (Milner, 1969).

Rat: Rats (sex and strain unspecified) were fed 10 mg/animal daily of *lead arsenate* (49 rats) or its arsenic equivalent of *calcium arsenate* (99 rats) for up to two years; there were 24 untreated controls. The numbers of survivors at one year were 27, 51 and 20, respectively; no evidence of carcinogenicity was obtained (Fairhall & Miller, 1941).

Groups of 50 male and female Bethesda black rats received *arsenic trioxide* either in tap-water or in 12% aqueous ethanol in the drinking-water. The starting level of 4 mg/l was increased monthly up to 34 mg/l and then held constant up to 24 months. The same numbers of controls received water or 12% aqueous ethanol. Fifteen to 33 rats lived for 21 months or more. No excess incidences of tumours were noted (Hueper & Payne, 1962).

In two-year feeding studies, either *sodium arsenite* (dietary concentrations corresponding to 0, 15.6, 31.2, 62.5, 125 or 250 mg/kg of diet arsenic) or *sodium arsenate* (0, 31.2, 62.5, 125, 250 or 400 mg/kg of diet arsenic) was given to groups of 25 male and 25 female Osborne-Mendel rats. The 4-15 survivors in each treated group developed no more tumours than did the 8-12 survivors in the untreated control groups. At the highest doses the survival rate was reduced (Byron *et al.*, 1967).

A group of 91 Long Evans rats of both sexes received 5 mg/l *sodium arsenite* in their drinking-water over their life-span. Tumour incidence was similar to that in untreated controls (Kanisawa & Schroeder, 1969) [The Working Group noted the very low dose used in this experiment].

Groups of 48-80 male and female Wistar rats were fed either *lead arsenate* at levels of 463 and 1850 mg/kg of diet or *sodium arsenate* at a level of 416 mg/kg of diet for 29 months. Two groups of 40 male and 40 female rats received either 463 mg/kg of diet lead arsenate or 416 mg/kg of diet sodium arsenate in combination with *N*-nitrosodiethylamine (NDEA) at a dose of 5 µg/animal by stomach tube on 5 days a week for up to 29 months. Two control groups of 110 male and female rats, either untreated or treated with NDEA, were used. The group fed 1850 mg/kg of diet lead arsenate showed a marked increase in mortality after 26 weeks of the experiment; and in the same group a cortical kidney adenoma and a bile-duct carcinoma were found. There were no differences among the other groups in the latency or incidence of tumours (Kroes *et al.*, 1974).

Dog: Eight groups, each of 3 male and 3 female beagle dogs, 6 months of age, received either *sodium arsenite* or *sodium arsenate* in the diet at concentrations corresponding to 5, 25, 50 or 125 mg/kg of diet arsenic for two years, at which time the survivors were killed. No tumours were seen. In the group treated with the highest level of sodium arsenite, weight loss and early mortality were recorded; 6 dogs given the highest level died by 19 months, and one female given 5 mg/kg died at 3 months (Byron *et al.*, 1967) [The Working Group noted the short duration of the experiment].

(b)   Skin application

Mouse: A group of 100 mice were painted thrice weekly with a solution of *potassium arsenite* in ethanol containing 1.8% *arsenic trioxide*, later reduced to 0.12% due to a high death rate. Of 33 mice that lived for three months, one developed a metastasizing squamous-cell carcinoma of the skin after 5.5 months (Leitch & Kennaway, 1922). Neubauer (1947) mentions various unsuccessful attempts to confirm the above finding.

In another experiment, 14 S mice were painted once weekly for 10 weeks with a 1% solution of *potassium arsenite* in methanol (total dose, 30 mg), and, starting 25 days later, with once-weekly applications of 0.17% or 0.085% croton oil in acetone. Three mice developed skin papillomas, but 4/19 controls that received treatment with croton oil alone also developed skin tumours (Salaman & Roe, 1956).

Two groups of 20 female Rockland all-purpose mice were used. Animals in the first group were painted 8 times with a 0.4% solution of *potassium arsenite* in 80% ethanol (total dose, 1.24 mg/animal) over 5 days, followed 2 days later by twice-weekly skin applications of 25 μl of 2% croton oil in benzene to test for tumour initiation. The second group was used to test for tumour promotion and received a single application of 75 μg DMBA in 25 μl acetone, followed one week later by twice-daily skin paintings of a 0.4% solution of potassium arsenite in 80% ethanol (total dose, 2.2 mg/animal per week) for 29 weeks. No cocarcinogenic effects were observed (Boutwell, 1963).

A group of 14 female and 54 male Swiss mice were painted with a 1.58% solution of *sodium arsenate* in water containing a 2.5% solution of Tween 60 twice weekly for up to 60 weeks (concentration of arsenic, 0.38%); a control group of 50 females and 19 males received 2.5% Tween 60 only. Two males developed a total of 3 papillomas, 2 of which regressed. Treatment with sodium arsenate in association with croton oil, DMBA or urethane did not result in higher tumour incidences (Baroni *et al.*, 1963).

(c)   Inhalation and/or intratracheal administration

Mouse: In an inhalation study reported as an abstract, aerosols of a 1% (w/w) aqueous solution of *sodium arsenite* were administered to 60 'tumour-susceptible' female mice. Exposure was for 20-40 min/day on 5 days/week for 55 weeks. Thirty cage mates and 30 controls were also used. No neoplasias were noted (Berteau *et al.*, 1978).

Rat: Groups of 14-23 male Wistar King rats received a total of 15 intratracheal instilla-tions (1 per week for 4 months) of 0.26 mg *arsenic trioxide*, 2.5 mg *copper ore* (containing 3.95% arsenic) or 2 mg *flue dust* (containing 10.5% arsenic), alone or in combination with 0.4 mg benzo[a]pyrene (BP). Average survival ranged from 372-670 days. No malignant lung tumours were observed in the rats treated with arsenic trioxide or copper ore alone, and no statistically significant increase in the incidence of malignant lung tumours was found when these compounds were given in combination with BP or when the incidence was compared with that in rats treated with BP alone. One adenocarcinoma of the lung occurred among 7 surviving rats given instillations of flue dust alone (Ishinishi *et al.*, 1977).

Nine male Wistar King rats, 10 weeks old, received 0.2 ml of an aqueous solution con-taining 1 mg/ml *arsenic trioxide* intratracheally once a week for 4 months (15 doses); 7 con-trol rats were treated with saline. The animals were observed for lifespan: 192-643 days after start of treatment (average, 413 days). One of the treated animals developed a lung adenoma and 4 had metaplasia and/or osteometaplasia of the alveolar cells or of the airway epithelial cells (Ishinishi *et al.*, 1976).

A group of 25 male BD IX rats, 12 weeks old at the start of the experiment, were given a single intratracheal instillation of 0.1 ml of an arsenic-containing mixture (*calcium arsenate*, copper sulphate and calcium hydroxide), which is also known as 'Bordeaux mixture' (dose of arsenic, 0.07 mg). Ten rats died within the first week after treatment; the remaining 15 were observed for lifetime (455-500 days), and 9 developed lung tumours (7 bronchogenic adeno-carcinomas and 2 bronchiolar-alveolar-cell carcinomas). No lung tumours occurred in 25 controls given intratracheal instillations of saline (Ivankovic *et al.*, 1979) [The Working Group noted that the name 'Bordeaux mixture' is used for a variety of formulations and that no copper-containing compound was tested alone].

(d) Subcutaneous and/or intramuscular administration

Mouse: Twenty-four female Swiss mice were given a daily s.c. injection of 0.5 mg/kg bw arsenic as a 0.005% aqueous solution of *sodium arsenate* throughout pregnancy (a total of 20 injections). Eleven of them developed lymphocytic leukaemia or lymphomas within 24 months after the start of the experiment. In contrast, none of 20 untreated females which died during the same period developed such tumours. Some of the progeny of the arsenate-treated mothers were left untreated, and others were given 20 once-weekly s.c. injections of 0.5 mg/kg bw arsenic as an aqueous sodium salt. All of the animals had been observed for up to 24 months at the time the experiment was reported; 12/71 untreated progeny and 7/97 arsenic-treated progeny were still alive at that time. During this period, 13/71 untreated progeny and 41/97 treated progeny developed lymphomas or lymphocytic leukaemia. Progeny of both sexes responded similarly, except that none of the arsenic-treated females lived for 24 months. Of 35 male and 20 female untreated, 4-week-old controls, 20 and 16, respectively, were dead at the time the report was published; and 3 males developed lymphocytic leukaemia or lymphomas. The age at death in mice with such tumours was in some instances, but not always, shorter in the treated animals than in untreated control males (Osswald & Goerttler, 1971) [This experiment is difficult to interpret since 19/55 control animals and some of the experimental animals were still alive at the time of reporting].

Groups of 18 male and 18 female (C57BL/6 x C3H/Anf)F_1 mice and 18 male and 18 female (C57BL/6 x AKR)F_1 mice were given a single s.c. injection of 464 mg/kg bw *dimethylarsinic acid* in water at 28 days of age. At 18 months, 10 males and 18 females of the first strain and 14 males and 15 females of the second strain were still alive. No increased incidence of tumours was observed compared with that in untreated and pooled controls (National Technical Information Service, 1968).

Rat: Paraffin pellets (250 mg) containing 30% *calcium arsenate* were implanted subcutaneously into 60 random-bred male albino rats. In an additional experiment, 100 mg calcium arsenate dissolved in 0.5 ml of sunflower oil were injected subcutaneously into 50 rats. No tumours were reported after 2.5 years (Arkhipov, 1968).

(e)   Intravenous administration

Mouse: Of 19 female Swiss mice, 11 developed lymphomas or lymphocytic leukaemia following 20 weekly i.v. injections of 0.5 mg/kg bw arsenic given as a 0.005% aqueous solution of *sodium arsenate* (Osswald & Goerttler, 1971).

(f)   Other experimental systems

Intramedullary injection: Of 25 male Osborne-Mendel *rats* given about 0.43 mg *metallic arsenic* as a suspension in lanolin by injection into the right femur, followed by a similar injection into the left femur 10 months later, 13 survived over one year, and one developed a spindle-cell sarcoma at the site of the injection after 21 months. In 19 controls alive after one year injected with lanolin alone, one developed a local fibrosarcoma (Hueper, 1954).

None of 6 *rabbits* given a single intramedullary injection of 0.64 mg *metallic arsenic* in lanolin developed a tumour. No local tumours occurred in 2 controls treated with lanolin alone, one of which lived up to 44 months (Hueper, 1954).

3.2 Other relevant biological data

(a) Experimental systems

Toxic effects

The toxicity and LD_{50} values observed for arsenic compounds vary greatly depending on the chemical form and oxidation state of the chemical involved: the toxicity of the tri-valent compounds is much greater than that of the pentavalent ones. The oral LD_{50} for arsenate (As[V]) in rats and mice has been found to be about 100 mg/kg, and that for arsenate (As[III]) about 10 mg/kg (Schroeder & Balassa, 1966). The 48-hr LD_{75} for arse-nate following i.p. administration in rats was 14-18 mg/kg bw (Franke & Moxon, 1936). The LD_{50} for sodium arsenite (As[III]) in mice by i.p. injection was about 5 mg/kg bw (Levvy, 1947). In rats, acute oral LD_{50} values of 23.6 mg/kg bw and 15.1 mg/kg bw were deter-mined for 'crude' and purified arsenic trioxide, respectively; the corresponding values in mice were 42.9 and 39.4 mg/kg bw (Harrisson et al., 1958).

Rats given 10 mg/kg bw per day arsenic trioxide by stomach tube for 40 days showed hair loss, then eczema, hyperplasia and hyperkeratosis of the skin. Clinical symptoms of bleeding, ulceration and crust formation occurred in some cases (Ishinishi et al., 1976). Oral administration of 0.125-62.5 mg/l arsenic trioxide to rats produced a dose-dependent pro-liferation in the bile duct, with chronic angiitis (Ishinishi et al., 1980).

The LC_{50} for arsine in mice by inhalation exposure has been estimated to be 0.67 mg/kg or 0.5 mg/l after 2.4 min (Levvy, 1947); a 30-minute exposure to 250 ppm (75 mg/m³) may be lethal (Luckey & Venugopal, 1977). The LD_{50} following i.p. injection in mice is about 2.5 mg/kg bw (Levvy, 1946).

The acute LD_{50} for technical methanearsonic acid, disodium salt in rats by oral adminis-tration is about 2800 mg/kg bw, and that of methanearsonic acid, monosodium salt is about 700 mg/kg bw (Berg, 1979). The i.p. LD_{50} for methanearsonic acid, disodium salt is 600 and 681 mg/kg bw in male and female mice, respectively, and 600 and 561 mg/kg bw in male and female rats, respectively. The i.p. LD_{50} for dimethylarsinic acid is 520 and 600 mg/kg bw in male and female mice and 720 and 520 mg/kg bw in male and female rats, respectively. The LC_{50} by inhalation exposure for dimethylarsinic acid in female rats is 3900 mg/m³ (Stevens et al., 1979).

A dose of 10 mg/kg bw methanearsonic acid, monosodium salt given orally for 10 days killed 4 of 5 cows (Dickinson, 1972). Long-term feeding of 50 mg/kg of diet methanearsonic acid, monosodium salt (1.5 mg/kg bw per day as As) to rabbits produced toxic hepatitis (Exon et al., 1974). The oral LD_{50} of arsanilic acid in rats was 216 mg/kg bw for 1-3-day-old rats and more than 1000 mg/kg bw for adult rats (Goldenthal, 1971).

Effects on reproduction and prenatal toxicity

A single i.p. injection of 45 mg/kg bw sodium arsenate to Swiss-Webster mice on one of days 6-11 of pregnancy resulted in an increased rate of foetal resorptions, growth retardation and a variety of malformations - predominantly fusion or forking of ribs, exencephaly, shortened jaw, open eyes, anophthalmia, etc. (Hood & Bishop, 1972).

When a single i.p. injection of 10 or 12 mg/kg bw sodium arsenite was given to Swiss-Webster mice on days 9-12 of pregnancy, there was a high rate of resorptions, and the surviving foetuses showed various malformations of the eyes, ribs, tail and brain (Hood, 1972).

Treatment with 50 mg/kg bw 2,3-dimercaptopropanol subcutaneously on day 9 of pregnancy either (i) 4 hrs before, (ii) concurrently with or (iii) 4 hrs after an i.p. injection of 40 mg/kg bw sodium arsenate reduced the frequency and severity of malformations in random-bred Swiss-Webster (SAF/ICR) mice when compared with arsenate treatment alone. With regard to skeletal malformations, the second regime was more effective than (i) or (iii). This difference in treatment schemes was less pronounced when total malformations were evaluated (Hood & Pike, 1972).

Random-bred CD-1 albino mice were treated with sodium arsenate on one of days 7-15 of gestation either intraperitoneally or by gastric intubation. A significantly increased rate of malformations was seen when 40 mg/kg bw were given intraperitoneally on days 9 or 10 of gestation; the abnormalities observed were predominantly short jaws, open eyes, kinked tails and exencephaly. Considerably fewer malformations were observed when 120 mg/kg bw arsenate were given by gastric intubation on the same day of pregnancy; but the number of resorptions was increased - especially when the arsenate was given on day 11 of pregnancy (Hood et al., 1978).

Oral doses of 10-40 mg/kg bw sodium arsenate given once on day 9, 10 or 11 of pregnancy increased the number of resorptions but did not significantly increase the number of malformations induced in ICR mice (Matsumoto et al., 1973).

When Wistar rats were treated with 20-40 mg/kg bw sodium arsenate intraperitoneally once on days 8-12 of pregnancy, a high percentage of malformed foetuses was observed. The main malformations were eye defects, exencephaly, gonadal or renal agenesis and rib or vertebral abnormalities. At higher doses, the rate of resorptions was increased dramatically (Beaudoin, 1974). Arsenate-induced renal agenesis was studied in detail in Wistar rat foetuses after a single i.p. injection of 45 mg/kg bw sodium arsenate on day 10 of pregnancy. Following treatment, the mesonephric duct failed to give rise to an uretric bud, with subsequent failure of induction of the metanephric blastema (Burk & Beaudoin, 1977).

Teratological data obtained with sodium arsenate in golden hamsters have been reviewed by Ferm (1977) . A high percentage of exencephaly was induced in golden hamsters injected intravenously with 20 mg/kg bw sodium arsenate on day 8 of gestation. A considerable increase in the resorption rate was also observed. A dose of 5 mg/kg bw had no teratogenic effect (Ferm & Carpenter, 1968). As could be expected, the type of malformations varied when 15-25 mg/kg bw sodium arsenate were administered intravenously to golden hamsters at different periods of pregnancy (day 8 at 9 a.m., 3 p.m. or 9 p.m.). Anencephaly, urogenital abnormalities and rib malformations were observed, and the rate of resorptions was substantial; the rates of resorption and of malformation increased with the dose (Ferm et al., 1971). The teratogenic effects produced in golden hamsters by i.v. administration of 20 mg/kg bw sodium arsenate on day 8 of pregnancy could be reduced significantly when 2 mg/kg bw sodium selenite were administered simultaneously or shortly before or after the arsenate treatment (Holmberg & Ferm, 1969).

Absorption, distribution, excretion and metabolism

Oral administration of 1 mg/kg bw As as arsenic trioxide to monkeys resulted in approximately 80% absorption from the gut; 75% of the administered dose was excreted within 14 days, primarily in urine (Charbonneau et al., 1978).

About 60% of arsine gas is absorbed by mice exposed to 0.025-2.5 mg/l by inhalation. In rabbits, highest concentrations were found in liver, lungs and kidneys. In mice, large amounts of arsenic were observed in the urine, associated with the initial haemoglobinuria, and smaller amounts were eliminated over longer periods (Levvy, 1947).

Administration of [14]C- and/or [74]As-dimethylarsinic acid to rats by oral, i.v. or intratracheal routes at doses of 120 μg/kg bw to 200 mg/kg bw showed that lung absorption was 92%, in comparison with 66% in the gastrointestinal tract. Highest concentrations were observed in blood, muscle, kidney, liver and lung. Total urinary excretion of either labelled form at 24 hours was found to be 71%, 60% and 25% when given by i.v., intratracheal and oral routes, respectively (Stevens et al., 1977).

Following dietary administration of 215 mg/kg of diet As as calcium arsenate or arsenic trioxide for up to 54 or 42 days in rats, highest arsenic levels (146-537 µg/g of dry tissue) were found in the kidneys and liver and relatively lower levels in hair, brain, bone, muscle and skin. Liver and kidney levels of arsenic were greater after administration of calcium arsenate than of arsenic trioxide (Morris & Wallace, 1938).

Arsenic is accumulated mainly in the liver and kidneys of mice (i.v. injection) (Deak *et al.*, 1976), rats (i.p. injection) (Lawton *et al.*, 1945) and rabbits (i.v. injection) (Du Pont *et al.*, 1942) following initial exposure to arsenite or arsenate. Livers and kidneys of mice (Bencko & Symon, 1969), rabbits (Bencko *et al.*, 1968) and dogs (Katsura, 1953) exposed chronically to arsenite or arsenic trioxide show early increases in arsenic content followed by a subsequent decrease. This decrease may occur in part as a result of an increase in the known biliary excretion of arsenic (Cikrt & Bencko, 1974; Klaassen, 1974) or enhanced bio-transformation of trivalent to pentavalent arsenic (Bencko *et al.*, 1976).

Following daily s.c. doses of ^{74}As- and ^{71}As-labelled potassium arsenite, Hunter *et al.* (1942) observed low blood levels of As and relatively higher tissue levels of As in rabbits, guinea-pigs and higher apes (two chimpanzees and one baboon). In contrast, rats showed higher arsenic levels in the blood than in major organs such as liver, kidneys, lungs and spleen. Some arsenic appeared to pass from the blood into the spinal fluid in apes.

Groups of 9 male and 9 female rats, 21 days of age, were given a diet containing 26.8 or 215 mg/kg of diet As as arsenic trioxide *ad libitum*. They were first mated when they were 90-110 days old, and the litters of the following 3 pregnancies were evaluated, as well as the first litter of the second generation. The amount of arsenic found in the newborns was lower in the 1st litter of the 1st generation (2.7 mg/kg dry weight) than in later litters (14.3 mg/kg and 20.0 mg/kg in the 3rd and 4th litters of the 1st generation) when 26.8 mg of arsenic were given per kg diet. Similar results were obtained with the high dose: an average of 70.4 mg/kg dry weight arsenic were present in the newborns of the 1st litter of the 1st generation, 109 mg/kg in the 4th litter of the 1st generation and 121 mg/kg in the 1st litter of the 2nd generation. The total content of arsenic per animal was the same at the age of 15 days as it was at birth; however, the arsenic content per kg dry weight was many times higher at birth than at 15 days of age (Morris *et al.*, 1938).

Following i.v. administration of ^{76}As as sodium arsenite to five rats and four rabbits, the urinary excretion of ^{76}As in the first 48 hours was <10% of the dose in rats and 30% in rabbits. Following i.p injection in mice, 75% of the dose was excreted within the first 24 hours. In all species tested, <10% of the total ^{76}As was excreted in the faeces. Unlike rabbits, rats retain most of the injected dose in the blood for a prolonged period. Tissue distribution studies revealed highest levels of ^{76}As in the blood and spleen of rats, in the liver, kidneys and lungs of rabbits and in the liver, kidneys and spleen of mice (Ducoff *et al.*, 1948).

In rabbits fed methanearsonic acid, monosodium salt for 12 weeks, 54% was eliminated in urine and 46% in faeces (Exon et al., 1974). Studies in which cows and dogs (Lakso & Peoples, 1975; Tam et al., 1978) were exposed to either arsenite or arsenate in the diet demonstrated that dimethylarsinic acid (90%) and methylarsonic acid are the primary chemical forms in which arsenic is excreted in urine.

Arsenate is metabolized in both fresh and salt water by bacteria and fungi to methylated compounds, predominantly to dimethylarsinic acid (Woolson, 1977).

Effects on intermediary metabolism

Exposure of mice to 50 mg/l arsenite in drinking-water inhibits hepatic respiration (Bencko, 1972; Bencko & Němečková, 1971). Similar findings have been reported in hepatic mitochondria of rats (Brown et al., 1976; Fowler et al., 1977, 1979) and mice (Fowler & Woods, 1979) exposed to 40 mg/l arsenate in drinking-water, and in renal mitochondria of rats exposed to 85 mg/l (Brown et al., 1976). Exposure to arsenate in these studies also decreased hepatic mitochondrial haem biosynthesis in both rats and mice but did not alter total microsomal cytochrome P-450 levels or oxidative demethylation directly (Woods & Fowler, 1978). These findings do not preclude the possibility of changes in other microsomal enzyme reactions, involving specific cytochrome P-450 or P-448 subpopulations, following exposure to arsenate.

Although there is a large body of additional information available on various metabolic reactions to arsenic in mammalian cells, only those studies concerned with nucleic acid metabolism are considered below.

Arsenic (as disodium arsenate) binds to thiol groups of the enzyme DNA polymerase, thus inhibiting DNA synthesis; the authors concluded that it interfered with DNA repair of damage induced by ultra-violet irradiation in human epidermal grafts (Jung & Trachsel, 1970; Jung et al., 1969). Sibatani (1959) found that arsenate inhibited incorporation of ^{32}P into DNA of rabbit lymphocytes to a greater degree than into RNA, suggesting inhibition of DNA repair or synthesis.

Disodium arsenate alters the metabolism of nucleosides and their derivatives in human lymphocytes cultured *in vitro* (Baron et al., 1975), and reduces the incorporation of labelled nucleosides into both RNA and DNA in cultured human peripheral lymphocytes (Petres et al., 1977).

Other studies, by Rossman et al. (1975), in bacteria have shown that sodium arsenite inhibits DNA repair in these organisms following ultra-violet irradiation (see section on mutagenicity below).

The mechanisms of arsine hemolysis appear to involve oxidation of arsine to arsenite *in vivo* with subsequent inhibition of sulphhydryl-containing enzymes (Gramar, 1955; Pernis & Magistretti, 1960). Studies concerning direct effects of arsine on kidney and liver slices have shown decreased tissue respiration (Hughes & Levvy, 1947).

Mutagenicity and other short-term tests

Arsenic has been tested in various bacterial tests, but usually only in single doses; thus, no dose-response data were available.

Sodium arsenite induced point mutations in two strains of *Escherichia coli* WP2 at doses of 0.16-0.8 mmol, allowing 40% survival of colony formation; negative results were obtained in a *recA⁻* strain. Arsenic trichloride and sodium arsenite gave positive results in a *rec* assay in *Bacillus subtilis* using 2.5 μmol/plate (Nishioka, 1975); the same test gave positive results with 0.05 M arsenic trioxide (Kada *et al.*, 1980). Arsenite (As[III]) (doses and compounds unspecified) was negative in the *Salmonella*/microsome test (Löfroth & Ames, 1978).

Sodium arsenite (0.1 mM) decreased mutation in and survival of ultra-violet-irradiated strains of *E. coli* WP2 proficient in recombination-repair, but had no effect on the survival of a deficient strain. It was therefore suggested that arsenicals inhibit certain kinds of repair to DNA damage induced by ultra-violet irradiation (Rossman *et al.*, 1975, 1977).

Potassium arsenite (0.5-1 μM) caused mitotic arrest and chromosomal aberrations (chromatid gaps, breaks, translocations, dicentrics and rings) in cultured human peripheral lymphocytes (Oppenheim & Fishbein, 1965).

Sodium arsenite, at concentrations ranging from 3×10^{-9} M to 6×10^{-8} M, caused chromosomal aberrations (chromatid breaks, chromatid exchanges) in cultured human peripheral lymphocytes and in human diploid fibroblast WI.38 and MRC5 cell lines (Paton & Allison, 1972).

Groups of 5 mice were given 10 or 100 mg/l sodium arsenite in their drinking-water for 8 weeks; some groups then received a single i.p. injection of 2 mg/kg bw tris(1-aziridinyl) phosphine oxide (TEPA). Arsenic treatment alone caused a slight increase in chromosomal aberrations in bone-marrow cells; the higher dose of arsenic potentiated the chromosome-damaging effects of TEPA. Administration of 100 mg/l sodium arsenite in drinking-water for 8 weeks also enhanced the occurrence of dominant lethals induced in male mice treated with 1 mg/kg bw TEPA; arsenic alone did not significantly increase the frequency (Šrám, 1976).

Administration of daily oral doses of 0.25, 0.5 and 1 mg/kg bw arsenite did not increase the incidence of pre-implantation, post-implantation or total dominant lethality in mice (Genčík *et al.*, 1977).

Arsenate (As[V]) (compounds and doses unspecified) was negative in the *Salmonella/* microsome test (Löfroth & Ames, 1978). Positive results were obtained in a *rec* assay in *B. subtilis* with 0.05 M arsenic pentoxide (Kada *et al.*, 1980); sodium methanearsonates were negative in this test (Shirasu *et al.*, 1976).

Sodium arsenate, at concentrations ranging from 6×10^{-9} M to 6×10^{-8} M, caused a small number of chromosomal aberrations (chromatid breaks, chromatid exchanges) in cultured human peripheral lymphocytes (Paton & Allison, 1972).

10^{-4} M sodium arsenite enhanced the morphological transformation of Syrian hamster secondary embryo cells by simian adenovirus SA7 (Casto *et al.*, 1979) [Transformed cells were not injected into suitable hosts to verify the occurrence of malignant transformation].

In an abstract, it was reported that methanearsonic acid, monosodium and disodium salts gave negative results in the *Salmonella*/microsome test, in DNA repair tests in *E. coli* and *B. subtilis* and in an assay for mitotic recombination in *Saccharomyces cerevisiae* (Simmon *et al.*, 1976). Methanearsonic acid, monosodium salt was one of a number of arsenic derivatives that were not mutagenic in the *Salmonella* spot test (without metabolic activation) (Andersen *et al.*, 1972).

(b) Humans

Acute toxic effects

Effects of arsenic compounds on humans have been reviewed by the National Academy of Sciences (1977), Nordberg *et al.* (1979), Pershagen & Vahter (1979) and the US Department of Health, Education, & Welfare (1975). Only a few aspects are described below.

The fatal dose of ingested arsenic trioxide in humans is reported to be in the range of 70-180 mg. Symptoms and signs observed in humans after large oral doses of inorganic arsenicals include severe gastrointestinal damage with vomiting and diarrhoea (often blood-tinged). Muscular cramps, facial oedema and cardiac abnormalities are also frequently present. Shock may develop rapidly, probably as a result of dehydration. Depending on the vehicle, the solubility and the particle size of the powder, symptoms may occur within minutes or be delayed for hours (Vallee *et al.*, 1960).

Exposure to arsenic trichloride, which has a vapour pressure at 25°C sufficient to produce an air concentration of 140,000 mg/m^3, can cause irritation or ulceration on contact or may be absorbed through the skin, with fatal results (Delepine, 1923; US Department of Heath, Education, & Welfare, 1975).

Oral exposures to inorganic arsenic sufficient to cause acute and delayed symptoms without systemic collapse have been reported; effects include gastrointestinal, cardiovascular, nervous and haematopoietic symptoms.

Effects on the peripheral nervous system have been reported by a number of authors (Garb & Hine, 1977; Heyman et al., 1956; Jenkins, 1966; O'Shaughnessy & Kraft, 1976). Histologically, Wallerian degeneration was found (Ohta, 1970).

Anaemia and leucopenia have been reported in patients poisoned by arsenic compounds (Feussner et al., 1979; Hamamoto, 1955; Heyman et al., 1956; Kyle & Pease, 1965). It was a general experience among physicians using Fowler's solution (containing arsenic tri-oxide) in the treatment of dermatological disorders that when an effective dose was reached the patient usually had a certain depression of the leucocyte count (Nordberg et al., 1979).

Changes in the electrocardiogram, including abnormalities in the Q-T interval and T-wave, have been reported in persons poisoned by arsenic (Barry & Herndon, 1962; Chhuttani et al., 1967; Hamamoto, 1955; Weinberg, 1960).

About twelve thousand Japanese infants were exposed to arsenic in 1955 (Morinaga incident) as a result of contamination of dry milk with inorganic arsenic compounds. Inges-tion was approximately 3.5 mg arsenic daily for 33 days. Fever, insomnia, anorexia, liver swelling and melanosis were the most common symptoms and signs; 130 deaths were re-ported (Hamamoto, 1955; Nordberg et al., 1979; Yamashita et al., 1972).

In 1956, more than 400 people were poisoned by soya sauce accidentally contaminated with an inorganic arsenic compound (probably calcium arsenate). Approximately 3 mg arsenic were ingested daily for 2-3 weeks. Facial oedema, anorexia, upper respiratory symptoms, skin lesions and peripheral neuropathy as well as enlarged livers were reported in these cases (Mizuta et al., 1956). Marked hepatic and renal damage have also been observed following ingestion of arsenic trioxide or sodium arsenate (Fréjaville et al., 1972; Gerhardt et al., 1978). Reynolds (1901) reported an incident in which 6000 persons in Manchester, UK were poisoned by beer containing 2-4 mg/l arsenic; 70 deaths occurred.

Exposure to airborne inorganic arsenic compounds (mainly arsenic trioxide) and other substances in a smelter caused irritation of the nasal mucosa (with perforation of the nasal septum), larynx and bronchi as well as conjunctivitis and dermatitis (Holmqvist, 1951; Pinto & McGill, 1953).

Acute exposure to arsine produces rapid haemolytic anaemia and clinical signs characterized by nausea, headache, anaemia, decreased haemoglobin levels, coppery skin pigmentation, icterus, haemoglobinuria and shock within 2-24 hours after exposure. Oliguria or anuria occur commonly after about 24 hours, due to blockage of the renal tubules by haemoglobin casts (Fowler & Weissberg, 1974; Levinsky et al., 1970; Levy et al., 1979; Parish et al., 1979; Pernis & Magistretti, 1960). One case of acute fatal intoxication due to arsine was reported in a foundry worker (Gramer, 1955).

Forestry workers exposed to dimethylarsinic acid herbicides (Tarrant & Allard, 1972; Wagner & Weswig, 1974) have elevated urinary levels of arsenic. No clinical signs of toxicity have been reported to date.

Chronic toxic effects

Effects on the respiratory system after long-term inhalation exposure to inorganic arsenic compounds have been reported, particularly in the smelting industry (Hine et al., 1977; Ishinishi, 1973; Lundgren, 1954; Pinto & McGill, 1953), where exposure levels in the 1950s were frequently about 0.5 mg/m^3 or even higher. Various symptoms and signs from the upper respiratory passages, including rhino-pharyngo-laryngitis and perforation of the nasal septum occurred in some groups of workers. Symptoms of tracheobronchitis and signs of pulmonary insufficiency due to emphysema were observed in other groups, particularly in those exposed to sulphur dioxide and other metals in addition to arsenic compounds (Lundgren, 1954).

Effects on the respiratory system as a result of exposure to arsenic in drinking-water were reported by Borgoño et al. (1977) in their studies in Antofagasta (Chile) [The Working Group considered that the role of arsenic compounds as immune-response suppressants (Gainer & Pry, 1972) should be considered when discussing the overfrequency of pulmonary fibrosis in the Antofagasta population].

Liver cirrhosis has been reported in humans who took Fowler's solution (Franklin et al., 1950) and in vine-dressers using arsenical herbicides (Lüchtrath, 1972; Roth, 1957a). In the latter case, consumption of alcohol cannot be excluded as a complicating factor. Butzengeiger (1940) also reported liver damage in vine-dressers and cellarmen exposed to arsenical insecticides. The homemade wine consumed by most of the workers was believed to be contaminated with arsenic, but most drank up to 2 litres daily.

Numerous reports indicate hyperpigmentation and keratoses in humans following chronic exposure to arsenicals (Alvarado et al., 1964; Borgoño et al., 1977; Tseng et al., 1968), and these lesions are used as clinical indicators of chronic arsenicism.

Peripheral neuropathy is an important manifestation of chronic arsenicism: chronic exposure to arsenicals produces peripheral neuropathy, with pseudoathetosis in advanced cases (Heyman et al., 1956; Robinson, 1975); chronic industrial exposure to arsenic in a copper smelter also induced peripheral neuropathy (Feldman et al., 1979). Hindmarsh et al. (1977) reported an increased incidence of electromyographic abnormalities in humans exposed to arsenic in well-water for prolonged periods.

Seven cases of arsenicism were reported among individuals who had lived near a mining factory and had been exposed to arsenic-containing effluents. One had malignant keratosis (Nakamura et al., 1976).

Cardiovascular disorders have also been reported in persons chronically exposed to arsenic compounds. Symptoms and signs of peripheral vascular disorders were found in vine-dressers with chronic arsenic poisoning (Butzengeiger, 1940), even many years after termination of exposure (Grobe, 1976). Lee & Fraumeni (1969) and Axelson et al. (1978) reported an increased mortality from cardiovascular disease in smelter workers exposed to high levels of airborne arsenic.

A high prevalence of a peripheral vascular disorder, the blackfoot disease, has been found in an area of Taiwan where high levels of arsenic occur in drinking-water (Tseng, 1977; Tseng et al., 1968) [Increased morbidity was related to calculated total amounts of arsenic ingested (in the range 10-50 g) by various subgroups of the population]. Peripheral vascular effects have also been reported in a population in Antofagasta (Chile) exposed to arsenic via drinking-water (Borgoño et al., 1977).

Chronic exposure of workers to arsine has been reported to produce haemoglobin values as low as 32 g/l and basophilic stippling, in the absence of other clinical signs (Bulmer et al., 1940).

Effects on reproduction and prenatal toxicity

A series of papers deals with a possibly embryotoxic hazard produced by a smelter which emits into the environment a number of 'potentially genotoxic' substances, such as lead, arsenic and sulphur dioxide. A significant reduction in birth weight was found in the offspring of employees (3391 ± 526 g, n = 323) and of the inhabitants of two small areas near the smelter (3394 ± 528 g, n = 1157 and 3411 ± 536 g, n = 689) in offspring of employees versus 3460 ± 554 g, n = 2700 in controls living in Umeå; $P < 0.05$). Later pregnancies were particularly affected. Moreover, a higher frequency of spontaneous abortion was noted in women living close to the smelter (10.1% of first pregnancies and 11% of all pregnancies) when compared with those living in an area further away from the smelter (5.1% of first pregnancies and 7.6% of all pregnancies). No correlation is possible with the type of toxic hazard involved. The frequency of multiple malformations also seemed to be higher in the 253 children born during the time of employment of their mothers (4 cases + 1 Down's syndrome: 20%) when compared with 4.6% in the 24,018 children of nonemployed women living in the area and with none in the 727 children born to current employees before or after their employment period at the smelter (Nordström et al., 1978a,b,c,d).

Absorption, distribution, excretion and metabolism

For data on the occurrence of arsenic in human tissues, see section 2.2(j).

Inorganic arsenic compounds are slightly absorbed through the skin when administered in a lipid vehicle, but parenterally-administered arsenic compounds are completely absorbed within 24 hours from i.m.- and s.c.-injected sites; 95-99% of the absorbed arsenic is found first in the red cells and then in the liver, kidney, lung, walls of the gastrointestinal tract and spleen. After two weeks, arsenic is stored in the hair, skin and bones (Oehme, 1972). Trivalent arsenic is more toxic than is pentavalent arsenic; the former is converted to the latter, which is rapidly excreted by the kidneys (Schroeder & Balassa, 1966).

At 20 hours after an i.v. injection of 4 mg of [76]As as sodium arsenite to one patient with terminal cancer, highest levels of arsenic were found in the liver and kidneys and relatively smaller levels in various other tissues. Excretion of [76]As in the first 24 hours after an i.v. injection of labelled sodium arsenite to 2 patients with terminal cancer was 16.7% of the injected dose; excretion was mainly *via* the urine (Ducoff et al., 1948).

Hunter et al. (1942) found that 33-50% of [74]As- and [71]As-labelled potassium arsenite given as 4 daily s.c. doses each of 1.4-1.5 mg to 2 healthy persons and to 1 terminal cancer patient was excreted in the urine within 2-3 days of the last dose; <1% of the total dose was excreted in the faeces.

Holland et al. (1959) reported that 5-9% of [74]As was taken up by 8 terminal cancer patients following inhalation of cigarette smoke containing labelled sodium arsenite. Approximately 45% of the inhaled arsenic was excreted in the urine and 2.5% in the faeces after 10 days. After oral exposure to arsenite, over 80% of the ingested dose was excreted within 60 hours (Bettley & O'Shea, 1975; Crecelius, 1977).

I.v. injection of radioactive arsenite to humans resulted in rapid clearance of arsenic from the plasma, with highest tissue accumulation in the liver and kidneys (Mealey et al., 1959).

A woman ingested approximately 30 ml of a rat poison containing 1.32% elemental arsenic as arsenic trioxide in the 30th week of pregnancy. She was given 150 mg dimercaprol intramuscularly 24 hours later; on the fourth day after the poisoning she was delivered of a live infant weighing 1100 g with a one-minute Apgar score of 4, who died 11 hours later. The following arsenic contents (calculated as arsenic trioxide) were found at autopsy: 7.4 mg/kg wet weight in liver, 1.5 mg/kg in kidneys and 0.2 mg/kg in brain. These data prove that the arsenic had reached the fetus at an extremely high concentration. The concentrations found in the newborn are considered by the authors to be almost 150 times reported normal values in adult tissues (Lugo et al., 1969).

Chemical speciation studies have shown that dimethylarsinic acid and methanearsonic acid are the primary forms of arsenic present in urine of humans exposed to arsenite by ingestion (Crecelius, 1977) or to arsenic trioxide by inhalation (Smith et al., 1977).

Mutagenicity and other short-term tests

A significantly increased incidence of chromosomal aberrations (secondary constrictions, chromatid gaps and breaks, acentrics and dicentrics) was found in cultured peripheral lymphocytes from 31 patients with extensive exposure to arsenic compounds (14 psoriatic patients, 17 vine-dressers) compared with 31 controls (14 psoriatics, 17 healthy volunteers). All those in the exposed group displayed typical arsenic hyperkeratosis, and several had had arsenic-induced skin carcinomas excised. In some cases, several decades had elapsed since the end of exposure to arsenic compounds (Petres et al., 1977).

Preliminary results showed that the frequency of chromosome aberrations in short-term cultured lymphocytes from 9 workers exposed to arsenic at a smelter was 87 in 819 mitoses, significantly increased as compared with that of 'apparently healthy individuals' who had 13 aberrations in 1012 mitoses. The authors pointed out that the workers were exposed simultaneously to other agents (Beckman et al., 1977).

Nordenson et al. (1978) reported an increase in chromosomal aberrations (gaps, and chromatid and chromosome aberrations) in cultured peripheral lymphocytes from 39 workers exposed to arsenic compounds at the same smelter. The urinary levels of arsenic ranged from 170-390 μg, but the correlation between frequency of aberrations and arsenic exposure was rather poor. The results suggested that both exposure to arsenic compounds and smoking contributed to the increases in chromosome aberrations.

Nordenson et al. (1979) examined the chromosomes of cultured peripheral lymphocytes (72-hr) from 16 psoriatics, 7 of whom had received total doses of 300-1200 mg and one an unknown dose of arsenic, 9-16 years before the start of the study. The average duration of psoriasis in treated patients was 29 years, and that in untreated psoriatics was 16 years.

Untreated psoriatics had significantly more chromatid gaps than healthy controls; and the frequency of gaps was significantly higher in arsenic-treated than in untreated patients. There was no significant difference bewteen the two groups in the frequency of chromatid or chromosome breaks; when data for chromatid and chromosome breaks were pooled, however, there was a significant increase in aberration frequency in the arsenic-treated group. The frequency of aberrations showed no apparent relationship to age, arsenic dose, time of treatment or frequency of psoriatic symptoms. There was no difference in the rate of sister chromatid exchange between the two groups of psoriatics.

An elevated rate of sister chromatid exchange was found in the cultured peripheral lymphocytes of 6 patients who had been exposed to 1% potassium arsenite (Fowler's solution) for asthma, psoriasis or anxiety for periods ranging from 4 months to 27 years; exposure had ceased 1-56 years from the time of the study. All 6 patients subsequently developed skin carcinomas and arsenic keratoses; 3 had a history of high X-ray exposure. The exposed group had, on average, 14 sister chromatid exchanges per mitosis, compared with 5.8 in 44 'normal' individuals. There was no difference in the incidence of chromosomal aberrations between the two groups (Burgdorf et al., 1977).

3.3 Case reports and epidemiological studies

(a) Arsenic drugs

A review is available (Schmähl et al., 1977).

Inorganic trivalent arsenic compounds, and particularly Fowler's solution, have been used widely for a variety of ailments (including skin diseases) and are still used in some countries. Large doses taken internally lead to chronic changes in the skin (arsenicism), such as hyperpigmentation and keratosis. The concurrence of chronic skin arsenicism with in situ and invasive carcinomas of the skin has been reviewed in 143 cases by Neubauer (1947) and by others (Bartak & Kejda, 1972; Ehlers, 1968; Jackson & Grainge, 1975; Minkowitz, 1964; Sanderson, 1963; Sommers & McManus, 1953). Characteristically, the skin cancers were multifocal, involved areas of the body unexposed to sunlight and occurred at atypical locations such as the palms and soles, while skin cancers not related to arsenicism are most often single lesions which occur on areas exposed to sunlight or at the site of application of, e.g., tar, X-rays or radium. The period from the beginning of treatment to the manifestation of tumours ranged from 5-60 years (average, 18 years), and most cancers occurred only after the drug had been taken for a relatively long time: 90% of cases had taken the drug for more than one year and 60% for more than five years. The average dose was 28 g (range, 0.2-121 g). The patients were relatively young when the cancers were noted: one-third were less than 40 years old, and almost three-quarters were less than 50. Aldick & Fabry (1973) reported a case of multifocal basal-cell carcinoma of the skin in a man whose mother had taken Fowler's solution during her pregnancy. Calnan (1954) reported one case of basal-cell epithelioma of the skin with bronchial carcinoma in a man treated for several years for psoriasis with Fowler's solution.

Fierz (1965) reviewed findings from 262 patients who had received Fowler's solution for the treatment of chronic skin disorders: 40% had hyperkeratosis on the palms and soles, and 8% had skin cancers. A dose-response relationship with total arsenic dose was observed for both conditions; the doses taken by patients with cancer ranged from 0.1-26 g arsenic, and tumours were observed at 6-26 years after treatment (average, 14 years).

Tay & Seah (1975) reported on the prevalence of cancer among 74 individuals with arsenic poisoning caused by ingestion of herbal preparations containing arsenic sulphide, taken mostly for the treatment of asthma. Six subjects were diagnosed for skin cancer; of 4 who had internal malignancies (2 with lung cancer, 1 with cancer of the gall bladder and 1 with haemangiosarcoma of the liver), 2 also had skin cancer. Three additional cases of angiosarcoma of the liver (Dalderup et al., 1976; Lander et al., 1975; Regelson et al., 1968; Roth, 1955) and one case of carcinoma of the liver with squamous-cell carcinoma of the lung (Goldman, 1973) have been reported in association with ingestion of Fowler's solution.

Isolated cases of cancers other than skin have been reported in patients who received Fowler's solution or other arsenic medication: Nurse (1978) reported one case of cancer of the neck and kidney, Prystowsky et al. (1978) one case of cancer of the nasopharynx, and Calnan (1954) and Robson & Jelliffe (1963) seven cases of lung cancer. Neubauer (1947) reported cases of skin cancers associated with cancers of the stomach, tongue and oral mucosa, uterus, ureter and bladder, oesophagus and breast, and one case each of breast cancer and pancreatic cancer without skin cancer [The Working Group considered that these reports do not provide evidence of an association between medicinal exposure to arsenic and tumours at these sites].

In a case-contol study, 419 patients (204 males and 215 females) with various histological types of skin cancer were compared with 200 control patients (100 of each sex) with no skin malignancies; the two groups were comparable for age, occupation and urban-rural residence. The proportion of those exposed to arsenic compounds was significantly greater in the group of patients with Bowen's disease (epithelioma) or superficial basal-cell carcinoma of the trunk (36%) than in the control group (14%); squamous-cell carcinomas were also seen. More than 85% of cases in all groups had been exposed to medicinal arsenic (Fritsch et al., 1971).

Reymann et al. (1978) studied a possible relationship between intake of arsenic compounds and incidence of internal malignant neoplasms (not further specified) by following up a group of patients with multiple basal-cell carcinomas, Bowen's disease, psoriasis, verruca plana or lichen planus who had been treated with arsenic drugs. The observed incidence was compared with the expected incidence of internal malignant neoplasms on the basis of national rates available from the Danish Cancer Registry. Except for one subgroup (women with multiple basal-cell carcinomas: 5 observed versus 1.2 expected), no statistically significant excess of internal malignant neoplasms was seen.

(b)   Arsenic in drinking-water

Basal-cell carcinomas and lesions of Bowen's disease developed in a man who was acutely intoxicated with arsenic after drinking well-water contaminated with arsenic (Degreef & Roelandts, 1974). Multiple basal-cell carcinomas (Wagner *et al.*, 1979) developed in a woman who had ingested well-water containing 1.2 mg/l arsenic for 4 months. Two males from the city of Antofagasta, Chile, who drank water containing an average of 0.6 mg/l (range, 0.05-0.96 mg/l) total arsenic for approximately 30 years (total dose, about 13 g arsenic), developed multiple, scattered squamous-cell carcinomas located in areas of the skin not exposed to sunlight (Zaldivar, 1974). One case of liver haemangioendothelioma has also been reported from the same area of Chile (Rennke *et al.*, 1971).

In certain other parts of the world (e.g., Reichenstein, Silesia and Cordoba, Argentina), the high levels of total arsenic found in drinking-water have been associated with a high rate of reporting of arsenicism and skin cancer cases (reviewed by Neubauer, 1947).

Tseng *et al.* (1968) and Tseng (1977) carried out a house-by-house survey of more than 40,000 people in an area of Taiwan who had drunk artesian well-water containing high levels of arsenic (average levels, about 0.5 mg/l; range, 0.01-1.8 mg/l) for more than 60 years. They found prevalence rates of skin cancer (10.6/1000), hyperpigmentation (184/1000), keratosis (71/1000) and a peripheral vascular disorder called 'blackfoot disease' (9/1000). No cases of any of these conditions were found among 7500 people in a neighbouring area with low arsenic levels in the drinking-water (0.001-0.02 mg/l). Skin cancer rates in areas of low (0.0-0.29 mg/l), medium (0.3-0.59 mg/l) and high ($\geq$0.6 mg/l) arsenic levels were 2.6/1000, 10.1/1000 and 21.4/1000, respectively. Similar dose-response relationships were seen for the other lesions. The skin cancers seen were atypical in that three-quarters of them were on areas of the body not exposed to sunlight; furthermore, virtually all the patients (99.5%) had more than one lesion.

Morton *et al.* (1976) found no excess of skin cancers in the population of a county in the US where there was a high arsenic content in the drinking-water; furthermore, the incidence of skin cancers within the county did not correlate with arsenic levels in the water. Mean arsenic levels (average, 16.5 μg/l; range, 0.0-2150 μg/l) were lower than those seen in the studies by Tseng (1977) and Tseng *et al.* (1968), however, and varied considerably throughout the county. Additionally, local dermatologists reported few cases of arsenical hyperkeratosis or hyperpigmentation, despite previous knowledge of the elevated arsenic levels.

[The Working Group noted that average arsenic levels were about 30 times greater in the study in Taiwan than in that in the US. The two reports are thus not necessarily contradictory.]

(c)   Air pollutants containing arsenic

Blot & Fraumeni (1975) found that average mortality rates from lung cancer for white males and females in the US in 1950-1969 were significantly increased in counties in which there were copper, lead or zinc smelting and refining industries (which are associated with substantial amounts of inorganic arsenic) but not in counties where aluminium or other non-ferrous ores (not associated with arsenic) were processed. When the data from 36 counties with copper, lead or zinc industries were pooled, the standardized mortality ratios (SMRs) for lung cancer were 112 for males and 110 for females. These could not be accounted for by differences in geographical region, population density, urbanization or socioeconomic status. Part of the excess can be attributed to the presence of smelter workers (who are at increased risk of lung cancer) in the death data for the counties. In over half of the counties, less than 1% of the total population was employed in smelters, and in almost 90% less than 3% were so employed. The authors calculated that the relative risk of lung cancer in smelter workers would have to be about 13 in order to account for the overall 12% increase seen in all the counties. They suggested that community air pollution from industrial emissions containing inorganic arsenic was the most likely cause of the increased lung cancer mortality.

In order to examine a possible association of the distance from a copper smelter with lung cancer incidence, a case-control study was undertaken using information from a population-based cancer registry. The cases consisted of all new cases of lung cancer registered during a certain period of time, while the control group consisted of all cases of lymphoma registered during the same period. No association was demonstrated between lung cancer and the distance between the smelter and place of residence for either men or women (Lyon *et al.*, 1977) [The Working Group noted that this study was conducted in a county in which the lung cancer mortality rate was one of the lowest of the 36 counties studied by Blot & Fraumeni (Stellman & Kabat, 1978). However, if lung cancer cases were associated with exposure to arsenic from the smelter, more cases than controls should have lived closer to the industry. This association was not observed. The use of lymphomas as a control group may have obscured an association, since lymphomas have been associated with arsenic exposure in at least one study (Ott *et al.*, 1974).

Mortality rates in an area around a large smelter in Sweden, which had emitted large amounts of arsenic during the processing of copper, lead, zinc and other nonferrous ores, were studied for a 14-year period and compared with those in a reference area whose population was similar with regard to urbanization, occupational profile and age distribution. No differences in mortality were found among either males or females for any causes of death other than lung cancer in men: the SMR for primary respiratory cancer in men in the exposed area was 250 (P=0.002) when compared with the reference area and 130 (not significant) when compared with national rates. This excess mortality was no longer significant (SMR=173) when those men occupationally exposed at the smelter were excluded. Smoking habits were not specifically studied; however, it was considered that they were unlikely to be substantially different in the two populations, which were similar with regard to several socioeconomic variables (Pershagen *et al.*, 1977).

Matanoski *et al.* (1980) studied cancer mortality in residents of an area in the US in which a pesticide plant was located, in comparison with that in other populations matched for race, sex, age and socioeconomic status. Arsenical products were produced at the plant from the early 1900s until 1973, and chlorinated and organophosphate pesticides were formulated from 1947. The population in the area where the plant was located demonstrated a significant excess of lung cancers (relative risk, 4) in males but not in females when compared with the matching populations; these comparisons were based on 25 deaths from lung cancer. The risk for lung cancer increased more rapidly in the exposed population than in the comparison group over the 17 years covered by the study. When the plant records of employees were reviewed, 2 lung cancer deaths were removed from the data, but the excess remained. A spot map indicated that the lung cancer cases were distributed in an area 8 city blocks wide and 9-12 blocks long, lying to the north and east of the plant. This area had the highest arsenic levels in soil, with a mean level of 63 mg/kg and a highest level of 695 mg/kg. The distribution of cases along a railroad line suggested that transportation routes might be the means of spreading arsenicals [The Working Group noted that interpretation of this study is made difficult by lack of information about other occupational exposures and about cigarette smoking. Furthermore, the lack of an effect in women suggests that factors other than environmental arsenic exposure are important].

(d) Occupational arsenic exposure

(i) Factories

Hamada *et al.* (1977) reported 3 cases of Bowen's disease among 28 workers who had been employed in the manufacture of lead arsenate from arsenic acid and lead oxide. In 2 of these 3, the duration of exposure to arsenic was relatively short, 2 or 3 years, while the time interval between the termination of exposure and the diagnosis of the disease was fairly long, both 24 years.

Two out of 26 patients reported to the New York State Tumor Registry with angiosarcoma of the liver had used arsenical pesticides for many years (Brady *et al.*, 1977) [The Working Group noted that it was not possible to determine from the paper whether one of the matched controls had also been exposed to arsenic].

Hill & Faning (1948) examined the proportionate mortality of workers involved in the manufacture of sheep-dip containing inorganic arsenicals, who, according to Perry *et al.* (1948), had median arsenic exposures ranging from 71-696 $\mu g/m^3$. Twenty-two of the 75 deaths in sheep-dip workers (29%) were due to cancer; comparable figures in other workers were 157 of 1216 deaths (13%). The excess of cancer in sheep-dip workers was limited to workers heavily exposed to arsenic (19/51, 37%), and no excess was seen in nonexposed workers (3/24, 12.5%). The excess cancer deaths were limited to respiratory (32% in exposed *versus* 16% in nonexposed) and skin cancers (14% in exposed *versus* 1% in nonexposed).

In a proportionate mortality study of deaths occurring in England and Wales between 1959 and 1963, Moss & Lee (1974) demonstrated a significant excess (11 *versus* 2.56 expected; $P<0.0001$) of oral and pharyngeal cancer in male textile workers engaged in fibre preparation. A further analysis of deaths from oral and pharyngeal cancer during the periods 1959-1963 and 1970-1971 by type of fibres used by fibre preparers indicated that 18/22 deaths occurred among those who had worked with wool, whereas only 56% of all fibre preparers had worked with this material. Thus, the risk for wool fibre preparers is even more significant than that calculated above. The following materials were reported to be present in raw wool: natural secretions and excretions, animal parasites, vegetable burrs and grass, soil, tar and paint, branding fluids, sheep-dips (which may have been contaminated with arsenic) and salves.

The proportional mortality of 173 workers who had been engaged in the production and packaging of arsenical insecticides was compared with that of 1809 dead workers who had worked in the same factory but had not been exposed to arsenic compounds (Ott *et al.*, 1974). Employees who had left the smelter prior to retirement were excluded from the analysis. Twenty-eight of the 173 deaths (16.2%) among the exposed group were due to respiratory cancers, while 104 of the 1809 deaths (5.7%) among the nonexposed workers were due to this cause. The only other excess was seen for cancers of the lymphatic and haematopoietic systems, other than leukaemia: 6/176 (3.5%) *versus* 25/1809 (1.4%). Less then 25% of workers were exposed to arsenic for more than one year; the remainder either left employment or were promoted to other jobs. Of the 173 deaths, 138 (80%) were in workers exposed for less than one year; and 16 of the 28 deaths due to lung cancer (57%) occurred in these workers. The ratio of observed to expected lung cancer deaths increased with total arsenic dose [The Working Group noted that only those workers who were employed until death or who retired from the company were considered. The loss of data on other workers, especially on those exposed to low levels of arsenic, may affect the results. This is supported by the fact that the relative risk remains around 2 with increasing exposure to arsenic over total arsenic doses of 0.12-1.6 mg, while risk increases regularly at doses above these levels]. A retrospective cohort analysis of a subset of the same population showed 20 observed deaths from respiratory cancer among the exposed workers, whereas 5.8 were expected on the basis of US white male mortality rates, giving a relative risk of 3.5. The ratio of observed to expected deaths due to malignant neoplasms of the lymphatic and haematopoietic tissues, except for leukaemia, was also considerably higher than expected: 5 observed, 1.3 expected, relative risk 3.9. The authors suggested that the smoking habits of the exposed workers were no different from those of the controls.

Mabuchi *et al.* (1979) studied mortality rates by cause in 1393 workers employed from 1946 to 1974 in a factory where pesticides were manufactured and formulated. Workers were exposed to many arsenic compounds as well as to copper sulphate, chlorinated hydrocarbons, organophosphates and carbamate and other organic herbicides. As of August 1977, 197 males and 43 females had died. The overall SMRs were close to one, and the only statistically significant excesses of mortality were seen for lung cancer in males (23 observed, 13.7 expected; SMR, 168) and anaemias in males (2 observed, 0.2 expected; SMR, 1000). A dose-response was demonstrated for lung cancer risk, which increased with duration of employment. Although based on small numbers of deaths, there was also a regular increase in lung cancer risk with increasing duration of exposure to arsenicals but not to nonarsenical products. There was also a slight excess of lymphomas in males (4 observed, 2.1 expected; P<0.05) [The Working Group noted that no data on smoking habits were available].

(ii)   Mines and smelters

Osburn (1957) reported an excessive proportionate mortality from cancer of the lung in an autopsy series of Rhodesian miners of gold-bearing ores containing large amounts of arsenic as arsenopyrite. The autopsy incidence of lung cancer was 5.8% (22 cases), which was reported by the authors to be more than double the rate for whites and 14 times the rate for non-whites in Johannesburg. Subsequently, Osburn (1969) re-examined hospital admissions for lung cancer in the gold-mining area and found an additional 37 lung cancers, one of which occurred in a nonminer. He calculated that the incidence of lung cancer among miners was 205.6/100,000, as compared with a rate of 33.8/ 100,000 in the general male population. He also found that 13/37 patients (35%) had palmar hyperkeratosis, indicative of chronic arsenicism. Seventy-six percent of the cases were cigarette smokers (all of the nonsmokers were underground miners), suggesting that the high rate of lung cancer in the area might be due to a combined effect of smoking and exposure to arsenical dust.

A proportionate mortality study showed no excess of cancer among current and retired workers who had been exposed to arsenic in a copper smelter during the period 1946-1960 (Pinto & Bennett, 1963). However, a more recent cohort mortality study of 527 male pensioners (aged 65 or more) from the same facility demonstrated a 12.2% excess of deaths from all causes (P<0.05; SMR=112.2), limited to deaths from respiratory cancers (SMR= 305). A clear linear dose-response effect was demonstrated (see Table 7) [χ^2 for trend, 7.86; P=0.005, calculated by the Working Group]. The excess risk of lung cancer could not be accounted for by smoking: the SMR for smokers was 287, and that for nonsmokers was 506 (Pinto *et al.*, 1978).

Table 7

Observed and expected numbers of deaths from respiratory cancer and standardized
mortality ratios in relation to arsenic exposure index[a]

Arsenic exposure index (arbitrary units)	No. of men	Deaths from respiratory cancer		
		Observed	Expected	SMR
0-1.9	36	1	0.9	111.1
2.0-2.9	109	4	2.1	190.5
3.0-5.9	205	11	3.9	282.0*
6.0-8.9	109	7	2.3	304.3*
9.0-11.9	38	4	0.7	571.4*
>12	29	5	0.6	833.3*

χ^2 trend = 7.86; P = 0.005[b]
χ^2 linearity = 1.78 (not significant)[b]

[a] From Pinto et al. (1978)

[b] Calculated by the Working Group

*P < 0.05

Milham & Strong (1974), using death certificates and company records, found 40 respiratory cancer deaths that had occurred between 1950 and 1971 in one copper smelting plant. 'Application of US mortality rates to the published population at risk in the smelter (Pinto & Bennett, 1963)' gave an expected number of 18 deaths from respiratory cancer (SMR=222; P<0.001) [The Working Group considered that the method of calculating expected deaths is inadequately described and that this study is thus difficult to interpret].

Lee & Fraumeni (1969) examined the mortality experience of 8047 men engaged in metal smelting during the period 1938-1963. Occupational exposure levels were categorized into 'heavy', 'medium' and 'light' for both arsenic trioxide and sulphur dioxide. As compared with the male population of the same states, smelter workers had an excess mortality from cancer of the respiratory system (147 observed *versus* 44.7 expected; SMR=329; P<0.01). This excess was as high as 8-fold for employees who had worked for more than 15 years and who were heavily exposed to arsenic. The risk also increased in proportion to the degree of exposure to arsenic and sulphur dioxide: SMRs were 239, 478 and 667 in those with light, medium and heavy arsenic exposure, respectively. The results were consistent with the view that inhaled arsenic is a respiratory carcinogen in humans; however, an influence of sulphur dioxide or unidentified agents, whose presence varied concomitantly with arsenic exposure, could not be discounted. When the data were examined by the method of proportionate mortality used in some of the previous studies, the percentage of deaths from respiratory cancer (7.8%) was not significantly different from figures reported in studies of other, nonmining occupations with exposure to arsenic, including those which had previously been considered to be negative (Pinto & Bennett, 1963; Snegireff & Lombard, 1951).

In a historical prospective study, Tokudome & Kuratsune (1976) observed a significantly increased mortality for lung cancer (ICD 7th revision = 162) (SMR=1189) among workers probably exposed to arsenic compounds in copper smelting operations in Japan, as compared with the national average. Significant excesses were also seen for colon cancer (3 observed *versus* 0.6 expected; SMR=508) and for liver cancer (11 *versus* 3.26; SMR=337). No significant excesses occurred in workers employed at the factory but not exposed to copper smelting. SMRs for lung cancer were 563, 735 and 1905 for employment durations of 1-9 years, 10-19 years and >20 years, respectively, and 635, 1250 and 1485 for employees in jobs with light, medium and heavy exposure to arsenic, respectively. The significantly elevated SMR for colon cancer in the smelter workers was not associated with a dose-response relationship. The average latent period for development of lung cancer was 37.6 years and was not related to level of exposure. Twenty-six of the 29 deaths from lung cancer occurred in workers after they had left the smelter. No information was given about the smoking habits of the workers; however, it is unlikely that smoking would account for differences of this magnitude.

Axelson *et al.* (1978) conducted a case-control study of deaths from lung cancer and from all other malignancies which had occurred in the area surrounding a copper smelter in Sweden. Controls were all deaths in the area, excluding those due to cancer, cardiovascular disease, cerebrovascular disease, cirrhosis of the liver and some other causes. Lung cancer rates among the workers exposed to arsenic in the smelter were higher than those among persons not so exposed (rate ratio = 4.6; 90% confidence interval, 2.2-9.6). A dose-response relationship between risk and exposure level was observed (although the trend was not significant) when exposures were estimated using a composite score of dose levels and duration of employment: rate ratios were 2.1, 5.9 and 8.8 in those with low, medium and high exposures, respectively. The excess of lung cancer did not correlate with exposure to nickel, lead, copper, selenium, bismuth, antimony or sulphur dioxide. No increased risk was observed for other malignancies, except for leukaemia and myelomas: 6 out of 7 of these cases (86%) had had exposure to arsenic, compared with 18 out of 32 among the controls (56%).

Rencher *et al.* (1977) carried out a proportional mortality study of men who were employed in the smelter, mine, concentrator and other operations of a copper corporation and who died between 1959 and 1969. Seven percent of deaths in workers in the smelter (where exposure to arsenic was high) were due to respiratory neoplasms, compared with 2.2% for those in the mine, 2.2% for those in the concentrator and 2.7% for those in the state in which the plant is located. The excess proportion at the smelter was statistically significant. It was also noted that the age-adjusted death rate for lung cancer of workers at the smelter was 4.8 times that of workers at the mine and 3.1 times that of the population of the state; however, no statistical test of significance was made since some approximations were required in calculating the rates. Smoking histories were available, and although smokers had an increased risk of lung cancer there was no evidence of an interaction with smoking. The cumulative exposure levels to sulphur dioxide, sulphuric acid mist, arsenic, lead and copper were calculated for each deceased smelter worker on the basis of duration and level of exposure. The subjects who died of lung cancer had considerably higher exposure indices for all of the above compounds than did those who died either of nonrespiratory cancer or of nonmalignant respiratory disease. These differences were statistically significant for sulphur dioxide, arsenic and lead; however, no reference was made to a dose-response relationship.

Newman *et al.* (1976) ascertained histological diagnoses for 143 lung tumours from which tissue had been saved by two local pathologists who work in an area of extensive copper mining and smelting. They found that 4/25 (16%) of cancers in smelter workers were well-differentiated epidermoid-cell tumours, while well- or moderately-differentiated tumours accounted for 27/54 (50%) of cancers in miners and for 21/45 (47%) in men not employed in copper industries. The proportions of poorly differentiated epidermoid cancers in these groups were 10/25 (40%), 6/54 (11%) and 6/45 (13%), respectively. The authors suggested that arsenic exposure may have been responsible for the excess of poorly-differentiated tumours in the smelter workers. The lower proportion in miners and the fact that the types of cancers were similar in miners and in men not employed in the copper industry were attributed to the lower levels of arsenic found in the mines compared with the smelter and to the high levels of arsenic pollution in the general community [The Working Group found that this study is difficult to interpret, since the sample was not random and the authors did not state what proportion their subjects represented of all lung cancers in the area. The non-random selection of certain tumours for study may have introduced bias by obviating a representative sample of all tumours].

(iii) Pesticide applicators

Vineyard workers in Germany and France have received heavy exposure to arsenical insecticides through inhalation of lead, calcium and copper arsenate dust and through ingestion of contaminated wine (Galy et al., 1963a, b; Latarjet et al., 1964; Liebegott, 1952). Clinical reports have described an association of chronic arsenicism with skin cancer in vineyard workers (Liebegott, 1952; Grobe, 1977). The concurrence of arsenicism and lung cancer was observed in post mortem studies of those vineyard workers who showed cutaneous stigmata of arsenic toxicity at death: lung cancer occurred in 12 out of 27 men autopsied and liver haemangioendothelioma in two (Roth, 1955, 1957a, b). Lung cancers were also reported by Galy et al. (1963a, b) and Latarjet et al. (1964). Liebegott (1952) described 3 liver carcinomas, 2 liver sarcomas and one oesphageal carcinoma among vineyard workers.

Seventeen vineyard workers with dermatological lesions due to arsenicism were estimated to have ingested an average total of 45 g arsenic (range, 5.6 to 132.9 g) for an average of 13 years (range 5-28 years). Ten of them had Bowen's disease, 6 had basal-cell carcinoma and 7 had squamous-cell carcinoma of the skin; cancer of the lung was seen in 4 patients, cancer of the larynx in one, and cancer of the vocal chords in one other. The average periods from exposure to development of disease were 35, 38, 39 and 39 years for Bowen's disease, basal-cell carcinoma, squamous-cell carcinoma of the skin and cancer of the lung, respectively (Wolf, 1974).

Poirier et al. (1973) reported squamous-cell carcinomas of the skin and of the lung in a vine-dresser who had used 'Bordeaux mixture' (lime and copper sulphate which did **not** contain arsenic) for 30 years and lead and calcium arsenate for 2 years, and who was a non-smoker. He also showed the skin lesions typical of chronic arsenicism.

Nelson *et al.* (1973) studied the mortality of residents in an apple-growing area who in 1938 had participated in a morbidity study of the health effects of lead arsenate spray. The 1231 cohort members were classified into three exposure groups, namely 'orchardists', who prepared and applied lead arsenate sprays, 'consumers' (eaters of apples), with no occupational contact with lead arsenate, and 'intermediates', who had infrequent exposure. The urinary level of total arsenic determined in 1938 showed that the orchardists had the heaviest exposure among the groups: mean urinary arsenic levels in men were 62.0, 71.0 and 140.5 µg/l in consumers, intermediates and orchardists, respectively; the levels in women were 56.3, 58.0 and 97.9 µg/l. However, no data were available about arsenic levels for individuals. The SMRs for all cancers were 0.65, 0.96 and 0.66 for consumers, intermediates and orchardists, respectively, indicating no excess mortality for all cancers as compared with the state average. Similar results were obtained for lung cancers. There was no evidence of increasing mortality with longer durations of exposure.

4. Summary of Data Reported and Evaluation

4.1 Experimental data

Arsanilic acid, arsenic trioxide, sodium arsenite, potassium arsenite (Fowler's solution) and dimethylarsinic acid were tested by the oral route in mice. Lead arsenate, calcium arsenate, arsenic trioxide, sodium arsenate and sodium arsenite were tested by the oral route in rats. Sodium arsenate and arsenite were tested orally in dogs.

Potassium arsenite, arsenic trioxide and sodium arsenate were tested by skin application in mice. Sodium arsenite was tested by inhalation in mice; and arsenic trioxide, a calcium arsenate-copper mixture and copper ore or flue dust containing arsenic were tested by intratracheal administration in rats. Sodium arsenate was tested by intravenous administration in mice. Dimethylarsinic acid was tested by subcutaneous injection in mice; and calcium arsenate was tested by subcutaneous injection in rats. Metallic arsenic was tested by intramedullary injection in rats and rabbits.

In addition, sodium arsenate was tested by subcutaneous injection in mice in an experimental model which included exposures extending from the prenatal to the postnatal period.

Of all these studies, only one involving the subcutaneous administration to mice of sodium arsenate throughout pregnancy and one involving the intratracheal administration of a calcium arsenate-copper mixture to rats provided some evidence of a carcinogenic effect. However, all of the studies, both positive and negative, suffer from some inadequacies.

There is evidence that arsenite and arsenate cross the placenta in mammals. Sodium arsenate and arsenite have embryolethal effects and a teratogenic potential in several mammalian species. A variety of malformations can be induced. When given orally, high doses of arsenate are required to induce a small percentage of abnormalities.

The evidence that arsenic compounds cause mutations and allied effects in bacteria is inconclusive. However, arsenic compounds induce chromosomal aberrations and morphological transformation in mammalian cells.

4.2 Human data

A large number of cases of skin cancer have been reported among people exposed to inorganic arsenic through drugs, drinking-water or pesticides. The clinical presentation and sites of these tumours are different from those of cancers caused by other known skin carcinogens, suggesting that they are causally associated with exposure to arsenic. In one epidemiological study, skin cancer was positively correlated with high arsenic levels in the drinking-water; a second study showed no such correlation, however, the water arsenic levels were substantially lower than those in the first study.

Three cohort studies of workers manufacturing arsenical pesticides showed an excess mortality from respiratory cancer. A further cohort study of workers exposed to lead arsenate during spraying showed no excess mortality from any cancer; however, these people may have been exposed to lower levels than were manufacturing workers.

Case-control and cohort studies in copper smelters demonstrated a significantly increased mortality from respiratory cancer among the workers; however, smelter workers are exposed not only to arsenic compounds but also to other factors in the working environment, some of which may be carcinogenic. An attempt was made to control for exposure to sulphur dioxide, copper, lead, nickel, selenium, antimony and bismuth in one case-control study, and the excess lung cancer remained. Smoking habits were examined in two of the studies and could not account for the excess.

The descriptive epidemiological studies on the mortality of people living in the neighbourhood of copper, lead and/or zinc smelters suggest increased mortality from respiratory cancer. One indicated excess mortality from lung cancer for both men and women, which was not associated with socioeconomic or geographical factors and could not be explained by occupational exposure alone. In the other, the excess mortality from respiratory cancer (which was present only for men) became insignificant when the deaths of workers in the smelter were excluded. These data are inadequate to evaluate the risk of nonoccupational exposure to low levels of airborne arsenic.

Four cases of haemangiosarcoma and one case of carcinoma of the liver have been reported in individuals exposed to medicinal arsenical preparations. One additional case of haemangiosarcoma of the liver was reported in association with general environmental exposure, and two further cases in workers exposed to arsenical pesticides; four cases of liver sarcoma and three of liver carcinoma were associated with vineyard exposure. An excess of lymphomas has been reported in workers in arsenic pesticide manufacture; and excesses of leukaemia, myeloma and colon and liver cancer have been found in smelter workers. An excess of oral cancers has been reported in a population exposed during the spinning of wool which may have been contaminated with arsenical sheep-dip.

Arsenite crosses the placenta. Smelter workers exposed during pregnancy to arsenic compounds (and possibly to other toxic substances) had an excess of infants with low birth weights, an increased frequency of abortions and an increased occurrence of multiple malformations.

An increased incidence of chromosomal aberrations was observed in patients treated with arsenical compounds and in workers exposed occupationally to arsenic compounds in a smelter environment.

4.3 Evaluation

There is inadequate evidence for the carcinogenicity of arsenic compounds in animals. There is *sufficient evidence* that inorganic arsenic compounds are skin and lung carcinogens in humans. The data suggesting an increased risk for cancer at other sites are inadequate for evaluation.

5. References

Airco Industrial Gases (1973) *Rare and Specialty Gases*, Murray Hill, NJ, pp. 12, 33

Aldick, H.J. & Fabry, H. (1973) Multiple basal cell carcinoma due to arsenic use during the fetal period (Ger.). *Der Hautarzt, 24,* 496

Alvarado, L.C., Viniegra, G., García, R.E. & Acevedo, J.A. (1964) Epidemiologic study of arsenicism in the colonies, Miguel Aleman and Eduardo Guerra, De Torreon, Coah. (Span.). *Salud Públ. Méx., 6,* 375-385

Anand, S.J.S. (1978) Determination of mercury, arsenic and cadmium in fish by neutron activation. *J. radioanal. Chem., 44,* 101-107

Andersen, K.J., Leighty, E.G. & Takahashi, M.T. (1972) Evaluation of herbicides for possible mutagenic properties. *J. agric. Food Chem., 20,* 649-656

Andreae, M.O. (1977) Determination of arsenic species in natural waters. *Anal. Chem., 49,* 820-823

Angino, E.E., Magnuson, L.M., Waugh, T.C., Galle, O.K. & Bredfeldt, J. (1970) Arsenic in detergents: possible danger and pollution hazard. *Science, 168,* 389-390

Arkhipov, G.N. (1968) Carcinogenicity of chemical poisons containing arsenic. *Vop. Pitan., 27,* 77

Aruscavage, P. (1977) Determination of arsenic, antimony, and selenium in coal by atomic absorption spectrometry with a graphite tube atomizer. *J. Res. US geol. Surv., 5,* 405-408

Atomergic Chemetals Company, *Product Catalog*, Carle Place, NY, p. 12

Axelson, O., Dahlgren, E., Jansson, C.-D. & Rehnlund, S.O. (1978) Arsenic exposure and mortality: a case-referent study from a Swedish copper smelter. *Br. J. ind. Med., 35,* 8-15

Baron, D., Kunick, I., Frischmuth, I. & Petres, J. (1975) Further *in vitro* studies on the biochemistry of the inhibition of nucleic acid and protein synthesis induced by arsenic. *Arch. Dermatol. Res., 253,* 15-22

Baroni, C., van Esch, G.J. & Saffiotti, U. (1963) Carcinogenesis tests of two inorganic arsenicals. *Arch. environ. Health, 7,* 668-674

Barry, K.G. & Herndon, E.G., Jr (1962) Electrocardiographic changes associated with acute arsenic poisoning. *Med. Ann. Dist. Columbia, 31,* 25-27, 65-66

Barták, P. & Kejda, J. (1972) Arsenic basal cell carcinoma of the skin in an adolescent (Ger.). *Der Hautarzt, 23,* 457-458

Beaudoin, A.R. (1974) Teratogenicity of sodium arsenate in rats. *Teratology, 10,* 153-157

Beckman, G., Beckman, L. & Nordenson, I. (1977) Chromosome aberrations in workers exposed to arsenic. *Environ. Health Perspect., 19,* 145-146

Bencko, V. (1972) Oxygen consumption by mouse liver homogenate during drinking water arsenic exposure. Part II. *J. Hyg. Epidemiol. Microbiol. Immunol., 16,* 42-46

Bencko, V. & Němečková, H. (1971) Oxygen consumption by mouse liver homogenate during drinking water arsenic exposure. Part I. *J. Hyg. Epidemiol. Microbiol. Immunol., 15,* 104-110

Bencko, V. & Symon, K. (1969) Dynamics of arsenic cumulation in hairless mice after peroral administration. *J. Hyg. Epidemiol. Microbiol. Immunol., 13,* 248-253

Bencko, V., Cmarko, V. & Palan, Š. (1968) The cumulation dynamics of arsenic in the tissues of rabbits exposed in the area of the ENO plant (Chekh.). *Cesk. Hyg., 13,* 18-22

Bencko, V., Beneš, B. & Cikrt, M. (1976) Biotransformation of As (III) to As (V) and arsenic tolerance. *Arch. Toxicol., 36,* 159-162

Berg, G.L., ed. (1979) *Farm Chemicals Handbook 1979,* Willoughby, OH, Meister, pp. D20-D21, D48-D49, D106-D107, D163, D 192-D193, D256-D257

Berteau, P.E., Flom, J.O., Dimmick, R.L. & Boyd, A.R. (1978) Long-term study of potential carcinogenicity of inorganic arsenic aerosols to mice (Abstract no. 243). *Toxicol. appl. Pharmacol., 45,* 323

Bettley, F.R. & O'Shea, J.A. (1975) The absorption of arsenic and its relation to carcinoma. *Br. J. Dermatol., 92,* 563-568

Birmingham, D.J., Key, M.M., Holaday, D.A. & Perone, V.B. (1965) An outbreak of arsenical dermatoses in a mining community. *Arch. Dermatol., 91,* 457-464

Blot, W.J. & Fraumeni, J.F., Jr (1975) Arsenical air pollution and lung cancer. *Lancet, ii,* 142-144

Borgoño, J.M., Vicent, P., Venturino, H. & Infante, A. (1977) Arsenic in the drinking water of the city of Antofagasta: epidemiological and clinical study before and after the installation of a treatment plant. *Environ. Health Perspect., 19,* 103-105

Boutwell, R.K. (1963) A carcinogenicity evaluation of potassium arsenite and arsanilic acid. *J. agric. Food Chem., 11,* 381-384

Brady, J., Liberatore, F., Harper, P., Greenwald, P., Burnett, W., Davies, J.N.P., Bishop, M., Polan, A. & Vianna, N. (1977) Angiosarcoma of the liver: an epidemiologic survey. *J. natl Cancer Inst., 59,* 1383-1385

Braman, R.S. (1975) *Arsenic in the environment.* In: Woolson, E.A., ed., *Arsenical Pesticides (ACS Symposium Series 7),* Washington DC, American Chemical Society, pp. 108-123

Braman, R.S. & Foreback, C.C. (1973) Methylated forms of arsenic in the environment. *Science, 182,* 1247-1249

Brown, E.J. & Button, D.K. (1979) A simple method of arsenic speciation. *Bull. environ. Contam. Toxicol., 21,* 37-42

Brown, R. & Taylor, H.E. (1975) *Trace Element Analysis of Normal Lung Tissue and Hilar Lymph Nodes in Spark Source Mass Spectrometry,* Accu-Labs Research, Inc., for National Institute for Occupational Safety and Health, Report No. NIOSH-75-129, Springfield, VA, National Technical Information Service

Brown, M.M., Rhyne, B.C., Goyer, R.A. & Fowler, B.A. (1976) Intracellular effects of chronic arsenic administration on renal proximal tubule cells. *J. Toxicol. environ. Health, 1,* 505-514

Bulmer, F.M.R., Rothwell, H.E., Polack, S.S. & Stewart, D.W. (1940) Chronic arsine poisoning among workers employed in the cyanide extraction of gold: a report of fourteen cases. *J. ind. Hyg. Toxicol., 22,* 111-124

Burgdorf, W., Kurvink, K. & Cervenka, J. (1977) Elevated sister chromatid exchange rate in lymphocytes of subjects treated with arsenic. *Hum. Genet., 36*, 69-72

Burk, D. & Beaudoin, A.R. (1977) Arsenate-induced renal agenesis in rats. *Teratology, 16*, 247-260

Burke, R.W. & Diamondstone, B.I. (1977) *Procedures for the determination of arsenic, copper, and nickel by molecular absorption spectrometry.* In: Mavrodineanu, R., ed., *Procedures Used at the National Bureau of Standards to Determine Selected Trace Elements in Biological and Botanical Materials,* US Department of Commerce, National Bureau of Standards, Washington DC, US Government Printing Office, pp. 73-79

Butzengeiger, K.H. (1940) On peripheral circulatory disorders during chronic arsenic intoxication (Ger.). *Klin. Wochenschr., 19*, 523-527

Byron, W.R., Bierbower, G.W., Brouwer, J.B. & Hansen, W.H. (1967) Pathological changes in rats and dogs from two-year feeding of sodium arsenite or sodium arsenate. *Toxicol. appl. Pharmacol., 10,* 132-147

Calnan, C.D. (1954) Arsenical keratoses and epithelioma with bronchial carcinoma (Abstract). *Proc. R. Acad. Med., 47,* 405-406

Carapella, S.C., Jr (1978) *Arsenic and arsenic alloys.* In: Kirk, R.E. & Othmer, D.F., eds, *Encyclopedia of Chemical Technology*, 3rd ed., Vol. 3, New York, John Wiley & Sons, Inc., pp. 243-250

Casto, B.C., Meyers, J. & DiPaolo, J.A. (1979) Enhancement of viral transformation for evaluation of the carcinogenic or mutagenic potential of inorganic metal salts. *Cancer Res., 39,* 193-198

Cawse, P.A. (1975) *A Survey of Atmospheric Trace Elements in the UK: Results for 1974,* Environmental and Medical Sciences Division, Harwell, Berks, Atomic Energy Research Establishment

Charbonneau, S.M., Spencer, K., Bryce, F. & Sandi, E. (1978) Arsenic excretion by monkeys dosed with arsenic-containing fish or with inorganic arsenic. *Bull. environ. Contam. Toxicol., 20,* 470-477

Chhuttani, P.N., Chawla, L.S. & Sharma, T.D. (1967) Arsenical neuropathy. *Neurology, 17,* 269-274

Cirkt, M. & Bencko, V. (1974) Fate of arsenic after parenteral administration to rats, with particular reference to excretion *via* bile. *J. Hyg. Epidemiol. Microbiol. Immunol., 18,* 129-136

Clement, W.H. & Faust, S.D. (1973) A new convenient method for determining arsenic (+3) in natural waters. *Environ. Lett., 5,* 155-164

Crecelius, E.A. (1977) Changes in the chemical speciation of arsenic following ingestion by man. *Environ. Health Perspect., 19,* 147-150

Curatola, C.J., Grunder, F.I. & Moffitt, A.E., Jr (1978) Hydride generation atomic absorption spectrophotometry for determination of arsenic in hair. *Am. ind. Hyg. Assoc. J., 39,* 933-938

Dalderup, L.M., Freni, S.C., Bras, G. & Bronckhorst, F.B. (1976) Angiosarcoma of the liver. *Lancet, i,* 246

Deak, S.T., Csaky, K.G. & Waddell, W.J. (1976) Localization and histochemical correlation of ^{73}As by whole-body autoradiography in mice. *J. Toxicol. environ. Health, 1,* 981-984

Degreef, H. & Roelandts, R. (1974) Arsenical intoxication due to pollution. *Arch. Belg. Dermatol., 30,* 35-38

Delèpine, S. (1923) Observation upon the effects of exposure to arsenic trichloride upon health. *J. ind. Hyg., 4,* 346-364, 410-423

D'Hondt, P., Lievens, P., Versieck, J. & Hoste, J. (1977) Determination of trace elements in animal and human muscle by semi-automated radiochemical neutron activation analysis. *Radiochem. radioanal. Lett., 31,* 231-240

Dickinson, J.O. (1972) Toxicity of the arsenical herbicide monosodium acid methanearsonate in cattle. *Am. J. vet. Res., 33,* 1889-1892

Doak, G.O., Long, G.G. & Freedman, L.D. (1978) *Arsenic compounds.* In: Kirk, R.E. & Othmer, D.F., eds, *Encyclopedia of Chemical Technology,* 3rd ed., Vol. 3, New York, John Wiley & Sons, Inc., pp. 251-266

Drever, J.I., Murphy, J.W. & Surdam, R.C. (1977) The distribution of As, Be, Cd, Cu, Hg, Mo, Pb, and U associated with the Wyodak coal seam, Powder River Basin, Wyoming. *Contrib. Geol. Univ. Wyoming, 15,* 93-101

Ducoff, H.S., Neal, W.B., Straube, R.L., Jacobson, L.O. & Brues, A.M. (1948) Biological studies with arsenic[76]. II. Excretion and tissue localization. *Proc. Soc. exp. Biol. (NY), 69*, 548-554

Du Pont, O., Ariel, I. & Warren, S.L. (1942) The distribution of radioactive arsenic in the normal and tumor-bearing (Brown-Pearce) rabbit. *Am. J. Syph. Gonorrhea Vener. Dis., 26,* 96-118

Durum, W.H., Hem, J.D. & Heidel, S.C. (1971) *Reconnaissance of Selected Minor Elements in Surface Waters of the United States, October 1970,* Geological Survey Circular 643, Washington DC, US Department of the Interior, pp. 1-3

Eccles, L.A. (1976) *Sources of Arsenic in Streams Tributary to Lake Crowley, California,* US Geological Survey, USGS/WRO/WRI-76/060, Springfield, VA, National Technical Information Service

EEC (1974) Council Directive of 17 December 1973 on the fixing of maximum permitted levels for undesirable substances and products in feeding stuffs. *Off. J. Eur. Comm., L 38,* 31-36

EEC (1975a) Proposal for a Council Directive relating to the quality of water for human consumption. *Off. J. Eur. Comm., C 214,* 2-17

EEC (1975b) Council Directive of 16 June 1975 concerning the quality required of surface water intended for the abstraction of drinking water in the Member States. *Off. J. Eur. Comm., L 194,* 26-31

EEC (1976) First Commission Directive of 15 December 1975 amending the Annex to Council Directive 74/63/EEC of 17 December 1973 on the fixing of maximum permitted levels for undesirable substances and products in feedingstuffs. *Off. J. Eur. Comm., L 4,* 24

Egan, A. & Spyrou, N.M. (1977) Determination of heavy metals in sewage-based fertilizer using short-lived isotopes. *J. radioanal. Chem., 37,* 775-784

Ehlers, G. (1968) Relationship between tumour and arsenic-containing drugs. Clinical and histological study (Ger.). *Zschr. Haut-Geschl. - Krkh., 43,* 763-774

Ehrlich, P. & Bertheim, O. (1907) *p*-Aminophenylarsinic acid. *Ber. dtsch. chem. Ges., 40,* 3292-3997 [*Chem. Abstr., 1,* 2715]

Exon, J.H., Harr, J.R. & Claeys, R.R. (1974) The effects of long term feeding of mono-
    sodium acid methanearsenate (MSMA) to rabbits. *Nutr. Rep. Int., 9*, 351-357

Fairhall, L.T. & Miller, J.W. (1941) A study of the relative toxicity of the molecular compo-
    nents of lead arsenate. *Publ. Health Rep. (Wash.), 56*, 1610-1625

Feldman, R.G., Niles, C.A., Kelly-Hayes, M., Sax, D.S., Dixon, W.J., Thompson, D.J. &
    Landau, E. (1979) Peripheral neuropathy in arsenic smelter workers. *Neurology,
    29,* 939-944

Ferm, V.H. (1977) Arsenic as a teratogenic agent. *Environ. Health Perspect., 19,* 215-217

Ferm, V.H. & Carpenter, S.J. (1968) Malformations induced by sodium arsenate. *J. Reprod.
    Fertil., 17,* 199-201

Ferm, V.H., Saxon, A. & Smith, B.M. (1971) The teratogenic profile of sodium arsenate in
    the golden hamster. *Arch. environ. Health, 22,* 557-560

Feussner, J.R., Shelburne, J.D., Bredehoeft, S. & Cohen, H.J. (1979) Arsenic-induced bone
    marrow toxicity: ultrastructural and electron-probe analysis. *Blood, 53,* 820-827

Fierz, U. (1965) Catamnestic study of the secondary effects of therapy with inorganic
    arsenic for skin disease (Ger.). *Dermatologica, 131,* 41-58

Filby, R.H. (1975) *Elemental Analysis of Human Lung Tissue and Other Selected Samples
    Utilizing Neutron Activation Analysis,* Report No. NIOSH-75-187, Nuclear Radiation
    Center, Washington State University, for National Institute for Occupational Safety
    and Health, Springfield, VA, National Technical Information Service

Fishbein, L. (1976) Environmental metallic carcinogens: an overview of exposure levels.
    J. Toxicol. environ. Health, 2, 77-109

Fisher, R.P. (1977) The NCASI inorganic priority pollutants analytical program: the
    analysis for thirteen priority pollutants in pulp and paper industry discharges by
    modern atomic absorption spectrometric methods. *Print Reprogr. Test Conference,*
    Publ. 77, Atlanta, GA, Technical Association of the Pulp and Paper Industry, pp. 217-
    225

Flanjak, J. (1978) Atomic absorption spectrometric determination of arsenic and selenium
    in offal and fish by hydride generation. *J. Assoc. anal. Chem., 61,* 1299-1303

Fowler, B.A., ed. (1977) Proceedings of the International Conference on Environmental Arsenic, Fort Lauderdale, FL, 1976. *Environ. Health Perspect, 19,* 1-242

Fowler, B.A. & Weissberg, J.B. (1974) Arsine poisoning. *New Engl. J. Med., 291,* 1171-1174

Fowler, B.A. & Woods, J.S. (1979) The effects of prolonged oral arsenate exposure on liver mitochondria of mice: morphometric and biochemical studies. *Toxicol. appl. Pharmacol., 50,* 177-187

Fowler, B.A., Woods, J.S. & Schiller, C.M. (1977) Ultrastructural and biochemical effects of prolonged oral arsenic exposure on liver mitochondria of rats. *Environ. Health Perspect., 19,* 197-204

Fowler, B.A., Woods, J.S. & Schiller, C.M. (1979) Studies of hepatic mitochondrial structure and function. Morphometric and biochemical evaluation of *in vivo* perturbation by arsenate. *Lab. Invest., 41,* 313-320

Franke, K.W. & Moxon, A.L. (1936) A comparison of the minimum fatal doses of selenium, tellurium, arsenic and vanadium. *J. Pharmacol. exp. Ther., 58,* 454-459

Franklin, M., Bean, W.B. & Hardin, R.C. (1950) Fowler's solution as an etiologic agent in cirrhosis. *Am. J. med. Sci., 219,* 589-596

Fréjaville, J.-P., Bescol, J., Leclerc, J.-P., Guillam, L., Crabie, P., Conso, F., Gervais, P. & Gaultier, M. (1972) Acute poisoning from arsenical derivatives (on the basis of 4 personal observations); haemostatic disturbances; ultramicroscopic study of the liver and kidney (Fr.). *Ann. intern. Med., 123,* 713-722

Fritsch, P., Schellander, F. & Konrad, K. (1971) Arsenic and epithelioma of the skin (Ger.). *Wien. klin. Wochenschr., 83,* 7-11

Gafafer, W.M., ed. (1964) *Occupational Diseases - A Guide to Their Recognition (Publication No. 1097),* US Department of Health, Education, & Welfare, Washington DC, Public Health Service, pp. 83-84

Gainer, J.H. & Pry, T.W. (1972) Effects of arsenicals on viral infections in mice. *Am. J. vet. Res., 33,* 2299-2307

Gallorinl, M., Greenberg, R.R. & Gills, T.E. (1978) Simultaneous determination of arsenic, antimony, cadmium, chromium, copper, and selenium in environmental material by radiochemical neutron activation analysis. *Anal. Chem., 50,* 1479-1481

Galy, P., Touraine, R., Brune, J., Gallois, P., Roudier, P., Loire, R., Lheureux, P. & Wiesendanger, T. (1963a) Bronchopulmonary cancer from chronic arsenical poisoning in Beaujolais vine-dressers (Fr.). *Lyon Méd., 43,* 735-744

Galy, P., Touraine, R., Brune, J., Roudier, R. & Gallois, P. (1963b) Pulmonary cancer of arsenical origin in Beaujolais vine-dressers (Fr.). *J. fr. Méd. Chir. thorac., 17,* 303-311

Garb, L.G. & Hine, C.H. (1977) Arsenical neuropathy: residual effects following acute industrial exposure. *J. occup. Med., 19,* 567-568

Genčík, A., Szokolayová, J. & Čerey, K. (1977) Dominant lethal test after peroral administration of arsenic (Chekh.). *Bratisl. lek. Listy, 67,* 179-187

Gerhardt, R.E., Hudson, J'B., Rao, R.N. & Sobel, R.E. (1978) Chronic renal insufficiency from cortical necrosis induced by arsenic poisoning. *Arch. int. Med., 138,* 1267-1269

Gills, T.E. (1977) *Determination of arsenic, antimony, chromium, copper, manganese, mercury, platinum, selenium, and vanadium. A. Determination of arsenic, antimony and copper in biological and botanical materials using neutron activation analysis.* In: Mavrodineanu, R., ed., *Procedures Used at the National Bureau of Standards to Determine Selected Trace Elements in Biological and Botanical Materials,* US Department of Commerce, National Bureau of Standards, Washington DC, US Government Printing Office, pp. 9-12

Goldenthal, E.I. (1971) A compilation of LD_{50} values in newborn and adult animals. *Toxicol. appl. Pharmacol., 18,* 185-207

Goldman, A.L. (1973) Lung cancer in Bowen's disease. *Am. Rev. resp. Dis., 108,* 1205-1207

Goode, S.R. & Matthews, R.J. (1978) Enzyme-catalyzed reaction-rate method for determination of arsenic in water. *Anal. Chem., 50,* 1608-1610

Gramer, L. (1955) One fatal case of acute arsine intoxication (Ger.). *Arch. Gewerbepathol. Gewerbehyg., 13,* 601-610

Grantham, D.A. & Jones, J.F. (1977) Arsenic contamination of water wells in Nova Scotia. *J. Am. Water Works Assoc.,* December, 653-657

Grobe, J.-W. (1976) Peripheral circulatory disorders and acrocyanosis in Moselle vine-dressers poisoned by arsenic (Ger.). *Berufsdermatosen, 24,* 78-84

Grobe, J.-W. (1977) Experts' opinions and therapeutic findings in vine-dressers with late lesions due to arsenic poisoning (Ger.). *Berufsdermatosen, 25,* 124-130

Hamada, T., Horiguchi, S. & Nakano, H. (1977) Cutaneous manifestations of occupational chronic arsenical poisoning (studies on lead arsenate poisoning, Part 3). *Osaka City med. J., 23,* 9-20

Hamamoto, E. (1955) Infant arsenic poisoning by powdered milk (Jpn.). *Nihon Iji Shimpo, 1649,* 3-12

Harrisson, J.W.E., Packman, E.W. & Abbott, D.D. (1958) Acute oral toxicity and chemical and physical properties of arsenic trioxides. *Arch. ind. Health, 17,* 118-123

Hawley, G.G., ed. (1977) *The Condensed Chemical Dictionary*, New York, Van Nostrand-Reinhold, p. 76

Henry, F.T., Kirch, T.O. & Thorpe, T.M. (1979) Determination of trace level arsenic (III), arsenic (V), and total inorganic arsenic by differential pulse polarography. *Anal. Chem., 51,* 215-218

Heyman, A., Pfeiffer, J.B., Willett, R.W. & Taylor, H.M. (1956) Peripheral neuropathy caused by arsenical intoxication. A study of 41 cases with observations on the effects of BAL (2,3-dimercapto-propanol). *New Engl. J. Med., 254,* 401-409

Hill, A.B. & Faning, E.L. (1948) Studies in the incidence of cancer in a factory handling inorganic compounds of arsenic. I. Mortality experience in the factory. *Br. J. ind. Med., 5,* 1-6

Hiltbold, A.E. (1975) *Behaviour of organoarsenicals in plants and soils.* In: Woolson, E.A., ed., *Arsenical Pesticides (ACS Symposium Series 7),* Washington DC, American Chemical Society, pp. 53-69

Hindmarsh, J.T., McLetchie, O.R., Heffernan, L.P.M., Hayne, O.A., Ellenberger, H.A., McCurdy, R.F. & Thiebaux, H.J. (1977) Electromyographic abnormalities in chronic environmental arsenicalism. *J. anal. Toxicol., 1,* 270-276

Hine, C.H., Pinto, S.S. & Nelson, K.W. (1977) Medical problems associated with arsenic exposure. *J. occup. Med., 19,* 391-396

Holland, R.H., McCall, M.S. & Lanz, H.C. (1959) A study of inhaled arsenic-74 in man. *Cancer Res., 19,* 1154-1156

Holmberg, R.E., Jr & Ferm, V.H. (1969) Interrelationships of selenium, cadmium, and arsenic in mammalian teratogenesis. *Arch. environ. Health, 18*, 873-877

Holmqvist, I. (1951) Occupational arsenical dermatitis. A study among employees at a copper ore smelting work including investigations of skin reactions to contact with arsenic compounds. *Acta dermato-venereol., 31* (Suppl. 26), 1-214

Hood, R.D. (1972) Effects of sodium arsenite on fetal development. *Bull. environ. Contam. Toxicol., 7*, 216-222

Hood, R.D. & Bishop, S.L. (1972) Teratogenic effects of sodium arsenate in mice. *Arch. environ. Health, 24*, 62-65

Hood, R.D. & Pike, C.T. (1972) BAL alleviation of arsenate-induced teratogenesis in mice. *Teratology, 6*, 235-238

Hood, R.D., Thacker, G.T., Patterson, B.L. & Szczech, G.M. (1978) Prenatal effects of oral *versus* intraperitoneal sodium arsenate in mice. *J. environ. Pathol. Toxicol., 1*, 857-864

Hueper, W.C. (1954) Experimental studies in metal cancerigenesis. VI. Tissue reactions in rats and rabbits after parenteral introduction of suspensions of arsenic, beryllium, or asbestos in lanolin. *J. natl Cancer Inst., 15*, 113-124

Hueper, W.C. & Payne, W.W. (1962) Experimental studies in metal carcinogenesis. Chromium, nickel, iron, arsenic. *Arch. environ. Health, 5*, 445-462

Hughes, W. & Levvy, G.A. (1947) The toxicity of arsine solutions for tissue slices. *Biochem. J., 41*, 8-11

Hunter, F.T., Kip, A.F. & Irvine, J.W., Jr (1942) Radioactive tracer studies on arsenic injected as potassium arsenite. I. Excretion and localization in tissues. *J. Pharmacol. exp. Ther., 76*, 207-220

IARC (1973) *IARC Monographs on the Evaluation of Carcinogenic Risk of Chemicals to Man*, Vol. 2, *Some Inorganic and Organometallic Compounds*, Lyon, pp. 48-73

Innes, J.R.M., Ulland, B.M., Valerio, M.G., Petrucelli, L., Fishbein, L., Hart, E.R., Pallotta, A.J., Bates, R.R., Falk, H.L., Gart, J.J., Klein, M., Mitchell, I. & Peters, J. (1969) Bioassay of pesticides and industrial chemicals for tumorigenicity in mice: a preliminary note. *J. natl Cancer Inst., 42*, 1101-1114

Interagency Regulatory Liaison Group (1978) *Hazardous Substances* (US Consumer Product Safety Commission, US Environmental Protection Agency, US Food & Drug Administration, US Occupational Safety & Health Administration), Washington DC, Bureau of National Affairs, pp. 65-72

Ishinishi, N. (1973) Review on toxicity of arsenic and arsenic compounds (Jpn.). *Nipp. Rinsho, 31,* 75-83

Ishinishi, N., Osato, K., Kodama, Y. & Kunitake, E. (1976) *Skin effects and carcinogenicity of arsenic trioxide: a preliminary experimental study in rats.* In: Nordberg, G.F., ed., *Effects and Dose-Response Relationships of Toxic Metals,* Amsterdam, Elsevier Scientific, pp. 471-479

Ishinishi, N., Kodama, Y., Nobutomo, K. & Hisanaga, A. (1977) Preliminary experimental study on carcinogenicity of arsenic trioxide in rat lung. *Environ. Health Perspect, 19,* 191-196

Ishinishi, N., Tomita, M. & Hisanaga, A. (1980) Study on chronic toxicity of arsenic trioxide in rats with special reference to the liver damages. *Fukuoka Acta med., 71,* 27-40

Ivankovic, S., Eisenbrand, G. & Preussmann, R. (1979) Lung carcinoma induction in BD rats after single intratracheal instillation of an arsenic-containing pesticide mixture formerly used in vineyards. *Int. J. Cancer, 24,* 786-788

Jackson, R. & Grainge, J.W. (1975) Arsenic and cancer. *Can. med. Assoc. J., 113,* 396-399

Japanese Society of Industrial Hygiene (1978) Recommendations for the concentrations permitted (Jpn.). *Jpn. J. ind. Health, 20,* 290-293

Jelinek, C.F. & Corneliussen, P.E. (1977) Levels of arsenic in the United States food supply. *Environ. Health Perspect., 19,* 83-87

Jenkins, R.B. (1966) Inorganic arsenic and the nervous system. *Brain, 89,* 479-498

Jiler, H., ed. (1975) *Commodity Year Book 1975,* New York, Commodity Research Bureau, Inc., p. 64

Johnson, D.L. & Pilson, M.E.Q. (1972) Arsenate in the western North Atlantic and adjacent regions. *J. Mar. Res., 30,* 140-149

Jung, E.G. & Trachsel, B. (1970) Molecular biology of arsenic carcinogenesis (Ger.). *Arch. klin. exp. Derm., 237,* 819-326

Jung, E.G., Trachsel, B. & Immich, H. (1969) Arsenic as an inhibitor of the enzymes concerned in cellular recovery (dark repair). *Ger. med. Mon., 14,* 614-616

Kada, T., Hirano, K. & Shirasu, Y. (1980) Screening of environmental chemical mutagens by the *rec*-assay system with *Bacillus subtilis. Chem. Mutagens, 6* (in press)

Kanisawa, M. & Schroeder, H.A. (1967) Life term studies on the effects of arsenic, germanium, tin, and vanadium on spontaneous tumors in mice. *Cancer Res., 27,* 1192-1195

Kanisawa, M. & Schroeder, H.A. (1969) Life term studies on the effect of trace elements on spontaneous tumors in mice and rats. *Cancer Res., 29,* 892-895

Katsura, K. (1953) Medicolegal studies of arsenic poisoning. II. Distribution of arsenic in visceral organs and arsenic concentrations of bone and hair in arsenic poisoning (Jpn.). *Shikoku Igaku Zasshi, 12,* 706-720

Kemp, K., Palmgren Jensen, F., Tscherning Møller, J. & Hansen, G. (1974) *Trace Multielement Analysis of Biological Tissue by Proton-induced X-ray Fluorescence Spectroscopy,* Risø, Roskilde, Denmark, Danish Atomic Energy Commission, Health Physics Department

Klaassen, C.D. (1974) Biliary excretion of arsenic in rats, rabbits and dogs. *Toxicol. appl. Pharmacol., 29,* 447-457

Kneip, T.J., Ajemian, R.S., Driscoll, J.N., Grunder, F.I., Kornreich, L., Loveland, J.W., Moyers, J.L. & Thompson, R.J. (1976) Analytical method for arsenic in urine and air. *Health Lab. Sci., 13,* 95-99

Knoth, W. (1966/67) Arsenic treatment (Ger.). *Arch. klin. exp. Derm., 227,* 228-234

Kobayashi, S. & Lee, G.F. (1978) Accumulation of arsenic in sediments of lakes treated with sodium arsenite. *Environ. Sci. Technol., 12,* 1195-1200

Korob, R.O., Cohen, I.M., Lage, M. & Milá, M.I. (1978) A procedure for simultaneous determination of arsenic, cadmium, copper, tin and zinc in beef extract by neutron activation analysis. *J. Radioanal. Chem., 42,* 121-131

Kroes, R., van Logten, M.J., Berkvens, J.M., de Vries, T. & van Esch, G.J. (1974) Study on the carcinogenicity of lead arsenate and sodium arsenate and on the possible synergistic effect of diethylnitrosamine. *Food Cosmet. Toxicol., 12,* 671-679

Kyle, R.A. & Pease, G.L. (1965) Hematologic aspects of arsenic intoxication. *New Engl. J. Med., 273,* 18-23

Ladwig, V.D. (1978) Swine disease guide. *Feedstuffs, 50,* 75-83

Lakso, J.U. & Peoples, S.A. (1975) Methylation of inorganic arsenic by mammals. *J. agric. Food Chem., 23,* 674-676

Lander, J.J., Stanley, R.J., Sumner, H.W., Boswell, D.C. & Aach, R.D. (1975) Angiosarcoma of the liver associated with Fowler's solution (potassium arsenite). *Gastroenterology, 68,* 1582-1586

Latarjet, R., Galy, P., Maret, G. & Gallois, P. (1964) Bronchopulmonary cancers and arsenical poisoning among Beaujolais vine-dressers (Fr.). *Mem. Acad. Chir. (Paris), 90,* 384-390

Lauwerys, R.R., Buchet, J.P. & Roels, H. (1979) The determination of trace levels of arsenic in human biological materials. *Arch. Toxicol., 41,* 239-247

Lawton, A.H., Ness, A.T., Brady, F.J. & Cowie, D.B. (1945) Distribution of radioactive arsenic following intraperitoneal injection of sodium arsenite into cotton rats injected with *Litomosoides carinii. Science, 102,* 120-122

Lee, A.M. & Fraumeni, J.F., Jr (1969) Arsenic and respiratory cancer in man: an occupational study. *J. natl Cancer Inst., 42,* 1045-1052

Leitch, A. & Kennaway, E.L. (1922) Experimental production of cancer by arsenic. *Br. med. J., ii,* 1107-1108

Léonard, A. & Lauwerys, R.R. (1980) Carcinogenicity, teratogenicity and mutagenicity of arsenic. *Mutat. Res., 75,* 49-62

Levinsky, W.J., Smalley, R.V., Hillyer, P.N. & Shindler, R.L. (1970) Arsine hemolysis. *Arch. environ. Health, 20,* 436-440

Levvy, G.A. (1946) The toxicity of arsine administered by intraperitoneal injection. *Br. J. Pharmacol., 1,* 287-290

Levvy, G.A. (1947) A study of arsine poisoning. *Q. J. exp. Physiol., 34,* 47-67

Levy, H., Lewin, J.R., Ninin, D.T., Schneider, H.R. & Milne, F.J. (1979) Asymptomatic arsine nephrotoxicity. *S. Afr. med. J., 56,* 192-194

Lewis, R.G. (1977) Determination of arsenic and arsenicals in foods and other biological materials. *Residue Rev., 68,* 123-149

Liebegott, G. (1952) Relationship between chronic arsenical intoxication and malignant tumours (Ger.). *Zentralbl. Arbeitsmed. Arbeittschutz., 2,* 15-16

Lindau, L. (1977) Emissions of arsenic in Sweden and their reduction. *Environ. Health Perspect., 19,* 25-29

Löfroth, G. & Ames, B.N. (1978) Mutagenicity of inorganic compounds in *Salmonella typhimurium*: arsenic, chromium and selenium (Abstract no. 1). *Mutat. Res., 53,* 65-66

Lüchtrath, H. (1972) Liver cirrhosis due to chronic arsenic intoxication in vintagers (Ger.). *Dtsch. med. Wschr., 97,* 21-22

Luckey, T.D. & Venugopal, B. (1977) *Metal Toxicity in Mammals,* Vol. 2, New York, Plenum Press, p. 209

Lugo, G., Cassady, G. & Palmisano. P. (1969) Acute maternal arsenic intoxication with neonatal death. *Am. J. Dis. Child., 117,* 328-330

Lunde, G. (1974) *The Analysis and Characterization of Trace Elements, in Particular Bromine, Selenium and Arsenic in Marine Organisms,* Blindern, Oslo, Norway, Central Institute for Industrial Research

Lundgren, K.D. (1954) Diseases of the respiratory organs of workers at a smelting work (Swed.). *Nord. Hyg. Tisdkr., 3,* 66-82

Lyon, J.L., Fillmore, J.L. & Klauber, M.R. (1977) Arsenical air pollution and lung cancer. *Lancet, ii,* 869

Mabuchi, K., Lilienfeld, A.M. & Snell, L.M. (1979) Lung cancer among pesticide workers exposed to inorganic arsenicals. *Arch. environ. Health, 34,* 312-320

Matanoski, G.M., Landau, E. & Seifter, J. (1980) Cancer mortality in an industrial area of Baltimore. *Environ. Prot. Agency tech. Rep.* (in press)

Matheson Company, Inc. (1979) *Matheson Catalog 50,* East Rutherford, NJ, pp. 66, 122-124, 128

Matsumoto, N., Okino, T., Katsunuma, H. & Iijima, S. (1973) Effects of Na-arsenate on the growth and development of the foetal mice (Abstract). *Teratology, 8,* 98

Mealey, J., Jr, Brownell, G.L. & Sweet, W.H. (1959) Radioarsenic in plasma, urine, normal tissues and intracranial neoplasms. *Arch. Neurol. Psychiatry, 81,* 310-320

Mellor, J.W. (1947) *A Comprehensive Treatise on Inorganic and Theoretical Chemistry,* Vol. 9, Chap. 51, *Arsenic,* London, Longmans, Green & Co., pp. 1-97

Metcalf, R.L. (1966) *Insecticides.* In: Kirk, R.E. & Othmer, D.F., eds, *Encyclopedia of Chemical Technology,* 2nd ed., Vol. 11, New York, John Wiley & Sons, Inc., pp. 677-738

Midwest Research Institute (1975) *Substitute Chemical Program. Initial Scientific Review of Cacodylic Acid,* for US Environmental Protection Agency, EPA-540-1-75-021, Springfield, VA, National Technical Information Service

Milham, S., Jr & Strong, T. (1974) Human arsenic exposure in relation to a copper smelter. *Environ. Res., 7,* 176-182

Milner, J.E. (1969) The effect of ingested arsenic on methylcholanthrene-induced skin tumors in mice. *Arch. environ. Health, 18,* 7-11

Ministry of Health & Welfare (1978) *Drinking Water Standards*, Tokyo

Minkowitz, S. (1964) Multiple carcinomata following ingestion of medicinal arsenic. *Ann. intern. Med., 61,* 296-299

Mizuta, N., Mizuta, M., Ito, F., Ito, T., Uchida, H., Watanabe, Y., Akama, H., Murakami, T., Hayashi, F., Nakamura, K., Yamaguchi, T., Mizuia, W., Oishi, S. & Matsumura, H. (1956) An outbreak of acute arsenic poisoning caused by arsenic contaminated soy-sauce (shoyu): a clinical report of 220 cases. *Bull. Yamaguchi med. School, 4,* 131-149

Modell, W., ed. (1977) *Drugs in Current Use and New Drugs,* New York, Springer, Part 1, pp. 11, 114

Morris, H.J. & Wallace, E.W. (1938) The storage of arsenic in rats fed a diet containing calcium arsenate and arsenic trioxide. *J. Pharmacol. exp. Ther., 64,* 411-419

Morris, H.P., Laug, E.P., Morris, H.J. & Grant, R.L. (1938) The growth and reproduction of rats fed diets containing lead acetate and arsenic trioxide and the lead and arsenic content of newborn and suckling rats. *J. Pharmacol. exp. Ther., 64,* 420-445

Morton, W., Starr, G., Pohl, D., Stoner, J., Wagner, S. & Weswig, P. (1976) Skin cancer and water arsenic in Lane county, Oregon. *Cancer, 37*, 2523-2532

Moss, E. & Lee, W.R. (1974) Occurrence of oral and pharyngeal cancers in textile workers. *Br. J. ind. Med., 31*, 224-232

Nakamura, I., Inoue, S., Ono, T., Kuwahara, H. & Kikuchi, I. (1976) Chronic arsenical poisoning due to environmental pollution. Seven cases among inhabitants near an abandoned mine. *Kumamoto med. J., 29*, 172-186

National Academy of Sciences (1977) *Arsenic. Medical and Biological Effects of Environmental Pollutants,* Division of Medical Sciences, Assembly of Life Sciences, National Research Council, Washington DC

National Institute for Occupational Safety & Health (1975) *Criteria for a Recommended Standard... Occupational Exposure to Inorganic Arsenic,* New Criteria, (NIOSH) 75-199, Washington DC, US Government Printing Office

National Technical Information Service (1968) *Evaluation of Carcinogenic, Teratogenic, and Mutagenic Activities of Selected Pesticides and Industrial Chemicals,* Vol. 1, *Carcinogenic Study,* Washington DC, US Department of Commerce

Nelson, W.C., Lykins, M.H., Mackey, J., Newill, V.A., Finklea, J.F. & Hammer, D.I. (1973) Mortality among orchard workers exposed to lead arsenate spray: a cohort study. *J. chron. Dis., 26*, 105-118

Neubauer, O. (1947) Arsenical cancer: a review. *Br. J. Cancer, 1*, 192-251

Newman, J.A., Archer, V.E., Saccomanno, G., Kuschner, M., Auerbach, O., Grondahl, R.D. & Wilson, J.C. (1976) Histologic types of bronchogenic carcinoma among members of copper-mining and smelting communities. *Ann. N.Y. Acad. Sci., 271*, 260-268

Nishioka, H. (1975) Mutagenic activities of metal compounds in bacteria. *Mutat. Res., 31*, 185-189

Nixon, D.E. (1976) *The Determination of Ultratrace Quantities of the Toxic Metals in Biomedical and Environmental Samples,* Doctoral Dissertation, Ames, IA, Iowa State University

Nordberg, G.F., Pershagen, G. & Lauwerys, R. (1979) *Inorganic Arsenic - Toxicology and Epidemiological Aspects,* Odense, Denmark, Department of Community Health and Environmental Medicine, Odense University

Nordenson, I., Beckman, G., Beckman, L. & Nordström, S., (1978) Occupational and environmental risks in and around a smelter in northern Sweden. II. Chromosomal aberrations in workers exposed to arsenic. *Hereditas, 88,* 47-50

Nordenson, I., Salmonsson, S., Brun, E. & Beckman, G. (1979) Chromosome aberrations in psoriatic patients treated with arsenic. *Human Genet., 48,* 1-6

Nordström, S., Beckman, L. & Nordenson, I. (1978a) Occupational and environmental risks in and around a smelter in northern Sweden. I. Variations in birth weight. *Hereditas, 88,* 43-46

Nordström, S., Beckman, L. & Nordenson, I. (1978b) Occupational and environmental risks in and around a smelter in northern Sweden. III. Frequences of spontaneous abortion. *Hereditas, 88,* 51-54

Nordström, S., Beckman, L. & Nordenson, I. (1979c). Occupational and environmental risks in and around a smelter in northern Sweden. V. Spontaneous abortion among female employees and decreased birth weight in their offspring. *Hereditas, 90,* 291-296

Nordström, S., Beckman, L. & Nordenson, I. (1979d) Occupational and environmental risks in and around a smelter in northern Sweden. VI. Congenital malformations. *Hereditas, 90,* 297-302

Nurse, D.S. (1978) Hazards of inorganic arsenic. *Med. J. Aust., i,* 102

Oehme, F.W. (1972) Mechanisms of heavy metal toxicities. *Clin. Toxicol., 5,* 151-167

Ohta, M. (1970) Ultrastructure of sural nerve in a case of arsenical neuropathy. *Acta neuropathol., 16,* 233-242

Oppenheim, J.J. & Fishbein, W.N. (1965) Induction of chromosome breaks in cultured normal human leukocytes by potassium arsenite, hydroxyurea and related compounds. *Cancer Res., 25,* 980-985

Osburn, H.S. (1957) Cancer of the lung in Gwanda. *Cent. Afr. J. Med., 3,* 215-223

Osburn, H.S. (1969) Lung cancer in a mining district in Rhodesia. *S. Afr. med. J., 43,* 1307-1312

O'Shaughnessy, E. & Kraft, G.H. (1976) Arsenic poisoning: long-term follow-up of a non-fatal case. *Arch. phys. Med. Rehabil., 57,* 403-406

Osswald, H. & Goerttler, K. (1971) Arsenic-induced leucoses in mice after diaplacental and postnatal application (Ger.). *Verh. dtsch. Gesellsch. Path., 55,* 289-293

Ott, M.G., Holder, B.B. & Gordon, H.L. (1974) Respiratory cancer and occupational exposure to arsenicals. *Arch. environ. Health, 29,* 250-255

Parish, G.G., Glass, R. & Kimbrough, R. (1979) Acute arsine poisoning in two workers cleaning a clogged drain. *Arch. environ. Health, 34,* 224-227

Paton, G.R. & Allison, A.C. (1972) Chromosome damage in human cell cultures induced by metal salts. *Mutat. Res., 16,* 332-336

Pernis, B. & Magistretti, M. (1960) A study of the mechanism of acute hemolytic anemia from arsine. *Med. Lavoro, 51,* 37-41

Perry, K., Bowler, R.G., Buckell, H.M., Druett, H.A. & Schilling, R.S.F. (1948) Studies in the incidence of cancer in a factory handling inorganic compounds of arsenic. II. Clinical and environmental investigations. *Br. J. ind. Med., 5,* 6-15

Pershagen, G. & Vahter, M. (1979) *Arsenic: a Toxicological and Epidemiological Appraisal,* Snv pm 1128, Stockholm, Sweden, The National Swedish Environment Protection Board

Pershagen, G., Ellnder, C.-G. & Bolander, A.-M. (1977) Mortality in a region surrounding an arsenic emitting plant. *Environ. Health Perspect., 19,* 133-137

Petres, J., Baron, D. & Hagedorn, M. (1977) Effects of arsenic cell metabolism and cell proliferation: cytogenetic and biochemical studies. *Environ. Health Perspect., 19,* 223-227

Pfaltz & Bauer, Inc. (1976) *Research Chemicals Catalog,* Stamford, CT, p. 341

Pinto, S.S. & Bennett, B.M. (1963) Effect of arsenic trioxide exposure on mortality. *Arch. environ. Health, 7,* 583-591

Pinto, S.S. & McGill, C.M. (1953) Arsenic trioxide exposure in industry. *Ind. Med. Surg., 22,* 281-287

Pinto, S.S., Henderson, V. & Enterline, P.E. (1978) Mortality experience of arsenic-exposed workers. *Arch. environ. Health, 33,* 325-332

Poirier, R., Favre, R., Kleisbauer, J.P., Ingenito, G., Paoli, J., Laval, P. & Serafino, X. (1973) Primary bronchial carcinoma in a vine-dresser. Role of arsenates (Fr.). *Nouv. Presse med., 2,* 91-92

Pomeroy, B.S. (1978) Poultry disease guide. *Feedstuffs, 50,* 97-104

Prager, B., Jacobson, P., Schmidt, P. & Stern, D., eds (1922) *Beilsteins Handbuch der Organischen Chemie,* 4th ed., Vol. 4, Syst. No. 411-414, pp. 610-615

Prystowsky, S.D., Elfenbein, G.J. & Lamberg, S.I. (1978) Nasopharyngeal carcinoma associated with long-term arsenic ingestion. *Arch. Dermatol., 114,* 602-603

Regelson, W., Kim, U., Ospina, J. & Holland, J.F. (1968) Hemangioendothelial sarcoma of liver from chronic arsenic intoxication by Fowler's solution. *Cancer, 21,* 514-522

Rencher, A.C, Carter, M.W. & McKee, D.W. (1977) A retrospective epidemiological study of mortality at a large western copper smelter. *J. occup. Med., 19,* 754-758

Rennke, H., Prat, G.A., Etcheverry, R.B., Katz, R.U. & Donoso, S. (1971) Malignant haemangioendothelioma of the liver and chronic arsenicism (Span.). *Rev. med. Chile, 99,* 664-668

Reymann, F., Møller, R. & Nielsen, A. (1978) Relationship between arsenic intake and internal malignant neoplasms. *Arch. Dermatol., 114,* 378-381

Reynolds, E.S. (1901) An account of the epidemic outbreak of arsenical poisoning occurring in beer-drinkers in the North of England and Midland counties in 1900. *Lancet, i,* 166-170

Robinson, T.J. (1975) Arsenical polyneuropathy due to caustic arsenical paste. *Br. med. J., ii,* 139

Robson, A.O. & Jelliffe, A.M. (1963) Medicinal arsenic poisoning and lung cancer. *Br. med. J., ii,* 207-209

Rossman, T., Meyn, M.S. & Troll, W. (1975) Effects of sodium arsenite on the survival of UV-irradiated *Escherichia coli*: inhibition of a *recA*- dependent function. *Mutat. Res., 30,* 157-162

Rossman, T.G., Meyn, M.S. & Troll, W. (1977) Effects of arsenite on DNA repair in *Escherichia coli*. *Environ. Health Perspect., 19,* 229-233

Roth, F. (1955) Haemangioendothelioma of the liver after chronic arsenic intoxication (Ger.). *Zentralbl. allgemein. Pathol. pathol. Anat., 93*, 424-425

Roth, F. (1957a) Late consequencies of chronic arsenicism in Moselle vine-dressers (Ger.). *Dtsch. med. Wochenschr., 82*, 211-217

Roth, F. (1957b) Arsenic-liver-tumours (haemangioendothelioma) (Ger.). *Z. Krebsforsch., 61*, 468-503

Safe Drinking Water Committee (1977) *Drinking Water and Health,* Advisory Center on Toxicology, Assembly of Life Sciences, National Research Council, Washington DC, National Academy of Sciences, pp. 316-344

Salaman, M.H. & Roe, F.J.C. (1956) Further tests for tumour-initiating activity: *N,N*-di-(2-chloroethyl)-*p*-aminophenylbutyric acid (CB1348) as an initiator of skin tumour formation in the mouse. *Br. J. Cancer, 10*, 363-377

Sanderson, K.V. (1961) Arsenic as a co-carcinogen in mice. *Br. Emp. Cancer Campaign, 39*, 628-629

Sanderson, K.V. (1963) Arsenic and skin cancer. *Trans. St John's Hosp. dermatol. Soc., 49*, 115-122

Sandhu, S.S., Warren, W.J. & Nelson, P. (1978) Trace inorganics in rural potable water and their correlation to possible sources. *Water Res., 12*, 257-261

Schmähl, D., Thomas, C. & Auer, R. (1977) *Iatrogenic Carcinogenesis,* Berlin, Springer, pp. 4-25

Schrauzer, G.N. & Ishmael, D. (1974) Effects of selenium and of arsenic on the genesis of spontaneous mammary tumors in inbred C3H mice. *Ann. clin. Lab. Sci., 4*, 441-447

Schrenk, H.H. & Schreibeis, L., Jr (1958) Urinary arsenic levels as an index of industrial exposure. *Am. ind. Hyg. Assoc. J., 19*, 225-228

Schroeder, H.A. & Balassa, J.J. (1966) Abnormal trace metals in man: arsenic. *J. chron. Dis., 19*, 85-106

Shirasu, Y., Moriya, M., Kato, K., Furuhashi, A. & Kada, T. (1976) Mutagenicity screening of pesticides in the microbial system. *Mutat. Res., 40*, 19-30

Shubik, P., Saffiotti, U., Lijinsky, W., Pietra, G., Rappaport, H., Toth, B., Raha, C.R., Tomatis, L., Feldman, R. & Ramahi, H. (1962) Studies on the toxicity of petroleum waxes. *Toxicol. appl. Pharmacol., 4 (Suppl.),* 1-62

Sibatani, A. (1959) *In vitro* incorporation of ^{32}P into nucleic acids of lymphatic cells. *Exp. Cell Res., 17,* 131-143

Siemer, D.D., Vitek, R.K., Koteel, P. & Houser, W.C. (1977) Determination of arsenic in beverages and foods by hydride generation atomic absorption spectroscopy. *Anal. Lett., 10,* 357-369

Simmon, V.F., Poole, D.C. & Newell, G.W. (1976) *In vitro* mutagenic studies of twenty pesticides (Abstract no. 42). *Toxicol. appl. Pharmacol., 37,* 109

Smith, T.J., Crecelius, E.A. & Reading J.C. (1977) Airborne arsenic exposure and excretion of methylated arsenic compounds. *Environ. Health Perspect., 19,* 89-93

Snegireff, L.S. & Lombard, O.M. (1951) Arsenic and cancer. Observations in the metallurgical industry. *Arch. ind. Hyg., 4,* 199-205

Snyder, C.A. & Isola, D.A. (1979) Assay of arsenic trioxide in air. *Anal. Chem., 51,* 1478-1480

Sommers, S.C. & McManus, R.G. (1953) Multiple arsenical cancers of skin and internal organs. *Cancer, 6,* 347-359

Spencer, E.Y. (1973) *Guide to the Chemicals Used in Crop Protection,* London, Ontario, Agriculture Canada, pp. 238-359

Šrám, R.J. (1976) Relationship between acute and chronic exposures in mutagenicity studies in mice. *Mutat. Res., 41,* 25-42

SRI International (1976) *NIOSH Analytical Methods for Set N,* PB-254 228, National Institute for Occupational Safety & Health, Springfield, VA, National Technical Information Service

Steinnes, E. (1977) A neutron activation method for the simultaneous determination of arsenic, mercury and selenium in soil. *Acta agric. scand., 27,* 110-112

Stellman, J.M. & Kabat, G.C. (1978) Arsenical air pollution and lung cancer. *Lancet, i,* 211

Stevens, J.T., Hall, L.L., Farmer, J.D., DiPasquale, L.C., Chernoff, N. & Durham, W.F. (1977) Disposition of ^{14}C and/or ^{74}As-cacodylic acid in rats after intravenous, intratracheal, or peroral administration. *Environ. Health Perspect., 19,* 151-157

Stevens, J.T., DiPasquale, L.C. & Farmer, J.D. (1979) The acute inhalation toxicology of the technical grade organoarsenical herbicides, cacodylic acid and disodium methanearsonic acid; a route comparison. *Bull. environ. Contam. Toxicol., 21,* 304-311

Suta, B.E. (1978) *Human Exposures to Atmospheric Arsenic,* for US Environmental Protection Agency, Contracts 68-01-4314 and 68-02-2835, Menlo Park, CA, SRI International, pp. 3-8, 39, 46-52, 76, 82, 85, 92

Talmi, Y. & Feldman, C. (1975) *The determination of traces of arsenic: a review.* In: Woolson, E.A., ed., *Arsenical Pesticides (ACS Symposium Series 7),* Washington DC, American Chemical Society, pp. 13-34

Tam, K.H., Charbonneau, S.M., Bryce, F. & Lacroix, G. (1978) Separation of arsenic metabolites in dog plasma and urine following intravenous injection of ^{74}As. *Anal. Biochem., 86,* 505-511

Tarrant, R.F. & Allard, J. (1972) Arsenic levels in urine of forest workers applying silvicides. *Arch. environ. Health, 24,* 277-280

Tay, C.-H. & Seah, C.-S. (1975) Arsenic poisoning from anti-asthmatic herbal preparations. *Med. J. Austr., 2,* 424-428

van Thoor, J.W., ed. (1968) *Chemical Technology: An Encyclopedic Treatment,* Vol. 1, New York, Barnes & Noble, pp. 393-400

Tokudome, S. & Kuratsune, M. (1976) A cohort study on mortality from cancer and other causes among workers at a metal refinery. *Int. J. Cancer., 17,* 310-317

Tridom/Fluka Company (1979) *Product Catalog,* Tridom Chemical Inc., Hauppauge, NY, p. 48

Tseng, W.P. (1977) Effects and dose-response relationships of skin cancer and blackfoot disease with arsenic. *Environ. Health Perspect., 19,* 109-119

Tseng, W.P., Chu, H.M., How, S.W., Fong, J.M., Lin, C.S. & Yeh, S. (1968) Prevalence of skin cancer in an endemic area of chronic arsenicism in Taiwan. *J. natl Cancer Inst., 40,* 453-463

UNEP/WHO (1980) *Environmental Health Criteria: Arsenic*, Nairobi, United Nations Environment Programme/Geneva, World Health Organization (in press)

US Bureau of the Census (1976) *Current Industrial Reports, Inorganic Chemicals, 1975,* Series M28A(75)-14, Washington DC, US Department of Commerce, p. 21

US Bureau of the Census (1978a) *Current Industrial Reports, Inorganic Chemicals, 1977,* Series M28A(77)-14, Washington DC, US Department of Commerce, p. 19

US Bureau of the Census (1978b) *US Imports of Chemical Elements, Inorganic and Organic Compounds, and Mixtures; and Drugs and Related Products (TSUSA Nos. 401.0200-440.000) for Consumption, December 1977,* IM 146, Schedule 4, Parts 1-3, US Department of Commerce, Springfield, VA, National Technical Information Service, p. 1222

US Bureau of the Census (1979a) *US Imports of Benzenoid Chemicals and Products; Chemical Elements, Inorganic and Organic Compounds, and Mixtures; and Drugs and Related Products for Consumption, December, 1978,* IM 146, Schedule 4, Parts 1-3, US Department of Commerce, Springfield, VA, National Technical Information Service, pp. 1747, 1347-1348, 1359

US Bureau of the Census (1979b) *US Exports, Schedule E Commodity Groupings, Schedule E Commodity by Country,* FT410/December 1978, US Department of Commerce, Washington DC, US Government Printing Office, pp. 2-107, 2-115, 2-167

US Bureau of Mines (1979) *Mineral Commodity Summaries, 1979,* Washington DC, US Department of the Interior, pp. 12-13

US Department of Health, Education, & Welfare (1964) *Occupational Diseases. A Guide to their Recognition*, Washington DC, US Public Health Service Publication, pp. 85-86

US Environmental Protection Agency (1975) *Environmental Protection Agency effluent guidelines and standards, 40 CFR 421 - Nonferrous metals.* In: *Environment Reporter Reference File*, Washington DC, Bureau of National Affairs, Inc., pp. 135:0503-135:0506

US Environmental Protection Agency (1976) *Environmental Protection Agency national interim primary drinking-water regulations, 40 CFR 141.* In: *Environment Reporter Reference File,* Washington DC, Bureau of National Affairs, Inc., pp. 132:0101-132:0107

US Environmental Protection Agency (1978) *Environmental Protection Agency effluent guidelines and standards for pesticides chemical manufacturing, 40 CFR 455 - Pesticide chemicals.* In: *Environment Reporter Reference File,* Washington DC, Bureau of National Affairs, Inc., pp. 135:1181-135:1183

US Occupational Safety & Health Administration (1978) Notice of permanent standard for inorganic arsenic. *Occup. Saf. Health Rep., 7,* 1842, 1881

US Occupational Safety & Health Administration (1979) *Occupational Safety and Health Standards, Subpart Z - Toxic and Hazardous Substances, 29 CFR 1910.* In: *Occupational Safety and Health Reporter Reference File,* Washington DC, Bureau of National Affairs, Inc., pp. 31:8301-31:8304, 31:8351-31:8358

US Tariff Commission (1956) *Synthetic Organic Chemicals, US Production and Sales, 1955,* Report No. 198, Second Series, Washington DC, US Government Printing Office, p. 138

US Tariff Commission (1961) *Synthetic Organic Chemicals, US Production and Sales, 1960,* TC Publication 34, Washington DC, US Government Printing Office, pp. 50, 162

US Tariff Commission (1969) *Synthetic Organic Chemicals, US Production and Sales, 1967,* TC Publication 295, Washington DC, US Government Printing Office, p. 164

Utidjian, H.M.D. (1974) Excerpts from Criteria for a Recommended Standard... Occupational Exposure to Inorganic Arsenic. 1. Recommendations for an inorganic arsenic standard. *J. occup. Med., 16,* 264-269

Vallee, B.L. (1973) *Arsenic.* In: *Air Quality Monographs, 73-18,* Washington DC, American Petroleum Institute

Vallee, B.L., Ulmer, D.D. & Wacker, W.E.C. (1960) Arsenic toxicology and biochemistry. *Arch. ind. Health, 21,* 132-151

Wade, A., ed. (1977) *Martindale: The Extra Pharmacopoeia,* 27th ed., London, The Pharmaceutical Press, pp. 1721-1723

Wagner, S.L. & Weswig, P. (1974) Arsenic in blood and urine of forest workers. *Arch. environ. Health, 28,* 77-79

Wagner, S.L., Maliner, J.S., Morton, W.E. & Braman, R.S. (1979) Skin cancer and arsenical intoxication from well water. *Arch. Dermatol., 115,* 1205-1207

Walsh, L.M. & Keeney, D.R. (1975) *Behavior and phytotoxicity of inorganic arsenicals in soils.* In: Woolson E.A., ed., *Arsenical Pesticides (ACS Symposium Series 7),* Washington DC, American Chemical Society, pp. 35-52

Walsh, L.M., Sumner, M.E. & Keeney, D.R. (1977) Occurrence and distribution of arsenic in soils and plants. *Environ. Health Perspect., 19,* 67-71

Watrous, R.M. & McCaughey, M.B. (1945) Occupational exposure to arsenic - in the manufacture of arsphenamine and related compounds. *Ind. Med., 14,* 639-646

Weast, R.C., ed., (1977) *CRC Handbook of Chemistry and Physics,* 58th ed., Cleveland, OH, The Chemical Rubber Company, pp. B-91, B-98, B-122, B-143, B-158, C-687

Webster, S.H. (1941) The lead and arsenic content of urines from 46 persons with no known exposure to lead or arsenic. *US Publ. Health Serv. Rep., 56,* 1953-1961

Weed Science Society of America (1979) *Herbicide Handbook,* 4th ed., Champaign, IL, pp. 252-255

Weers, C.A., Hoede, D. & Das, H.A. (1978) Application of selective evaporation in the determination of arsenic and bromine in dry biological material by thermal neutron activation analysis. *J. Radioanal. Chem., 42,* 113-119

Weinberg, S.L. (1960) The electrocardiogram in acute arsenic poisoning. *Am. Heart J., 60,* 971-975

Weiss, H.V. & Bertine, K.K. (1973) Simultaneous determination of manganese, copper, arsenic, cadmium, antimony and mercury in glacial ice by radioactivation. *Anal. chim. Acta, 65,* 253-259

Whanger, P.D., Weswig, P.H. & Stoner, J.C. (1977) Arsenic levels in Oregon waters. *Environ. Health Perspect., 19,* 139-143

WHO (1970) *European Standards for Drinking-Water*, 2nd ed., Geneva, World Health Organization, p. 33

WHO (1971) *International Standards for Drinking-Water*, 3rd ed., Geneva, World Health Organization, p. 32

WHO (1973) Trace elements in human nutrition. Report of a WHO Expert Committee. *World Health Org. tech. Rep. Ser., No. 532,* 49-50

WHO (1977) *International Pharmacopoeia*, Vol. 2, Geneva, p. 298

Windholz, M., ed. (1976) *The Merck Index*, 9th ed., Rahway, NJ, Merck & Co., pp. 106-109, 204, 209, 709, 988, 1108-1111

Winell, M. (1975) An international comparison of hygienic standards for chemicals in the work environment. *Ambio, 4*, 34-36

Wolf, R. (1974) Occupational arsenic lesions in vine-growers (Ger.). *Berufsdermatosen, 22*, 34-47

Woods, J.S. & Fowler, B.A. (1978) Altered regulation of mammalian hepatic heme biosynthesis and urinary porphyrin excretion during prolonged exposure to sodium arsenate. *Toxicol. appl. Pharmacol., 43,* 361-371

Woolson, E.A., ed. (1975a) *Arsenical Pesticides (ACS Symposium Series 7)*, Washington DC, American Chemical Society

Woolson, E.A., (1975b) The persistence and chemical distribution of arsanilic acid in three soils. *J. agric. Food Chem., 23,* 677-681

Woolson, E.A. (1977) Fate of arsenicals in different environmental substrates. *Environ. Health Perspect., 19,* 73-81

Yamashita, N., Doi, M., Nishio, M., Hojo, H. & Tanaka, M. (1972) Recent observations of Kyoto children poisoned by arsenic tainted 'Morinaga dry milk' (Jpn.). *Jpn. J. Hyg., 27,* 364-402

Yoakum, A.M. (1976) *Analysis of Blood, Hair, Urine, and Dust Samples for Heavy Metals*, Report No. EPA-600/1-76-029, Stewart Laboratories, Inc., Knoxville, TN, for US Environmental Protection Agency, Springfield, VA, National Technical Information Service

Zaldívar, R. (1974) Arsenic contamination of drinking water and foodstuffs causing endemic chronic poisoning. *Beitr. Pathol., 151,* 384-400

BERYLLIUM and BERYLLIUM COMPOUNDS

Beryllium and beryllium compounds were first considered by an IARC Working Group in 1971 (IARC, 1972). Since that time, new data have become available, and these are included in the present monograph and have been taken into consideration in the evaluation.

1. Chemical and Physical Data

1.1 Synonyms, trade names and molecular formulae

Table 1. Synonyms (Chemical Abstracts Services names are given in bold), trade names and atomic or molecular formulae of pure beryllium and beryllium compounds[a]

Chemical name	Chem. Abstr. Reg. Serial	Synonyms and trade names	Formula
Beryllium	7440-41-7	Beryllium-9; glucinium; glucinum	Be
Beryllium acetate	543-81-7	**Acetic acid, beryllium salt**; beryllium acetate normal	$Be(C_2H_3O_2)_2$
Beryllium acetate, basic	19049-40-2	**Hexakis [μ-acetato-0:0'] -μ_4 -oxotetraberyllium**; beryllium oxide acetate	$Be_4O(C_2H_3O_2)_6$
Beryllium carbonate[b]	66104-24-3	Beryllium carbonate, basic; beryllium oxide carbonate; **bis[carbonato(2-)] dihydroxytriberyllium**	$(BeCO_3)_2.Be(OH)_2$
Beryllium chloride	7787-47-5	Beryllium dichloride	$BeCl_2$
Beryllium fluoride	7787-49-7	Beryllium difluoride	BeF_2
Beryllium hydroxide	13327-32-7	Beryllium dihydroxide; beryllium hydrate	$Be(OH)_2$
Beryllium oxide	1304-56-9	Beryllia; beryllium monoxide Thermalox[®]	BeO
Beryllium phosphate	13598-15-7	Beryllium hydrogen phosphate; **phosphoric acid, beryllium salt (1:1)**	$BeHPO_4$
Beryllium silicate	13598-00-0	Beryllium silicic acid ; *ortho*silicate; phenacite; **phenakite**	Be_2SiO_4

Table 1 (contd)

Chemical name	Chem. Abstr. Reg. Serial No.	Synonyms and trade names	Formula
Beryllium sulphate	13510-49-1	Sulfuric acid, beryllium salt (1:1)	$BeSO_4$
Beryllium sulphate tetrahydrate	7787-56-6	Beryllium sulfate tetrahydrate; sulfuric acid, beryllium salt (1:1), tetrahydrate	$BeSO_4.4H_2O$
Zinc beryllium silicate	39413-47-3	Silicic acid, beryllium zinc salt [beryllium zinc salt of silicic acid]	Exact composition unknown or undetermined

[a]See also Table 4, p. 162

[b]Chemical Abstracts name and serial number shown were selected as being the closest to the formula given by Weast (1977). Related compounds registered by Chemical Abstracts (none of which is entirely distinct from that listed] are: carbonic acid, beryllium salt (1:1) tetrahydrate, $BeCO_3.4H_2O$ [60883-64-9]; carbonic acid, beryllium salt (1:1), $BeCO_3$ [13106-47-3]; and bis[carbonato(2-)] oxodiberyllium, $(CO_3)_2B_2O$ [66104-25-4].

Table 1a. Synonyms (Chemical Abstracts Services names are given in bold), trade names and molecular formulae of impure beryllium compounds

Chemical name	Chem. Abstr. Reg. Serial No.	Synonyms and trade names	Formula
Bertrandite	12161-82-9	**Bertrandite [Be$_4$(H$_2$Si$_2$O$_9$)]**; beryllium silicate hydrate	4 BeO.2SiO$_2$.H$_2$O
Beryllium-aluminium alloy	12770-50-2	Aluminum beryllium alloy; **aluminum alloy, Al, Be**; aluminium-beryllium alloy Lockalloy	-
Beryllium-copper alloy	11133-98-5	Beryllium copper; **copper alloy, Cu, Be**	-
Beryllium-copper-cobalt alloy	55158-44-6	Cobalt-beryllium copper; **copper alloy, Cu, Be, Co**	-
Beryllium-nickel alloy	37227-61-5	Nickel-beryllium alloy; **nickel alloy, Ni, Be**	-
Beryl ore	1302-52-9	**Beryl [Be$_3$(AlSi$_3$O$_9$)$_2$]**; beryllium aluminium silicate; beryllium alumino-silicate; beryllium aluminum silicate	3BeO.Al$_2$O$_3$.6SiO$_2$

1.2 Chemical and physical properties

Physical properties of the beryllium compounds considered in this monograph are given, when available, in tables 2 and 2a. Information on the solubility of pure compounds, from Weast (1977), unless otherwise specified, is given below.

Beryllium - reacts with hot water, alkali and dilute acids

Beryllium acetate - insoluble in cold water, ethanol, diethyl ether and carbon tetra-chloride; dissolves slowly with hydrolysis in boiling-water (Windholz, 1976)

Beryllium acetate, basic - decomposes in water; soluble in chloroform and acetic acid; slightly soluble in ethanol and diethyl ether

Beryllium carbonate - insoluble in cold water; decomposes in hot water; soluble in acids and alkali

Beryllium chloride - very soluble in water, ethanol (151.1 g/l at 20°C) (Stephen & Stephen, 1963) and diethyl ether; slightly soluble in benzene and chloroform

Beryllium fluoride - very soluble in water; soluble in sulphuric acid; slightly soluble in ethanol

Beryllium hydroxide - very slightly soluble in water and dilute alkali; soluble in hot, concentrated sodium hydroxide and acids (Windholz, 1976)

Beryllium oxide - practically insoluble in water (2×10^{-4} g/l at 20°C); reacts with concentrated sulphuric acid (Weast, 1977) and with water vapour at elevated temperatures (Pinto & Greenspan, 1968)

Beryllium phosphate - poorly soluble in water (Schepers, 1964)

Beryllium silicate - insoluble in most mineral acids

Beryllium sulphate - insoluble in cold water; converted to the tetrahydrate in hot water

Beryllium sulphate tetrahydrate - soluble in water (425 g/l at 20°C); practically in-soluble in ethanol; slightly soluble in concentrated sulphuric acid

Zinc beryllium silicate - no information available

Table 2. Physical properties of pure beryllium and beryllium compounds [a]

Chemical name	Atomic/molecular weight	Melting-point (°C)	Boiling-point (°C)	Density (g/cm³)	Crystal system
Beryllium	9.01	1278±5	2970 (5mm)	1.85^{20}	α - close-packed hexagonal[b]; β - body-centred cubic
Beryllium acetate	127.10	300 (dec.)	—	—	plates
Beryllium acetate, basic	406.32	284	331	1.36^{4}	octahedral
Beryllium carbonate	181.03	—	—	—	—
Beryllium chloride	79.92	405	520	1.899^{25}	needles
Beryllium fluoride	47.01	544[c]; 800 (subl.)	1160[c]	1.986^{25}	amorphous
Beryllium hydroxide	43.03[e]	—	—	1.92^{d}	powder or crystals[d]
Beryllium oxide	25.01	2530±30	~3900	3.01	hexagonal
Beryllium phosphate	—	—	—	—	—
Beryllium silicate	110.11	—	—	3.0	triclinic
Beryllium sulphate	105.07	550–600 (dec.)	—	2.443	—
Beryllium sulphate tetrahydrate	177.14	100 ($-2H_2O$)	400 ($-4H_2O$)	$1.713^{10.5}$	tetrahedric
Zinc beryllium silicate	—	—	—	—	—

[a] From Weast (1977), unless otherwise specified
[b] Ballance et al. (1978)
[c] Dean (1973)
[d] Windholz (1976)

Table 2a. Physical properties of impure beryllium compounds and alloys

Chemical name	Molecular weight	Melting-point (^{o}C)	Specific gravity	Crystal system
Bertrandite	238.23[a]	–	2.6[b]	rhombohedric[a]
Beryllium-aluminium alloy	–	–	–	–
Beryllium-copper alloy Copper Alloys Nos 170, 172 and 173	–	865-980[c]	8.26[2][c]	–
Copper Alloy No. 175	–	1029-1068[c]	8.75[2][c]	–
Beryllium-copper-cobalt alloy	–	–	–	–
Beryllium-nickel alloy	–	–	–	–
Beryl ore	537.51[a]	1410±100[a]	2.66[a]	hexagonal[a]

[a]Weast (1977)

[b]Pough (1960)

[c]Copper Development Association, Inc. (1973)

1.3 Technical products and impurities

Beryllium metal is available in the US as a commercial grade with 97% minimum purity (Petkof, 1979). Electrorefined beryllium metal is also available; maximum impurities are as follows (mg/kg): iron, 300; aluminium, 100; silicon, 100; carbon, 300; nickel, 200; magnesium, 60; and copper, 50 (Ballance *et al.*, 1978).

The purity of beryllium metal available in Japan is typically over 98.0%, with 1.8% maximum beryllium oxide.

Typical chemical composition and impurity limits for *beryllium acetate, basic, beryllium carbonate, beryllium chloride, beryllium fluoride* and *beryllium sulphate* (Kawecki Berylco Industries, Inc., 1968) are given in Table 3. *Beryllium hydroxide* contains different levels of several impurities depending on whether it is made from beryl ore or bertrandite ore. Typical impurity levels for the two materials (Ballance *et al.*, 1978) are also given in Table 3.

Beryllium oxide is available in the US as a commercial grade, with a purity of approximately 99.5% and a specific gravity of 2.86-2.91 (Walsh & Rees, 1978). Typical commercial beryllium oxide contains 0.02-0.08% sulphur and the following levels (mg/kg) of other impurities: silicon, 50; aluminium, 40; calcium, <30; sodium and magnesium, 25; iron, 20; chromium, 5; nickel, 3; copper, lead and manganese, 2 or less; and boron, cadmium, cobalt, lithium and silver, <1 (Brush Wellman, Inc., undated). Technical grades of beryllium oxide that were available formerly were produced as intermediate products in the production of beryllium metal and beryllium-copper alloys; these contained major amounts of impurities such as sodium, calcium and aluminium salts and iron, magnesium and lithium (Schwenzfeier, 1964).

Beryl ore is available in commercial grades of varying purities, containing 10-13% beryllium oxide, 16-19% aluminium oxide, 64-70% silicon dioxide, 1-2% alkali metal oxides and 1-2% iron and other oxides (Ballance *et al.*, 1978).

Beryllium-aluminium alloy is available in the US as a grade containing 62% beryllium and 38% aluminium (van Oss, 1970).

Beryllium-copper alloy is available in the US as high-strength and high-conducting alloys, with the following specifications (% permitted) (Ballance *et al.*, 1978; Copper Development Association, Inc., 1973).

	High-strength alloys			High-conductivity alloys	
Copper Alloy No.	170	172	173	175	176
copper	98.3	98.1	97.7	96.9	-
beryllium	1.6-1.79	1.82-2.0	1.8-2.0	0.4-0.7	0.3-0.8
nickel and cobalt	0.2 min	0.2 min	0.2 min		
nickel, iron and cobalt	0.6 max	0.6 max	0.6 max		
lead			0.2-0.6		
iron				0.1 max	
cobalt				2.4-2.7	1.4-1.7
silver					1.0

Beryllium-copper master alloy (used for subsequent refining into commercial alloys) contains 3.75-4.5% beryllium, 0.72% max of other elements and the remainder consists of copper (Petkof, 1975).

Beryllium-nickel alloy contains 2-3% beryllium and up to 4% other additives, such as carbon, magnesium, titanium and chromium; the rest consists of nickel (Ballance *et al.*, 1978).

Bertrandite contains 42.1% beryllium oxide, 50.3% silicon dioxide and 7.6% water (Pough, 1960).

2. Production, Use, Occurrence and Analysis

Four reviews on beryllium have been published (Ballance *et al.*, 1978; Drury *et al.*, 1978; Hurlbut, 1974; Pinto & Greenspan, 1968).

2.1 Production and use

BERYLLIUM

(a) Production

Beryllium was discovered by Vauquelin in 1798 as a constituent of the mineral beryl. The metal was isolated in 1828, independently by Wohler and by Bussy, by the reduction of

Table 3. Typical chemical composition and impurity limits for certain beryllium compounds

	Anhydrous beryllium chloride powder	Anhydrous beryllium fluoride discs	Beryllium acetate, basic	Beryllium carbonate	Beryllium sulphate crystals	Beryllium hydroxide	
						Beryl-derived	Bertrandite-derived
Beryllium (%)	11.2	19.0	8.7	6.2	4.6		
(mg/kg)							
Aluminium	50	75	10	30	20	2200	400
Iron	100	75	10	100	10	400	50
Silicon	30	-	40	150	20	400	250
Sodium	-	-	-	-	10	2500	100
Cadmium	10	-	-	-	-	-	-
Nickel	120	40	-	-	-	100	5
Copper	10	10	-	-	-	-	-
Cobalt	10	-	-	-	-	20	<1
Zinc	10	-	-	-	-	-	-
Chromium	10	-	-	-	-	60	20
Manganese	10	-	-	-	-	1500	10
Magnesium	150	-	-	-	-	3000	50
Calcium	-	-	-	-	-	5000	50
Lithium	-	-	-	-	-	200	<20

beryllium chloride with potassium. Beryllium metal is produced commercially in the US by either the thermal reduction of beryllium fluoride with metallic magnesium or the electro-refining of beryllium metal pebble or scrap carried out in a fused salt bath (Ballance *et al.*, 1978).

Beryllium has been produced commercially in the US since the 1940s (Ballance *et al.*, 1978). In 1979, two companies were reported to have been producing beryllium (Bureau of National Affairs, Inc., 1979a). Prior to 1965, 45.4-68 thousand kg were produced annually (Drury *et al.*, 1978).

In 1978, 660 kg of beryllium (unwrought, waste and scrap) were imported into the US, primarily from Mexico and France (US Department of Commerce, 1979). Exports of beryl-lium and beryllium alloys (wrought or unwrought, waste and scrap) amounted to 72.8 thousand kg in 1977, primarily to Japan, France and the UK (US Department of Commerce, 1978).

Beryllium has been produced commercially in Japan since about 1955 by the chlori-nation of beryllium oxide in the presence of carbon, followed by reduction and electrolysis of the intermediate chloride. In 1978, one Japanese manufacturer produced an estimated 100 kg of beryllium. No information was available on whether it is produced elsewhere.

World production of beryllium, excluding the US, was 97.1 thousand kg in 1977, down from 320 thousand kg in 1969 (US Bureau of Mines, 1979a).

(b) Use

US consumption of *beryllium* decreased from about 200 thousand kg in 1974 to 63 thousand kg in 1978. The decrease is attributed to reductions in defence and aerospace pro-grammes (US Bureau of Mines, 1979b). In 1977, beryllium was used as follows: electrical uses (other than components), 37.3%; nuclear reactors, 19.4%; aerospace applications, 17.9%; electrical components, 16.4%; and other uses, 9% (US Bureau of Mines, 1979a). Estimated percentages used in various beryllium products in 1978 were as follows: beryl-lium-copper and other alloys, 70-80%; beryllium metal, 15-20%; and beryllium oxide, 5-10% (Farkas, 1979).

Beryllium metal is used extensively as a window material for X-ray tubes, a moderator material for nuclear weapons, and a neutron reflector in high-flux test reactors. Aero-space applications include the production of heat sink material in low-weight, high-per-formance aircraft brakes, and mirror components of satellite optical systems (Ballance *et al.*, 1978; Farkas, 1979).

In Japan, of the 100 kg beryllium used in 1978 most was for audio equipment such as loudspeakers.

BERYLLIUM ACETATE AND BERYLLIUM ACETATE, BASIC

(a) Production

Beryllium acetate was first prepared by the reaction of basic beryllium acetate with glacial acetic acid and excess acetic anhydride (Steinmetz, 1907). Basic beryllium acetate was prepared in 1901 by Urbain and Lacombe (Windholz, 1976). It was first prepared commercially by the combination of beryllium oxide and acetic anhydride (Kawecki, 1953). It is currently produced either by this method or by the reaction of glacial acetic acid with beryllium oxide or hydroxide.

Beryllium acetate is not produced commercially in the US; only one US company produces an undisclosed amount of basic beryllium acetate (see preamble, p. 20). Separate data on US imports and exports are not reported. No information was available on whether it is produced elsewhere.

(b) Use

Beryllium acetate has no known commercial uses. The basic acetate is used as an intermediate in the production (normally on the laboratory scale) of high purity beryllium salts.

BERYLLIUM CARBONATE

(a) Production

Although the synthesis of beryllium carbonate tetrahydrate was reported by Klatzs in 1869, by passing a stream of carbon dioxide through a suspension of beryllium hydroxide in water (Mellor, 1946), it is doubtful that the tetrahydrate was recovered, since it is only stable under carbon dioxide pressure (Walsh & Rees, 1978). The stable carbonate, beryllium oxide carbonate (or basic beryllium carbonate), is produced as a precipitate when sodium carbonate is variable in composition, depending on the identity of the initial beryllium salt employed and the reaction conditions. The precipitate is usually a mixture consisting of 2-5 molecules of the hydroxide for each molecule of the carbonate (Walsh & Rees, 1978).

Only one US company produces an undisclosed amount of basic beryllium carbonate (see preamble, p. 20). US imports of beryllium carbonate are believed to be negligible, and separate export data are not reported. No information was available on whether it is produced elsewhere.

(b)   Use

Beryllium carbonate is used primarily on a laboratory scale as an intermediate in the preparation of other beryllium salts.

BERYLLIUM CHLORIDE

(a)   Production

This compound was prepared by Rose in 1828 by the reaction of chlorine with a mixture of carbon and beryllium oxide (Mellor, 1946). Essentially the same method was used for commercial production in the US in 1978 (Walsh & Rees, 1978).

One company in the US produces an undisclosed amount of this chemical (see preamble, p.   20   ). Available information indicated that it is also produced by one company in the UK, although it may be produced elsewhere as well.

(b)   Use

The major use of beryllium chloride is in the laboratory manufacture of beryllium metal by electrolysis. In the anhydrous form, beryllium chloride is used as an acid catalyst in organic reactions (Windholz, 1976).

BERYLLIUM FLUORIDE

(a)   Production

This compound was produced by Lebeau in 1898 by heating ammonium fluoro-beryllate in a stream of dry carbon dioxide or by the action of hydrogen fluoride on beryllium carbide (Mellor, 1946). Commercial production involves the thermal decomposition of the diammonium tetrafluoroberyllate (Walsh & Rees, 1978).

Beryllium fluoride is believed to have been produced commercially in the US since the 1940s. Two companies in the US produce an undisclosed amount of this chemical (see preamble, p.   20).   No information was available on whether it is produced elsewhere as well.

(b)   Use

The major use of beryllium fluoride is as a chemical intermediate in the commercial production of beryllium metal and beryllium alloys. It is also used in the manufacture of glass and nuclear reactors (Windholz, 1976).

BERYLLIUM HYDROXIDE

(a)   Production

This compound was prepared by Weeren in 1854 by the reaction of beryllium oxide with potassium hydroxide (Mellor, 1946). It is produced commercially by either: (1) the sulphuric acid extraction of beryl ore, in which the ore is fused into beryl glass and reacted with sulphuric acid, and the resulting beryllium sulphate is treated with organic chelating agents and sodium hydroxide; or (2) the bertrandite process, in which the wet-milled ore is reacted with sulphuric acid, followed by extraction of beryllium with di(2-ethylhexyl)-phosphate in kerosene, then treatment with ammonium carbonate solution, and finally heating to form the hydroxide (Ballance *et al.*, 1978).

Beryllium hydroxide is believed to have been produced commercially in the US since the 1940s; two companies in the US produce an undisclosed amount from beryl ore (see preamble, p. 20).

No information was available on whether it is produced elsewhere as well.

(b)   Use

The major use of beryllium hydroxide is as a chemical intermediate in the commercial production of beryllium metal, beryllium-copper and other alloys, and beryllium oxide (Ballance *et al.*, 1978; Windholz, 1976).

BERYLLIUM OXIDE

(a)   Production

This compound was prepared by Ebelmen in 1853 by heating beryllium silicate with an excess of potassium carbonate (Mellor, 1946). It is produced commercially by dissolving technical-grade beryllium hydroxide in sulphuric acid and calcining the isolated high purity beryllium sulphate tetrahydrate at selected temperatures ranging from 1150-1450°C, depending upon the desired properties of the beryllium oxide product. In a less important commercial process, the solution of technical-grade beryllium hydroxide in sulphuric acid is filtered, and an organic chelating agent is added before ammonium hydroxide is used to pre-cipitate high-purity beryllium hydroxide, which is selectively calcined to beryllium oxide powder (Walsh & Rees, 1978).

Beryllium oxide has been produced commercially in the US since about 1958; and two companies in the US produce an undisclosed amount (see preamble, p. 20   ). In 1978, combined US imports of beryllium oxide and carbonate were 3.06 thousand kg (US Depart-ment of Commerce, 1979).

Beryllium oxide was first produced commercially in Japan in about 1955. However, production virtually ceased in 1976; and in 1978 only minor amounts were believed to have been produced by one producer. Imports were approximately 15.6 thousand kg in 1974 and 32.5 thousand kg in 1978.

No information was available on whether it is produced elsewhere as well.

(b) Use

The major use for beryllium oxide is in the manufacture of ceramics, since it has high thermal conductivity and heat capacity combined with high electrical resistivity. Beryllium oxide ceramic parts are often used in electronic and microelectronic applications (such as semiconductor devices and integrated circuits requiring thermal dissipation), in microwave tubes and in lasers (Farkas, 1979; Walsh & Rees, 1978).

Beryllium oxide has also been used as a moderator and/or reflector in nuclear reactors (Boland, 1958).

An estimated 32.5 thousand kg of beryllium oxide were used in Japan in 1978, pri-marily for the production of beryllium-copper alloy; 2-3% was used to produce metallic beryllium.

BERYLLIUM PHOSPHATE

(a) Production

The preparation of various hydrated forms of beryllium phosphate has been reported, including reaction of disodium hydrophosphate with a beryllium salt solution and reaction of beryllium hydroxide solution with phosphoric acid (Mellor, 1946). Production of bery-llium phosphate was reported in the US in 1978; however, it is not believed to be produced there currently.

No information was available on whether it is produced elsewhere as well.

(b)   Use

No data were available to the Working Group.

BERYLLIUM SILICATE

(a)   Production

Production of beryllium silicate was reported in the US in 1978;   however, it is not believed to be produced there currently.   No information was available on whether it is produced elsewhere as well.

(b)   Use

No data were available to the Working Group.

BERYLLIUM SULPHATES

(a)   Production

Beryllium sulphate tetrahydrate was prepared by Vauquelin in 1798 by the action of sulphuric acid on beryllium oxide (Mellor, 1946).   It is produced commercially in a highly purified state by fractional crystallization from a beryllium sulphate solution prepared by the reaction of beryllium hydroxide with sulphuric acid.   The dihydrate beryllium sulphate is obtained by heating the tetrahydrate to $92^{\circ}C$, and anhydrous beryllium sulphate by heating the dihydrate to $400^{\circ}C$ (Walsh & Rees, 1978).

Beryllium sulphate tetrahydrate has been produced commercially in the US since the 1940s;   and two companies currently produce an undisclosed amount (see preamble, p. 20). Available information indicated that it is also produced by one company in the UK, although it may be produced elsewhere as well.

(b)   Use

Beryllium sulphate tetrahydrate is used as a chemical intermediate in the processing of beryl and bertrandite ores, from which all commercially significant beryllium and beryllium compounds are produced (Ballance *et al.*, 1978).

ZINC BERYLLIUM SILICATE

(a)   Production

No data were available on current commercial production.

(b)   Use

Zinc beryllium silicate was used as an oxygen-dominated phosphor in luminescent materials (Fonda, 1952).

BERTRANDITE

(a)   Production

Bertrandite, a naturally occurring mineral, is mined by open-pit methods by one company in the US. Although it is the principal beryllium mineral produced in the US (Petkof, 1975), production data are not reported (see preamble, p. 20). Separate data on US imports and exports were not available.

(b)   Use

Bertrandite is used as a mineral source of beryllium. It is milled and processed into technical-grade beryllium hydroxide for processing into beryllium-containing materials. In the US, it is the primary source of beryllium products; but in the rest of the world, beryl is the principal source of beryllium mineral (Petkof, 1975).

BERYL ORE

(a)   Production

The only commercial mineral sources of beryllium are beryl ore and, since 1969, bertrandite ore. In 1973, about 7.89 million kg of beryl ore (including some bertrandite ore) were processed in the US. In 1978, beryl ore was mined in the US by only one company. In 1977, 677 thousand kg of beryl ore were imported into the US, 63% of which came from Brazil, 24% from Argentina and lesser amounts from the Republic of South Africa, Mozambique, Australia and Spain (Petkof, 1979).

Japanese imports of beryl ore were approximately 262 thousand kg in 1974 and 91 thousand in 1975. No imports have been reported more recently.

World production, excluding the US, of beryl ore in 1977 was 2.41 million kg, down from 2.9 in 1975 and 3.6 million in 1973. The USSR, Brazil and Argentina produced 70.4, 17.7 and 4.1%, respectively, of the 1977 total; lesser amounts were produced in Southern Rhodesia, Rwanda, Uganda, Madagascar, Mozambique, and the Republic of South Africa (Petkof, 1979). No information was available on whether it is produced elsewhere as well.

(b)   Use

Use of beryl ore (including bertrandite ore, calculated as equivalent of beryl ore) in the US in 1977 was 3.78 million kg, down from 7.89 million kg in 1973. The US and the USSR were the major users in 1977 (Petkof, 1979). In Japan, an estimated 262 thousand kg of beryl ore were used in 1975, entirely in the production of beryllium oxide.

BERYLLIUM-ALUMINIUM ALLOY

(a)   Production

Although beryllium-aluminium alloys were some of the earliest alloys of beryllium developed (Beaver, 1963), they are not believed to be produced for commercial use.

(b)   Use

Beryllium-aluminium alloys have been tested in metallurgical laboratories. Addition of beryllium to aluminium casting alloys refines the grain size, resulting in better surface polishing;   this treatment reduces melt losses and improves casting fluidity (Ballance *et al.*, 1978).

BERYLLIUM-COPPER ALLOY

(a)   Production

Beryllium-copper alloy was first prepared in the early 1920s by adding beryllium to copper. It is currently produced by the reduction of beryllium oxide by carbon in the presence of molten copper in an arc furnace at 1800-2000°C (Ballance *et al.*, 1978). After further refining, this master alloy is diluted with copper to a wide variety of commercial alloys (Petkof, 1975).

Beryllium-copper alloy is believed to be produced by 2 companies in the US, but data on the amounts produced were not available (see preamble, p.   20   ). Separate data on US imports and exports are not reported.

(b)   Use

The high-strength beryllium-copper alloys are widely used for small electrical contacts, springs, pen and pencil clips, switches, bellows, Bourdon pressure gauges and injection moulds for plastics (Ballance *et al.*, 1978). The high-conductivity alloys are used in electrical springs, switches and contacts, and in discs and tips for welding. Other electrical applications are in connectors, circuit-breaker parts, fuse clips and high-frequency connector plugs (Roskill Information Services, 1975).

In 1974, the US national stockpile contained 6.7 million kg beryllium-copper master alloy. In 1976, the US government issued new goals for a strategic stockpile of 15.2 million kg (Petkof, 1976).

BERYLLIUM-COPPER-COBALT ALLOY

(a) Production

Beryllium-copper-cobalt alloy is produced by precipitation-hardening (heating followed by quenching) of copper and age-hardening by a second heat treatment at a lower temperature (Roskill Information Services, 1975). No data on production, imports or exports were available to the Working Group.

(b) Use

Beryllium-copper-cobalt alloy is used in resistance-welding electrodes and holders, nozzles for gas and oil burners, plunger tips for die-casting machines, bushings, bearings, soldering iron tips, current-carrying springs and electrical contacts, clips, connectors and circuit-breaker parts (Roskill Information Services, 1975).

BERYLLIUM-NICKEL ALLOY

(a) Production

Beryllium nickel alloy is produced by precipitation-hardening with solution annealing, quenching and ageing (Ballance et al., 1978). No data on production, imports or exports were available to the Working Group.

(b) Use

Beryllium nickel alloys are used in electrical connections when high temperatures prevent the use of beryllium-copper alloys (Farkas, 1979; Pinto & Greenspan, 1968). They are used in strip form as springs and electrical connectors and in related high-temperature applications, and by the glass industry in various glass-moulding functions (Ballance et al., 1978).

2.2 Regulatory status (see also preamble, p. 21)

In 1949, to control exposure to beryllium in the beryllium refining industry, the US Atomic Energy Commission adopted a limit for beryllium concentrations in community air of 0.01 $\mu g/m^3$ averaged over a 30-day period (National Institute for Occupational Safety & Health, 1979; US Environmental Protection Agency, 1973).

The US Occupational Safety and Health Administration's health standards require that an employee's exposure to beryllium and beryllium compounds at no time exceed an 8-hour time-weighted average of 2 $\mu g/m^3$, an acceptable ceiling concentration of 5 $\mu g/m^3$ or an acceptable maximum peak concentration above the acceptable ceiling concentration for an 8-hour shift of 25 $\mu g/m^3$ for a maximum of 30 min (Bureau of National Affairs, Inc., 1979b).

The US Environmental Protection Agency requires that emissions of beryllium to the air from a beryllium facility not exceed 10 g over a 24-hr period or 0.01 $\mu g/m^3$ as a monthly average (US Environmental Protection Agency, 1978). The maximum allowable concentration for beryllium in various countries varies from 0-2 $\mu g/m^3$ (Japanese Society of Industrial Hygiene, 1978; Winell, 1975).

2.3 Occurrence

(a) Natural environment

Beryllium ranks 44th in abundance among the elements, constituting about 0.0006% of the earth's crust (Drury et al., 1978). Of the beryllium compounds (other than beryl ore and bertrandite) included in this monograph, only beryllium silicate is known to occur naturally in mineral form as phenakite (Windholz, 1976).

Bertrandite occurs in beryl pegmatite. Bertrandite crystals have been found at Mt Antero, Colorado; small crystals are found in the cleavelandite feldspar at Portland, Connecticut, coating beryl at Bedford, New York, and associated with apatite at Stoneham, Maine. Bertrandite plates have been found in a pegmatite in Jefferson County, Colarado, and in the state of Rio Grande do Norte in Brazil (Pough, 1960).

Known resources of beryllium in the US consist primary of bertrandite located at Spor Mountain and Gold Hill, Utah, and in the Seward Peninsula, Alaska (Petkof, 1976).

The natural sources of beryllium are listed in Table 4.

Beryl, the major beryllium ore, contains 3-5% beryllium. Beryllium is also obtained from bertrandite ore, which contains about 15% (Drury et al., 1978). Beryllium concentrations in rocks and minerals range from 0.038-11.4 mg/kg (Table 5). The beryllium content of mineral oils has been estimated to be less than 100 $\mu g/l$ (Drury et al., 1978; Reeves, 1978a).

Table 4. Representative natural mineral sources of beryllium[a]

Mineral	Composition	Geological occurrence	Geographical distribution
Beryl	$3BeO.Al_2O_3.6SiO_2$	Pegmatite	US (Kentucky, Texas, Arizona, Nevada, Idaho), Argentina, Brazil, India, Madagascar
Beryllonite	$NaBePO_4$	Pegmatite	US (Maine)
Bertrandite	$4BeO.2 SiO_2.H_2O$	Pegmatite	US (Colorado, Maine), France, Bohemia
Bromellite	BeO	Veins	Sweden
Chrysoberyl	$Be(AlO_2)_2$	Pegmatite	Brazil, Ceylon, Ural Mountains, US (New York)
Euclase	$BeHAl SiO_5$	Pegmatite	Brazil, Ural Mountains, Austrian Alps
Hambergite	$Be_2(OH)BO_3$	Pegmatite	Norway, Madagascar
Helvite	$Mn_4 Be_3 Si_3 O_{12} S$	Pegmatite, veins	US (New Mexico), Norway, USSR, Australia, Canada, Brazil
Herderite	$CaBePO_4(OH,F)$	Pegmatite	US (Maine)
Leucophanite	$(Ca,Na)_2 BeSi_2(O,OH,F)$	Pegmatite	Norway
Phenakite	Be_2SiO_4	Pegmatite	US (Colorado), Ural Mountains, Vosges Mountains

[a]From Drury et al. (1978)

Table 5. Concentrations of beryllium in rocks and minerals[a]

Rock type or mineral	Beryllium content (mg/kg)
Igneous	6
Ultrabasic	0.2
Basalt	0.3
Nepheline syenite	0.65
Diorites	1.6
Diorite and gabbro-diorite	1.8
Granite	3.6
Shales	3.6
Shale and clay	7
Earth's crust	10
Upper part of the lithosphere	2
Talc	0.065
Asbestos	0.24
Kaolin	7.4
Monazite	0.059
Phosphate	0.08-3.75
Mafic	< 1
Silicic	6.5
Alkalic	11.4
Meteorites	0.038
Sandstones and limestones	< 1

[a]From Drury et al. (1978)

World coals contain 0.1-1000 mg/kg beryllium (Drury *et al.*, 1978). In one study in the US, the beryllium concentration in coal ranged from 1.46-1.52 mg/kg (Wicks & Burke, 1977). An analysis of coal samples from seven countries showed the following beryllium concentrations: Australia, 15 mg/kg; US, <5-13 mg/kg; and the Federal Republic of Germany, Norway, Poland, the UK and the USSR, <5 mg/kg (Lövblad, 1977).

(b)   Air

The atmospheric background level of beryllium is usually <0.0001 $\mu g/m^3$. It was not detectable in most of the 100 cities sampled by the National Air Surveillance Network, and a maximum of 0.003 $\mu g/m^3$ was found in a survey of the air of more than 30 metropolitan areas. This concurs with the findings of a 1958 study of suspended particulate samples from Houston, Texas, Denver, Colorado and Louisville, Kentucky (Drury *et al.*, 1978).

Atmospheric beryllium concentrations are often higher than normal near beryllium processing plants. A mean concentration of 0.0155 $\mu g/m^3$ and a maximum concentration of 0.0827 $\mu g/m^3$ were reported near a Pennsylvania factory; background samples from several locations in the area averaged only 0.0002 $\mu g/m^3$. During a partial shutdown of the factory, the beryllium concentration was reduced to 0.0047 $\mu g/m^3$; a two-week shutdown resulted in an average of 0.0015 $\mu g/m^3$ (Drury *et al.*, 1978).

The range of beryllium concentrations measured in Ohio ambient air particulates at a rural site was 2.7-5.8 $\mu g/m^3$, that at an industrialized urban site, 10.4-19.5 $\mu g/m^3$, and that at a suburban site 4-7.2 $\mu g/m^3$ (Ross *et al.*., 1977).

(c)   Cigarette smoke

In a study of three brands of cigarettes, beryllium concentrations of 0.47, 0.68 and 0.74 μg/cigarette were found; 4.5, 1.6 and 10.0% of the beryllium content, respectively, escaped into the smoke during smoking (Drury *et al.*, 1978).

(d)   Occupational exposure

According to the National Institute for Occupational Safety & Health (1972), beryllium metal and those of its compounds that are used industrially cause both acute and chronic respiratory disease. Prior to 1950, many cases of beryllium disease were associated with the manufacture and use of fluorescent tubes, and particularly with the disposal of broken tubes. The use of beryllium phosphors in such tubes was discontinued in 1949. Since 1950, use of beryllium in industry has increased, and the range of industrial processes that could lead to occupational exposure has been expanded. Industrial plants vary widely in size and operation. Processing and manufacturing activities include mining, extraction, refining, alloy manufacture, metallurgical operations, manufacture of ceramics, electronic equipment, non-ferrous foundry products, aerospace equipment, tools and dies, beryllium-alloy machining, moulding, grinding, cutting and fabrication as well as processes in the electroplating and atomic energy industries.

In 1970, the National Institute for Occupational Safety and Health indicated that 30,000 workers potentially had exposure to the dust or fumes of beryllium, of which 2500 were employed in its production. In view of the widespread use of this metal and its compounds, the total estimate is probably very conservative. Actual worker exposure to beryllium varies considerably: a study of a beryllium-alloy plant conducted in 1947-1948 showed concentrations of beryllium in air ranging from 411 $\mu g/m^3$ in the general air surrounding the mix operation to 43,300 $\mu g/m^3$ in the breathing zone of alloy operatives (National Institute for Occupational Safety & Health, 1972).

According to the National Institute for Occupational Safety & Health (1972), control measures were introduced throughout the US in 1949, and exposure levels in beryllium facilities were reduced markedly. Extraction plants, for example, were able to maintain exposure levels of 2 $\mu g/m^3$ or less; machine shops achieved even lower levels (0.1 $\mu g/m^3$). Certain foundry operations, however, continued to generate beryllium into the air in concentrations consistently in excess of 2 $\mu g/m^3$; current values that exceed 50 $\mu g/m^3$ probably indicate failure of control methods due either to inadequate protection or to accidental breakdown of equipment. It is of note that in some plants that fail to achieve consistent ambient beryllium levels of less than 2 $\mu g/m^3$, elevated concentrations are not confined to production areas but may be found throughout the plant (National Institute for Occupational Safety & Health, 1972).

(e) Water and sediments

Less than 1 $\mu g/l$ beryllium was found in fresh water and 0.6 ng/l in seawater. The average beryllium content of the Pacific Ocean was 0.57 ng/l, 68% of which was in solution and 32% in particulate form. Sediments contained 2-3 mg/kg (Drury *et al.*, 1978).

Beryllium concentrations in 15 major US river basins ranged from 0.01-1.22 $\mu g/l$, with a mean of 0.19 $\mu g/l$ (Safe Drinking Water Committee, 1977). Samples taken from various areas near the Seward Peninsula in Alaska showed beryllium concentrations of 0.034-2.4 $\mu g/l$ in water samples and 4.4-2700 $\mu g/kg$ in sediment (Gosink, 1976). Beryllium was one of several trace elements found in bottom sediments in lakes of southern Illinois, in concentrations ranging from 1.4-7.4 mg/kg (Dreher *et al.*, 1977). In the eastern US and in Siberia, surface water contains beryllium in concentrations ranging from 0.1-0.9 $\mu g/l$. It has been found in US drinking-water at levels of 0.01-0.7 $\mu g/l$, with a mean of 0.013 $\mu g/l$ (Safe Drinking Water Committee, 1977).

Beryllium concentrations in effluents from metals industries, power plants and from industrial and municipal wastes in the US ranged from 18-21 μg/l (US Environmental Protection Agency, 1977). Typical concentrations in treated pulp and paper mill effluents are <0.6 μg/l (Fisher, 1978).

(f) Soils and plants

Due to its prevalence in rocks, beryllium occurs in most soils. The beryllium contents of soil samples in various locations have been reported as follows: world-wide, 0.1-40 mg/kg (average, 6 mg/kg); US, 0.13-0.88 mg/kg (average, 0.37 mg/kg); and Kenya, 0.04-1.45 mg/kg (Drury *et al.*, 1978).

Plant leaves generally contain more beryllium than either twigs or fruit, except for certain desert shrubs in the southwestern US which contain more beryllium in their twigs than in their leaves (Griffitts *et al.*, 1977). Beryllium concentrations in orchard leaves in the US were about 0.026 mg/kg (Wicks & Burke, 1977).

Levels of beryllium found in various trees and shrubs are as follows: hickory, 1 mg/kg dry weight and 30 mg/kg in plant ash; dogwood and other broad-leaved trees and shrubs, >0.1 mg/kg dry weight; conifers, 0.1 mg/kg dry weight and <1 mg/kg in plant ash; lodgepole pine, Englemann spruce and Douglas fir in Colorado and Idaho, <1 mg/kg in plant ash (Griffitts *et al.*, 1977).

Average levels of beryllium found in various plants in Australia are as follows (mg/kg ash weight): acacia, 0.46; angiosperms, 0.69; field lupine seeds, 0.02; grass, 0.26-0.35; and tobacco, 0.24-0.25 (Meehan & Smythe, 1967).

(g) Food

The beryllium concentrations of various foodstuffs collected in New South Wales, Australia, ranged from 0.01-0.12 mg/kg, with oyster flesh and mushrooms containing the most (Meehan & Smythe, 1967). Green head lettuce contained the highest beryllium level in other foods tested (0.33 mg/kg on a dried basis); potatoes, tomatoes, bread and rice contained 0.08-0.24 mg/kg on a dried basis (Drury *et al.*, 1978).

(h) Animals

Beryllium concentrations in bovine liver in the US ranged from 0.013-0.021 mg/kg (Wicks & Burke, 1977).

(i)   Human tissues and secretions

The concentrations of beryllium found in normal human body tissues and in tissues taken from people with known exposure to beryllium have been reviewed (Hurlbut, 1974). Results are reported for concentrations in brain, muscle, vertebrae, bone, kidney, liver, heart, hair, lung, blood, urine and spleen as determined by a variety of methods, carried out between 1961 and 1970. Since the beryllium content varied significantly for certain tissue samples, the author suggested that there could be doubt about the validity of the analytical data: values varied from 0.04 μg/kg to 0.06 mg/kg for nonexposed people and from 0.02 μg/kg to 40 mg/kg for exposed people.

Beryllium concentrations in lung have been reported for cases of berylliosis and autopsied humans with no known exposure to beryllium (DeNardi et al., 1952; Meehan & Smythe, 1967). Values reported from lung tissue from cases of berylliosis varied from a fraction of a μg/g to more than 1 mg/g; while, in general, lower values were found in lung tissue from nonexposed individuals, although values as high as those in cases of berylliosis were found in some.

Random urine samples from 16 employees exposed to beryllium showed beryllium concentrations of <10 μg/l (4.8-5.8 μg/l); the content in samples from 120 people living in urban California ranged from 0.40-1.0 μg/l (Grewal & Kearns, 1977).

2.4 Analysis (see also preamble, p. 21)

Methods for sampling beryllium-containing materials and for the separation, concentration and analysis of beryllium, and comparisons of analytical procedures have been reviewed (Drury et al., 1978; Hurlbut, 1974). Manual methods for measuring beryllium in stationary source emissions have been described (Coulson & Haynes, 1972). Techniques for analysing beryllium in copper alloys utilize atomic absorption and gamma activation (Ballance et al., 1978). Bertrandite can be identified in mineral samples by the properties that it whitens but does not fuse on charcoal and that it turns blue in the cobalt nitrate test (Pough, 1960).

Typical methods for analysis for determining levels of beryllium in environmental samples are summarized in Table 6. Abbreviations are: AAS, atomic absorption spectrometry; FAAS, flameless atomic absorption spectrometry; FAES, flameless atomic emission spectrometry; GC/EC, gas chromatography/electron capture; and UV, ultra-violet spectrometry.

Table 6. Analytical methods for beryllium and beryllium compounds

Sample matrix	Sample preparation	Assay procedure	Sensitivity or limit of detection	Reference
Bulk chemical	Add solutions of uramil-N,N-diacetic acid, acetate buffer and water	UV (267 nm)	-	Presas-Barrosa et al. (1977)
	Add solutions of chromal blue G, cetyltrimethylammonium chloride and acetate buffer; dilute; allow colour to develop	Spectrophotometry (626 nm)	-	Uesugi & Miyawaki (1976)
	Add hydroxynaphthol blue solution; allow to stand 5 min	Spectrophotometry	2.7 μg	Brittain (1978)
Formulations				
β-Alumina ceramics	Grind; dissolve in strong phosphoric acid solution	AAS	0.02 mg/kg	Havezov & Tamnev (1978)
Technological solution	-	Aerosol-Spark spectrography	0.001 mg/l	Gusarskii et al. (1977)
Copper-beryllium alloy	Make complex with sodium (ethylenedinitrilo) tetraacetate; precipitate beryllium as phosphate; ignite; weigh as pyrophosphate	Gravimetry	-	Ballance et al. (1978)
	Add ammonium aurintricarboxylate to form a red lake	Photometry	-	Ballance et al. (1978)
Air	Dissolve collection filter matrix in hydrofluoric acid; add nitric acid and water; boil ; dilute	FAAS AAS	0.05 ng/m^3 2.5 ng/m^3	Zdrojewski et al. (1976)

Table 6 (contd)

Sample matrix	Sample preparation	Assay procedure	Sensitivity or limit of detection	Reference
Air (contd)	Dry collection filter; add nitric and sulphuric acids and distilled, deionized water; reflux at 80°C for 7 hrs ; add EDTA-buffer solution and sodium hydroxide to pH 6; add trifluoroacetyl-acetone:benzene solution (1:1); desiccant chelate; wash with sodium hydroxide	GC/EC	-	Ross et al. (1977)
	Extract filter with sulphuric acid; add chrome Azurol S solution, gum arabic solution and EDTA; adjust pH to 2.0; add cetylpyridinium bromide and hexamine solution; adjust to pH 5	Spectrophotometry (605 nm)	-	Mulwani & Sathe (1977)
	Ash collection filter strips; reflux with mixture of nitric and hydrochloric acids containing 55.5 μg/ml indium and yttrium; concentrate extraction liquid; add nitric acid; centrifuge; add 40% lithium chloride solution containing 20% nitric acid and 200 μg/ml indium and yttrium	Optical emission spectroscopy	5.3 mg/m^3	Scott et al. (1976)
Water [Chemical procedures were developed to simulate natural water matrix]				
Standard Reference Material 1643 (natural fresh water)	Acidify with nitric acid to stabilize solution	FAAS (234.9 nm) FAES (234.9 nm)	0.06 μg/l 2 μg/l	Epstein et al. (1978)

Table 6 (contd)

Sample matrix	Sample preparation	Assay procedure	Sensitivity or limit of detection	Reference
Pond water	Evaporate and dry residue at 80°C for 48 hrs; mix with graphite (1:1) and grind	Optical emission spectroscopy	0.06 mg/l	Cowgill (1976)
Surface water, tap-water	Acidify with nitric acid to pH 2	FAAS	0.01 µg/l	Lagas (1978)
Biological samples				
Standard Reference Material 1571 (orchard leaves)	Wet-ash dried tissue in mixture of nitric:perchloric acids (1:1); add water, EDTA solution and phenol red; adjust pH to 7-8; add acetylacetone solution; extract (chloroform); perform a series of acidifications and evaporations; add water, cyclohexane-diaminetetra-acetic acid solution and phenol red; adjust pH to 7-8; add buffer solution and 2-hydroxy-3-naphthoic acid reagent	Fluorescence spectrometry	-	Wicks & Burke (1977)
Standard Reference Material 1577 (bovine liver)	Wet-ash dried tissue in mixture of nitric:perchloric acids (1:1); add water, EDTA solution and phenol red; adjust pH to 7-8; add acetylacetone solution; extract (chloroform); perform a series of acidifications and evaporations; add water, cyclohexane-diaminetetraacetic acid solution and phenol red; adjust pH to 7-8; add buffer solution and 2-hydroxy-3-naphthoic acid reagent	Fluorescence spectrometry	-	Wicks & Burke (1977)

Table 6 (contd)

Sample matrix	Sample preparation	Assay procedure	Sensitivity or limit of detection	Reference
Human blood plasma	Extract [chloroform and 2,4-dioxo-4-(4-hydroxy-6-methyl-2-pyrone-3-yl) butyric acid ethyl ester]; dilute chloroform layer with ethanol	Fluorescence spectrometry	0.5 μg	Drevenkar *et al.* (1976)
Dog blood, rat liver homogenate	Add sodium hydroxide; dissolve by heating; dilute and wash with nitric acid; neutralize with sodium hydroxide to a phenolphthalein endpoint, adding solutions of sodium EDTA and acetate buffer; add trifluoroacetyl-acetone-benzene solution; wash benzene aliquots with ammonium hydroxide solution	GC/EC	-	Frame & Ford (1974)
Urine	Add nitric acid containing lanthanum or add nitric acid and excess ammonium hydroxide; centrifuge; decant solution; heat to 80°C	FAAS	0.01 μg/l	Hurlbut (1978)
Urine	-	FAAS	0.5 μg/l	Grewal & Kearns (1977)
Human and rat urine	Add EDTA to aqueous sample; adjust to pH 6; add trifluoroacetylacetone in benzene; extract	GC/EC	1 μg/l	Foreman *et al.* (1970)
Faecal sample	Add nitric acid; apply heat; add hydrogen peroxide and nitric acid; bring mixture to a boil; add ferrous chloride, controlling the foaming by adding water, nitric acid or octanol; evaporate; heat; dissolve residue in nitric acid containing lanthanum	FAAS	1 μg/kg	Hurlbut (1978)

Table 6 (contd)

Sample matrix	Sample preparation	Assay procedure	Sensitivity or limit of detection	Reference
Hair	Clean (acetone, distilled water, detergent, nitric acid); dry with nitric acid, then again with nitric acid:perchloric acid (1:1); add nitric acid containing lanthanum	FAAS	< 1 μg/kg	Hurlbut (1978)
Fingernails	Clean; dry; digest as for hair sample above	FAAS	< 1 μg/kg	Hurlbut (1978)
Lung tissue, hilar lymph node	Ash homogenized samples; mix with graphite and an indium internal standard; compact mixture into electrodes	Spark source mass spectrometry	-	Brown & Taylor (1975)
Other				
Coal	Dry and char sample	FAAS	0.005 ng	Gladney (1977)

3. Biological Data Relevant to the Evaluation
of Carcinogenic Risk to Humans

A review is available (National Institute for Occupational Safety & Health, 1972).

3.1 Carcinogenicity studies in animals

Summaries of the scientific literature on beryllium carcinogenesis in experimental animals have been compiled by Groth (1980), Infante & Wagoner (1975), Reeves (1978b), Schepers (1961) and Sunderman (1971, 1977).

(a) Oral administration

Rat: *Beryllium sulphate* was administered to 52 male and 52 female Long-Evans rats in the drinking-water (5 mg/l Be) from weaning until death. Longevity of beryllium-treated rats did not differ significantly from that of an equal number of controls, but some rats in the treated and control groups died during an epidemic of pneumonia. Malignant tumours were found in 12/50 treated rats and in 10/50 control rats that were autopsied (Schroeder & Mitchener, 1975) [The Working Group noted the low dose of beryllium sulphate used and that the types and locations of tumours in treated and control rats were not specified].

In a study reported as an abstract, addition of *beryllium sulphate* to the diet of Wistar rats at concentrations of 5, 50 or 500 mg/kg of diet for 2 years did not affect tumour incidence (Morgareidge *et al.*, 1977) [The Working Group noted that this brief report does not specify the numbers of rats in the treatment and control groups, nor the numbers and types of tumours that were found].

(b) Inhalation and/or intratracheal administration

Rat: It was reported in an abstract that pulmonary carcinomas (adeno- and epidermoid carcinomas) developed in albino rats that were exposed by chronic inhalation to an aqueous aerosol of *beryllium sulphate* for 7 hrs/day on 5½ days/week for 13-18 months. Metastases were noted occasionally (Vorwald *et al.*, 1955) [The Working Group noted that the strain, the numbers of rats treated, the use of controls and the atmospheric concentrations of beryllium sulphate used were unspecified].

A group of 52 albino Sherman and Wistar rats were exposed to an aqueous aerosol of *beryllium sulphate tetrahydrate* by inhalation, to give a concentration of 1 $\mu g/ft^3$ Be (35.7 $\mu g/m^3$), for 8 hrs/day on 5½ days/week for 6 months. The rats were maintained thereafter without treatment for periods up to 18 months. Lung tumours (76), often multiple, and including carcinomas, were found in treated rats and none in 139 control rats (Schepers *et al.*, 1957).

Groups of 75 male and 75 female Sprague-Dawley CD rats were exposed by continuous inhalation of an aqueous aerosol of *beryllium sulphate tetrahydrate,* to give a concentration of 34 $\mu g/m^3$ Be, for periods up to 56 weeks. Subgroups of animals were killed each month up to that time and at weekly intervals from 72-77 weeks after start of exposure. Metaplastic changes in alveolar epithelium were seen at 20-32 weeks; from 36 weeks, alveolar adenocarcinomas were found and were seen in all 43 rats killed 52 weeks after the start of exposure. No lung tumours were found in 150 unexposed controls (Reeves *et al.*, 1967).

Albino (Charles River CD and Greenacres Controlled Flora) male rats were exposed by chronic inhalation of *beryl ore* (median particle diameter, 0.64 μm) or *bertrandite ore* (median particle diameter, 0.27 μm) as 15 mg/m^3 dust for 6 hrs/day on 5 days/week; the bertrandite chamber contained 210 $\mu g/m^3$ Be and the beryl chamber, 620 $\mu g/m^3$ Be. By 17 months, 18/19 rats exposed to beryl ore dust had developed pulmonary tumours, including 9 adenocarcinomas. Most of the tumours were of microscopic dimensions, but 4 were identified by gross examination at necropsy. No metastases were found. Lung changes, including granulomatous lesions, but no tumours were seen in rats exposed to bertrandite ore dust (Wagner *et al.*, 1969).

Beryllium chloride was administered by intratracheal instillation to 3 groups of 30 albino random-bred rats of both sexes. No tumours were observed in the group that received 5 mg beryllium chloride suspended in 0.3 ml polyglucine 3 times at 2-week intervals. However, one adeno- and one squamous-cell bronchogenic carcinoma were found within 15½ months in 2/16 animals that received 3 mg beryllium chloride in polyglucine with 3 mg India-ink powder at the same schedule; and one squamous-cell bronchogenic carcinoma was found within 15 months in 1/14 animals of the group that received 3 mg beryllium chloride plus 3 mg 7, 12-dimethylbenz[a]anthracene plus 3 mg India-ink powder in polyglucine at the same schedule. No lung tumours were found in untreated control rats (Griciute, 1971).

In a study reported as an abstract, intratracheal administration of *beryl ore, beryllium oxide, beryllium hydroxide, beryllium metal* or *beryllium-aluminium alloy* induced pulmonary tumours in rats (Groth *et al.*, 1972) [The Working Group noted that insufficient details were given to permit evaluation of these observations.

Four groups of 20 male, white, random-bred rats were exposed to *beryllium fluoride* at mean concentrations of 0.4 mg/m^3 Be or 0.04 mg/m^3 Be and to *beryllium chloride* at mean concentrations of 0.2 mg/m^3 Be or 0.02 mg m^3 Be. Animals were exposed for 1 hr on 5 days /week for 4 months; the maximal length of observation was 22 months after the beginning of treatment. The first neoplasms were observed after 16 months; lung tumours (1 adenoma, 2 squamous-cell carcinomas and 5 adenocarcinomas) developed in 8/14 animals that received 0.4 mg/m^3 Be as beryllium fluoride or 0.2 mg/m^3 Be as beryllium chloride. Liver metastases were found in 2 of the rats with pulmonary adenocarcinomas. Five lung tumours (2 adenomas and 3 adenocarcinomas) developed in 18 animals that received 0.04 mg/m^3 as beryllium fluoride or 0.02 mg/m^3 Be as beryllium chloride. No tumours were observed in 20 control rats (Litvinov *et al.*, 1975) [The Working Group noted that certain inadequacies in the reporting of the data made it impossible to distinguish the various treated groups].

Submicron-sized, high-fired *beryllium oxide* particles were administered as dry dust to 184 female Wistar rats by single exposures *via* the nose only for periods ranging from 0.5-3 hrs. The initial alveolar depositions of beryllium ranged from 1-91 µg/rat; the biological half-life of beryllium in the lung was 325 days. Within 20 months, 1 rat which had received the highest level of beryllium exposure had developed a lung tumour (an adenocarcinoma). No lung tumours developed in 128 unexposed rats during the 2-year observation period (Sanders *et al.*, 1978).

Groups of 35 female Wistar rats, 3 months old, received single intratracheal instillations of saline suspensions of 0.5 or 2.5 mg/rat *beryllium metal* (100% Be), *passivated beryllium metal* (99% Be, containing 0.26% chromium), *beryllium-aluminium alloy* (62% Be), *beryllium-copper alloy* (4% Be), *beryllium-nickel alloy* (2.2% Be) or *beryllium-copper-cobalt alloy* (2.4% Be). The size of the various particles varied from 1-2 µm. Forty controls were injected with saline alone. The rats were sacrificed at various intervals from 1-18 months. No lung tumours were found in 39 controls, nor in 30 or 33 receiving the beryllium-copper-cobalt alloy, nor in 27 or 28 receiving the beryllium-nickel alloy, nor in 24 or 28 receiving the beryllium-copper alloy, at the two dose levels, respectively. In rats treated with beryllium metal, lung tumours were observed in 9/16 at the higher dose and in 2/21 at the lower dose. Lung tumours were also observed in rats treated with the passivated metal (9/26 at the higher dose and 7/20 at the lower dose) and in rats treated with the beryllium-aluminium alloy (4/24 at the higher dose and 1/21 at the lower dose) (Groth *et al.*, 1980).

A group of 35 female Wistar rats received single intratracheal instillations of 50 µg *beryllium hydroxide* in water suspension, followed 10 months later by a second instillation of 25 µg. Of 25 rats sacrificed at 19 months, 6 had adenomas of the lung and 7 had adeno-carcinomas of the lung; bronchiolar alveolar-cell tumours were seen in all 25 animals

(Groth *et al.*, 1980) [The Working Group noted the unusual schedule of dose and treatment, resulting in a high incidence of tumours, and considered that this observation would be strengthened by confirmatory studies].

It was reported in an abstract that rats (sex and strain unspecified) were given intra-tracheal administrations of *beryllium oxide*, produced by calcining beryllium hydroxide for 10 hrs at 500°C (dose unspecified); lung tumours developed after 7-8 months. In contrast, the lungs of rats treated with beryllium oxide produced by calcining beryllium hydroxide for 10 hrs at 1600°C (dose unspecified) showed minimal pathological changes (Spencer *et al.*, 1965).

Hamster: Bronchial alveolar hyperplasia, but no neoplasms, was seen in 2 groups of 65 male Syrian golden hamsters following inhalation of *beryl* or *bertrandite ore* dusts at 15 mg/m^3 for 6 hrs/day on 5 days/week for up to 17 months (Wagner *et al.*, 1969).

Rabbit: A group of 19 albino rabbits were exposed to aqueous aerosols of *beryllium oxide* by inhalation (particle diameter, 0.28 µm) at doses of 1, 6 or 30 mg/m^3 Be for 5 hrs/day on 5 days/week for 9-13 months. One osteosarcoma, located in the inferior ramus of the left pubis, developed in a rabbit exposed 255 times during 11 months to 6 mg/m^3 Be (Dutra *et al.*, 1951).

Monkey: Two groups of 14-16 male squirrel monkeys (*Saimiri sciurea*) were exposed by inhalation of *beryl ore* (median particle diameter, 0.64 µm) or *bertrandite ore* (median parti-cle diameter, 0.27 µm) as 15 mg/m^3 dust for 6 hrs/day on 5 days/week for up to 23 months, when all animals were killed. No preneoplastic or neoplastic lesions were seen in the lungs (Wagner *et al.*, 1969)   [The Working Group noted the short duration of observation].

A group of 10 rhesus monkeys *(Macaca mulatta)* were exposed intermittently by inhala-tion of *beryllium sulphate* aerosol to give a concentration of 39 µg/m^3 Be. Over approxi-mately 10 years of observation, 2 monkeys developed pulmonary anaplastic carcinomas (Vorwald, 1967; Vorwald *et al.*, 1966). In a later publication, Vorwald (1968) reported pul-monary anaplastic carcinomas in 8/11 animals.

(c)   Intravenous administration

Mouse: In a study reported as an abstract, malignant bone tumours were seen in mice that had received 20-22 twice-weekly i.v. injections of *zinc beryllium silicate* (total dose, 0.26 mg Be/mouse) but not in those that had received similar injections of *beryllium oxide* (total dose, 1.54 mg Be/mouse) or zinc silicate (Cloudman *et al.*, 1949) [The Working Group noted that the mouse strain, number of mice and incidence of tumours were unspecified].

Rabbit: In a study reported as an abstract, i.v. injections of *zinc beryllium silicate* or *beryllium oxide* suspended in an unspecified vehicle induced osteosarcomas in rabbits. The compounds were administered into ear veins as suspensions of particles with diameters ⩽ 3 µm. Osteosarcomas developed in all of 7 rabbits that survived 7 or more months after treatment with zinc beryllium silicate (20 doses totalling 1 g/rabbit, over a 6-week period); visceral metastases were present in 4 of the 7. One sarcoma was seen in a rabbit killed one year after injection of beryllium oxide. Administration of 65 other minerals, including zinc silicate, zinc oxide and silicic acid, in the same way to rabbits failed to produce tumours (Gardner & Heslington, 1946).

Osteosarcomas were produced in rabbits by i.v. administration of *zinc beryllium silicate* (20-22 twice-weekly injections; total dose, 17 mg Be/rabbit) but not by similar i.v. administration of *beryllium oxide* (390 mg/rabbit) or zinc silicate (Cloudman *et al.*, 1949) [The Working Group noted that the numbers of rabbits in the experimental groups, the injection vehicle and the incidence of osteosarcomas in rabbits that received zinc beryllium silicate were not specified].

Barnes (1950), Barnes *et al.* (1950) and Sissons (1950) found osteosarcomas in 6/17 rabbits that survived repeated i.v. injections of an aqueous suspension of *zinc beryllium silicate* (total dose, 1-2.1 g/rabbit) and in 1 of 11 survivors given an aqueous suspension of *beryllium silicate* (total dose, 1-1.2 g/rabbit). Tumours arose between 39 and 83 weeks after the end of treatment. Metastases were common. No tumours were seen in 8 rabbits that survived 14-120 weeks after i.v. injection of an aqueous suspension of zinc silicate (average total dose, 1.2 g/rabbit). Two of 24 rabbits that received i.v. injections of an aqueous suspension of *beryllium metal* (total dose, 40 mg/rabbit) developed osteosarcomas (Barnes *et al.*, 1950).

Osteosarcomas were observed in 6/6 rabbits within 11-24 months after i.v. administration of *zinc beryllium silicate* as a 1% suspension in saline (0.2-1 g/rabbit in divided doses); 1 osteosarcoma was observed 16 months after similar administration of *beryllium oxide* to 9 rabbits. No tumours arose in 5 rabbits given i.v. injections of *beryllium phosphate* (0.1% suspension in saline) (Hoagland *et al.*, 1950). Nash (1950) independently reported the results of some of the same experiments described by Hoagland *et al.* (1950).

Osteosarcomas were observed in 4/6 rabbits treated with a 1% isotonic saline suspension of *beryllium oxide* (360-700 mg Be/rabbit in 20-26 i.v. injections, 3 times/week) and in 2/3 rabbits treated with an isotonic saline suspension of *zinc beryllium silicate* (64-90 mg Be/rabbit in 17-25 i.v. injections, 3 times/week) (Dutra & Largent, 1950).

Osteosarcomas were found in 2/4 rabbits within 18 months after a single i.v. injection of 1 g/rabbit *beryllium phosphate*. No tumours were found in 3 rabbits that received 1 g *beryllium oxide* by i.v. injection. When mixtures of these beryllium compounds with zinc oxide, manganese oxide and/or silicon oxide were injected, osteosarcomas developed in 9/31 rabbits (Araki *et al.*, 1954).

Osteosarcomas were induced in 3/20 rabbits 15-18 months after single i.v. injections of *beryllium oxide* (total dose, 1 g/rabbit as a 1% suspension in saline) (Komitowski, 1968).

Osteogenic sarcomas (often multiple) were observed in 5/10 male rabbits 9-11 months after they received 20 i.v. injections of 5 ml of a 1% suspension of *zinc beryllium silicate* twice weekly for 10 weeks (total dose, 1 g). No controls were used (Janes *et al.*, 1954) [The Working Group noted that the same authors (Janes *et al.*, 1975) were later unable to obtain the same results using different batches of zinc beryllium silicate. They advanced the hypothesis that this might be due to the different batches used].

Fodor (1977), Higgins *et al.* (1964), Kelly *et al.* (1961) and Peterson *et al.* (1964) have also induced osteosarcomas in rabbits by i.v. injections of *zinc beryllium silicate* or *beryllium oxide*.

(d) Other experimental systems

Intrabronchial and/or bronchomural injections: A group of 20 young rhesus *monkeys* were given single intrabronchial and/or bronchomural injections of a 5% suspension of *beryllium oxide* in isotonic saline. During approximately 10 years' observation, 3/20 monkeys developed pulmonary anaplastic carcinomas (Vorwald, 1967; Vorwald *et al.*, 1966) [The results presented above are those retabulated by Reeves (1978b), one of the authors of the original paper by Vorwald *et al.* (1966)].

Intramedullary or subperiosteal administration: A group of 30 Wistar *rats* received a single injection into the medullary canal of the tibia of 33 mg/rat *zinc beryllium silicate* suspended in 0.5 ml gelatin. No sarcomas deveoped subsequently at the injection site (Mazabraud, 1975) [The Working Group noted that the period of observation was not specified].

A high incidence of osteosarcoma was reported in *rabbits* after 1-43 injections of 20 mg *beryllium oxide* into the right femur marrow. The injections were given twice weekly in isotonic saline. Of 55 treated rabbits, one developed a chondroma, 3 developed osteomas, 15 developed osteosarcomas, 2 developed chondrosarcomas and 7 developed osteochondrosarcomas. The average time between the last injection and the appearance of a tumour was 85 days. The period of observation was 1-2 years (Yamaguchi, 1963).

Osteosarcomas were observed in 8/40 rabbits that received implants in the bone-marrow cavity of gelatin pellets containing 25 mg *beryllium metal* and i.v. injections of 1%

beryllium metal suspended in saline. No controls were used (Komitowski, 1971) [It is not clear from the text whether the same animals received both treatments or not].

Osteosarcomas were induced in *rabbits* of mixed breeds and both sexes following a single injection of 20 mg/rabbit *zinc beryllium silicate* suspended in 0.5 ml water into the medullary cavity of the right tibia. Local osteosarcomas developed in 4/12 animals within 12-15 months after the injection; all 4 tumours metastasized to the lungs. No tumours arose at the site of intramedullary injection of 20 mg zinc oxide into the opposite tibias of the same rabbits (Tapp, 1966).

Osteosarcomas were also induced following subperiosteal injections of 10 mg *zinc beryllium silicate, beryllium silicate* or *beryllium oxide* to 3 groups of 6 *rabbits*. Eight rabbits were killed between 10 and 18 months when X-ray photographs or physical examination suggested that a tumour might have developed. Osteosarcomas arose at the upper end of the right tibia near the site of the injection, 10-25 months after the operation, in 2 rabbits that received beryllium oxide, in 1 rabbit that received beryllium silicate, and in 1 rabbit that received zinc beryllium silicate (Tapp, 1969a,b).

An unspecified quantity of *beryllium oxide* powder in gelatin suspension was injected into the medullary cavity of rabbits. Osteosarcomas developed in 5/20 animals within 24 months; all of the tumours metastasized to the lungs (Komitowski, 1974).

Osteosarcomas developed in 30/173 *rabbits* administered 0.5 ml of a 2% saline suspension of *beryllium carbonate* by intramedullary injection once weekly for a total of 30 weeks, but in 0/10 rabbits administered the same dosage of *beryllium acetate* (Matsuura, 1974).

Zinc beryllium silicate was administered to 65 *rabbits* as a single injection into a femoral or tibial epiphysis, as 33 mg Be in 0.5 ml gelatin. Osteosarcomas subsequently developed at the injection site in 45 rabbits (Mazabraud, 1975).

3.2 Other relevant biological data

Beryllium oxide and other beryllium compounds are produced in forms the physical and chemical characteristics of which depend on the details of the process involved. There is also evidence that the biological activity of the various forms is similarly affected (and may decay with time). It should be noted, however, that in most studies the exact chemical and physical properties of the substances investigated are unspecified.

Toxic effects

For beryllium fluoride, the acute oral LD_{50} in mice and rats is about 100 mg/kg bw; the s.c. LD_{50} in mice is 20 mg/kg bw; the i.v. LD_{50} in mice is 1.8 mg/kg bw (Luckey & Venugopal, 1977); and the i.p. LD_{50} in hamsters is 20 mg/kg bw (Vacher *et al.*, 1973). The i.v. LD_{50} of beryllium hydroxide in rats is 3.8 mg/kg bw. For beryllium chloride, the i.m. LD_{50} in mice is 12 mg/kg bw; the oral LD_{50} in rats is 86 mg/kg bw; and the i.p. LD_{50} is 4.4 mg/kg bw in rats and 50 mg/kg bw in guinea-pigs. For beryllium sulphate, the oral LD_{50} in rats and mice is 80 mg/kg bw; the s.c. LD_{50} in rats and mice is 1.5 mg/kg bw; the i.p. LD_{50} in rats is 18 mg/kg bw; the i.v. LD_{50} is 7.2 mg/kg bw in rats and 0.6 mg/kg bw in monkeys; and the s.c. LD_{50} in rabbits is 1.5 mg/kg bw. For beryllium phosphate, in rats, the oral LD_{50} is 82 mg/kg bw and the i.v. LD_{50} is 4.2 mg/kg bw (Luckey & Venugopal, 1977); and for mice the i.v. LD_{50} is 1.4 mg/kg bw (Vacher *et al.* 1973). For beryllium acetate, the i.p. LD_{50} in rats is 317 mg/kg bw. For beryllium carbonate, the i.p. LD_{50} in guinea-pigs is 50 mg/kg bw (Luckey & Venugopal, 1977). The i.v. LD_{50} of beryllium sulphate tetrahydrate in mice is 265 μg/kg bw (as Be) (Vacher *et al*, 1973).

It was reported in an abstract that when a washed suspension of finely divided beryllium metal in water was injected intravenously into young rabbits, to give a dose of 40 mg/animal Be, 9/24 died within 7 days and 10 more during the next month with acute liver necrosis. Of the remaining 5 rabbits, 2 died from pulmonary infections, and 2 developed characteristic bone sarcomas (Barnes, 1950).

Skilleter & Price (1978) studied the uptake of beryllium in parenchymal and non-parenchymal liver cells of rats after i.v. injection of 12.5-250 μmol/kg bw particulate beryllium phosphate or of 12.5-85 μmol/kg bw beryllium sulphate. Beryllium phosphate was removed from the blood predominantly by the non-parenchymal (sinusoidal) cells and later distributed partly to parenchymal cells and partly to the spleen. After administration of beryllium sulphate (which forms beryllium phosphate in plasma), a greater proportion of beryllium is taken up by parenchymal cells. The differences in behaviour were suggested by the authors to be related to the smaller size of the beryllium phosphate particles formed in plasma.

Vacher *et al.* (1973) observed that beryllium phosphate blocked the functioning of the reticuloendothelial system of mice after i.v. injection of 12 μg/kg bw (as Be) and that beryllium sulphate did so in a dose of 75 μg/kg bw (as Be).

Fodor (1977), studying the histogenesis of beryllium oxide-induced osteosarcomas in rabbits, found that injected insoluble beryllium particles were accumulated primarily in reticuloendothelial cells of the bone marrow. He suggested that beryllium oxide exerts a prolonged local action during slow dissolution of beryllium particles in the bone marrow.

Groups of 4 female *Macaca mulatta* monkeys were exposed to aerosol concentrations of various beryllium salts: (i) 27 $\mu g/ft^3$ (964 $\mu g/m^3$) beryllium fluoride; (ii) 66 $\mu g/ft^3$ (2.357 mg/m^3) beryllium sulphate; (iii) 66 $\mu g/ft^3$ (2.357 mg/m^3) beryllium phosphate; (iv) 373 $\mu g/ft^3$ (13.3 mg/m^3) beryllium phosphate; and (v) 2750 $\mu g/ft^3$ (98.2 mg/m^3) beryllium phosphate for 6 hrs per day over 7-30 days, followed by an observation period of 7-270 days in air. All animals of group (v) died of pneumonitis within 20 days and all those of group (iv) within 92 days except for one which died of peritonitis; 1 animal of each of groups (iii) and (ii) and 2 of group (i) died of pneumonitis. Beryllium fluoride and the higher concentrations of beryllium phosphate caused severe and universal pulmonary reactions (including desquamation, hyperplasia of bronchial epithelium and oedema of the mucosa) and evoked changes in the liver (hepatocyte degeneration, sinusoid distension), kidneys (glomerular reaction and tubular degeneration), adrenals, pancreas, thyroid and spleen. Some of these damages were reversible, and others appeared to be progressive. The authors stressed the similarity between the lesions seen in the monkeys and those reported in patients who died from acute and subacute berylliotic pneumonitis (Schepers, 1964).

Granulomatous pulmonary lesions, resembling to some extent the 'berylliosis' seen in humans, has been produced after exposure of guinea-pigs (Policard, 1950) or rats (Lloyd Davies & Harding, 1950) to beryllium oxide. Effects on the skeleton, in the form of beryllium rickets, were reported by Guyatt *et al.* (1933) in rats fed beryllium carbonate. Cloudman *et al.* (1949) observed osteosclerosis in rabbits and mice injected intravenously with beryllium oxide or zinc beryllium silicate. Necrotic liver lesions were reported in rats and rabbits by Aldridge *et al.* (1950) following single i.v. injections of beryllium sulphate.

Dutra (1951) observed that least-calcined beryllium oxide was more effective than other forms in producing granulomas of the skin in pigs after implantation.

No data on the prenatal toxicity of beryllium or beryllium compounds were available.

Absorption, distribution and excretion

Absorption *via* inhalation was studied in rats exposed to beryllium sulphate tetrahydrate. Pulmonary beryllium concentrations reached a plateau related to the inhalation concentration after approximately 36 weeks: after 12 weeks, 2.5 μg Be were present in whole lung; at 20 weeks, 6 μg Be; at 28 weeks, 8 μg Be; and at 36 weeks, 12 μg Be (Reeves, 1979). Clearance from the lungs was multiphasic: after discontinuation of the exposure, the beryllium concentration in the lung decreased to half in about 2 weeks; later, the clearance rate decreased, and a small proportion of the initial concentration remained in the lungs for many months (Reeves & Vorwald, 1967).

Radioactive [7]Be-beryllium chloride when administered in a carrier (unspecified) by intratracheal injection to rats showed a pulmonary half-life of 20 days; when it was administered without a carrier, its half-life was 24 hrs (Kuznetsov et al., 1974). Further studies by the same group (Bugryshev et al., 1976) demonstrated that the highest concentrations of beryllium were found in the skeleton (42-55%), with 6-15% in liver, 4-15% in spleen and none detectable in lung 15 min after i.v., i.m. or i.p. injection of carrier-free [7]Be-beryllium chloride. The highest concentration 15 min after intratracheal administration was found in the lungs (72%), with 36% in the skeleton; after 94 days, most of the radioactivity was still present in the lungs (20%).

Organ distribution of beryllium appears to be dose-dependent: 2.5 hrs after their i.v. injection to rats, small doses (<50 μg/kg bw Be) were taken up preferentially in the skeleton, and higher doses (up to 500 μg/kg bw Be) preferentially in the liver. Beryllium was later mobilized from the liver and transfered to the skeleton (Reeves, 1979).

When beryllium sulphate was injected intratracheally to rats, 70% of the retained dose remained in the lung at 16 days. About half the total amount eliminated was *via* the faeces. After 16 days, lung retention dropped sharply and the particulates moved into the hilar and peritracheal nodes and trunks. Deposition in liver, spleen and, particularly, the skeleton was concluded to involve the blood stream (Van Cleave & Kaylor, 1955).

According to an abstract, the distribution of beryllium oxide in the body varies with the method of its preparation. After intratracheal instillation of beryllium oxide prepared by calcining α-beryllium hydroxide for 10 hrs at 500°C, it was found in high concentrations in the liver, kidneys and bones of rats; whereas an oxide prepared by calcining α-beryllium hydroxide for 10 hrs at 1600°C remained mainly in the lungs (Spencer et al., 1965) [No data on doses were given].

Beryllium is excreted partly in urine. Because of colloidal binding in plasma, beryllium does not cross the glomerular membrane, and it is excreted *via* the tubules. The proportion of intratracheally injected beryllium excreted in urine was 20-69% (Reeves, 1979; Van Cleave & Kaylor, 1955).

Faecal and urinary contents of beryllium and concentrations in various organs of rats were studied after ingestion of beryllium sulphate tetrahydrate as 0.16 and 1.66 mg/l Be in drinking-water. Absorption was approximately 20%, since 60-90% of the ingested beryllium sulphate passed unabsorbed into the faeces. Only 1% of the administered Be was found in the urine (Reeves, 1965). After absorption, beryllium is transported mainly in the form of a colloidal phosphate, probably adsorbed on plasma α-globulin (Feldman et al., 1953; Reeves & Vorwald, 1961; Vacher & Stoner, 1968).

Placental passage of various γ-emitting isotopes as saline solutions of 1 μCi/ml was studied in rats 30 min to 2 hrs after i.v. injection on the 14th, 17th and 20th day of gestation. [7]Be was included in these studies, and its placental transfer was compared with that of [47]Ca. Under these experimental conditions, the incorporation of [47]Ca into the foetus was found to increase as gestation advanced: 0.06 % dose/g on day 14, 0.13 % dose/g on day 17, and 0.23 % dose/g on day 20 of gestation. The placenta contained 0.12% dose/g on day 14 and 0.11 % dose/g at day 20. Although very similar data were obtained for placental tissue after the ingestion of [7]Be (0.14 on day 14 and 0.16 on day 20), the content of the foetus was only 0.006 % dose/g on the 14th day of gestation and 0.017 % dose/g on the 20th day. When compared with [47]Ca, the relative uptake of [7]Be was only 0.16 ± 0.02 on day 14 and 0.07 ± 0.04 on day 20 of gestation. The low rate of placental transfer of [7]Be in these studies was similar to that found with [115]mCd or [203]Hg (Schulert et al., 1969).

Effects on intermediary metabolism

Ionic beryllium has been shown to inhibit a number of enzymes *in vitro*, e.g., various phosphatases, phosphoglucomutase, hexokinase, deoxythymidine kinase, lactate dehydrogenase and amylase (review by Reeves, 1979).

In a series of studies on the livers of partially hepatectomized rats, beryllium sulphate tetrahydrate, injected intravenously at 30 μmol/kg bw had a marked affinity for rat liver nuclei and inhibited DNA synthesis, but had little effect on RNA or protein biosynthesis (Marcotte & Witschi, 1972; Witschi, 1968, 1970).

Mutagenicity and other short-term tests

Changes in various physico-chemical properties of purified DNA treated with beryllium suggest an interaction of beryllium with DNA (Kubinski et al., 1977; Truhaut et al., 1968).

Beryllium chloride (1-10 mM) increased the misincorporation of nucleoside triphosphates during polymerization of poly-d(A-T) by *Micrococcus luteus* DNA polymerase, and strongly inhibited the 3 → 5 exonuclease activity of this enzyme (Luke et al., 1975). In a similar system, beryllium chloride reduced the fidelity of DNA synthesis in an *in vitro* assay containing avian myeloblastosis virus DNA polymerase, a synthetic prime-template, and complementary and noncomplementary nucleotide triphosphates. This effect was dose-related (2-10 mM) and was ascribed to the non-covalent binding of ionic divalent beryllium to the DNA polymerase (Sirover & Loeb, 1976).

Beryllium sulphate was inactive in the following short-term tests: (i) assays for point mutations in *Salmonella typhimurium* strains TA1535, TA1536, TA1537, TA1538, TA98 and TA100 (Rosenkranz & Poirier, 1979; Simmon, 1979a); (ii) *Escherichia coli* pol[+]/pol[-] assay for DNA-modifying effects (Rosenkranz & Poirier, 1979); *Saccharomyces cerevisiae*

D3 assay for mitotic recombination (Simmon, 1979b); and (iii) i.p. host-mediated assay, using adult male Swiss-Webster mice and *S. typhimurium* strains TA1530, TA1535 and TA1538 and *S. cerevisiae* D3 (Simmon *et al.*, 1979).

Beryllium sulphate was positive in the *Bacillus subtilis rec* assay at 10 mM (Kada *et al.*, 1980). No effect was seen in a *rec* assay (spot test) using 50 mM beryllium chloride (Nishioka, 1975).

Beryllium chloride (0.5-10 mM) caused chromosome aberrations (stickiness, chromatid gaps and breaks, and fragments) and mitotic delay in cultured peripheral lymphocytes and primary kidney cells of the domestic pig (Talluri & Guiggiani, 1967). No chromosome aberrations were noted with 0.01 and 1 μM beryllium sulphate in human diploid fibroblasts and human leucocytes *in vitro* (Paton & Allison, 1972).

Beryllium sulphate (2.5 and 5 μg/ml) induced morphological transformation of Syrian hamster secondary embryo cells (DiPaolo & Casto, 1979) and (at 0.56 mM) enhanced the morphological transformation of these cells by simian adenovirus SA7 (Casto *et al.*, 1979) [In neither of these studies were transformed cells injected into suitable hosts to verify the occurrence of malignant transformation].

(b) Humans

Acute toxicity

Beryllium dermatitis of exposed skin and granulomatous ulcerations of the skin at sites where insoluble beryllium compounds were embedded, and conjunctivitis, have been described (Curtis, 1951; Nishimura, 1966; Van Ordstrand *et al.*, 1945).

Acute effects on the respiratory system, with signs and symptoms of rhinitis, pharyngitis, tracheobronchitis and pneumonitis, have been observed following inhalation of high concentrations of soluble beryllium compounds, including the fluoride. The estimated range of concentrations required to produce such effects is reported to be 30 mg/m^3 for the high-fired oxide, 1-3 mg/m^3 for the low-fired oxide and 0.1-0.5 mg/m^3 for beryllium sulphate. Although fatalities have occurred, recovery usually takes place weeks or months after acute berylliosis (review by Reeves, 1979; Van Orstrand *et al.*, 1943).

Saxén & Pasila (1978) described a recent case of acute beryllium disease following intense exposure to broken fluorescent light tubes, probably containing zinc beryllium silicate, in spite of the fact that use of this material was discontinued many years ago. The first symptoms were seen 3 months after exposure and granulomas another 3 months afterwards.

Chronic toxicity

A chronic pulmonary condition known as 'berylliosis', which is frequently fatal, was first described by Hardy & Tabershaw (1946). Pulmonary X-rays demonstrated a miliary mottling, and interstitial granulomatosis was diagnosed upon histopathological examination. The condition is considered to be caused by beryllium compounds of low solubility, and particularly the low-fired oxide. There is no established dose-response relationship; very slightly exposed individuals, such as 'neighbourhood cases', sometimes show severe clinical forms of the disease (DeNardi *et al.*, 1949, 1952; Hardy & Tepper, 1959; Reeves, 1979; Sterner & Eisenbud, 1951). The following studies illustrate the generally recognized, wide individual variation in sensitivity regarding development of berylliosis; one explanation that has been proposed for this variation is that the disease involves an immune reaction.

Jones William (1977) reviewed the pathology and diagnosis of beryllium disease and emphasized the usefulness of *in vitro* methods of hypersensitivity detection (macrophage migration inhibition by sensitized thymic lymphocytes) in its diagnosis and prevention. Ermakova & Vasilieva (1978) observed increased rosette-formation in patients with berylliosis compared with persons not exposed to beryllium. Constantinidis (1978) described a case of beryllium disease and reviewed the literature on both acute and chronic beryllium disease. Lieben *et al.* (1964) reported 2 cases of berylliosis in two subjects exposed to beryllium-copper alloys for 20 and 27 years at concentrations probably between 0.3-12 $\mu g/m^3$ Be and a third case of a subject who had been exposed for 2 years to concentrations of less than 1 $\mu g/m^3$. Cianciara & Swiatkowski (1978) found radiological changes and changes in respiratory volumes over 4-12 months in workers exposed for about 24 months to beryllium in concentrations less than the MAC value (0.001 mg/m^3).

Beryllium is stored in the body over long periods of time: 22 and 23 years after last employment exposure to beryllium, analysis of lung tissue showed 'elevated beryllium' in 2 workers who died of lung cancer (Mancuso, 1979a).

3.3 Case reports and epidemiological studies

(a) Case reports

Among the nineteen malignant neoplasms reported to the Beryllium Case Registry as the cause of death in beryllium workers (Infante *et al.*, 1980), one was a bone sarcoma (Hardy, 1976).

(b) Epidemiological studies

Acute and chronic pulmonary disease due to exposure to beryllium has been described for over 30 years. Although 'neighbourhood' cases have occurred, most of the affected individuals worked in industries processing or using beryllium. In the US, a Beryllium Case Registry was established in 1051 which has continued to acquire new cases of beryllium poisoning submitted on a voluntary basis.

Four epidemiological studies were considered by an earlier Working Group (IARC, 1972) to be inadequate to evaluate the carcinogenic effects of beryllium; a brief review of these follows. Hardy *et al*. (1967), in their review of the US Beryllium Case Registry data for the period 1952-1966, did not primarily address the question of carcinogenesis. However, in reviewing the methods and usefulness of the Registry, they noted that during the period in question there was no evidence that suggested that beryllium was carcinogenic. Stoeckle *et al*. (1969) reviewed 60 selected cases of chronic beryllium disease (of both occupational and non-occupational origin) which had been followed for up to 25 years. There were 17 deaths, none of which were reported as being due to cancer. Mancuso & El-Attar (1969) studied the incidence of cancer in workers employed at 2 separate companies manufacturing beryllium products. The study was inconclusive, and the authors stated that 'at present, the carcinogenic challenge, in terms of quality and/or quantity of beryllium exposure is unknown'. Mancuso (1970) extended his review of the same 2 cohorts of workers. He noted that the highest death rate from lung cancer occurred among those employees with the shortest duration of employment and that prior occurrence of 'chemical respiratory illness' seemed to be linked with a higher risk of subsequent development of lung cancer [The Working Group noted that short exposure to beryllium and chemical respiratory illness may be closely correlated].

Since the last report (IARC, 1972), 3 further epidemiological studies have been reported. The reports on the 2 cohorts studied by Mancuso (1970) and Mancuso & El-Attar (1969) have been updated (Mancuso, 1980a,b), and one of the 2 cohorts has been studied separately by Wagoner *et al*. (1980). Data from the Beryllium Case Registry (which collects clinical cases of beryllium disease from a wider variety of sources than the 2 beryllium plants) has been reanalysed by Infante *et al*. (1980). These 4 studies are summarized in Table 7.

Wagoner *et al*. (1980) conducted a follow-up study of a cohort of 3055 white males identified through employment records who were working sometime during the period 1 January 1942 - 30 September 1968. Work at the plant, situated in Pennsylvania, was in the extraction, processing and fabrication of beryllium. The vital status of all but 79 (3%) of the cohort was established, and death certificates were obtained for all but 12 deceased workers (0.4%). Using a modified life-table technique, a comparison was made between observed numbers of deaths and those expected in the general white male population of the US. For the period 1968-1975, expected deaths were calculated by applying US mortality rates for the years 1965-1967. No data on smoking prior to 1967 were available (as is common to

TABLE 7

Four recent epidemiological studies on beryllium exposure

Reference/Description	Result	No. of people	Duration
Wagoner *et al.* (1980) Retrospective cohort study; beryllium refining; in Pennsylvania; compared with US white males	Lung cancer: 47 observed/34.29 expected; SMR 137; P < 0.05 (20 observed/10.79 expected; SMR 185; P < 0.01 for lung cancer 25 years or more after onset of beryllium exposure) irrespective of duration of exposure	3055 white males	Employment 1942-1948 Follow-up 1968-1975
Mancuso (1980a) Cohort study; beryllium production; in Pennsylvania (cf Wagoner) and Ohio; compared with US white polulation	**Ohio:** lung cancer: 25 observed/12.52 expected; SMR 199; P < 0.01 **Pennsylvania:** lung cancer: 40 observed/29.11 expected; SMR 137	1222 white males 2044 white males	Employment 1942-1948 Follow-up: Ohio - 1974; Pennsylvania - 1975
Mancuso (1980b) Cohort study; beryllium production; in Pennsylvania and Ohio; compared with viscose rayon workers	Lung cancer: 80 observed/57.06 expected; SMR 140; P < 0.01	3685 white males	Employment 1937-1948 Follow-up - 1976
Infante *et al.* (1980) Beryllium Case Registry; compared with US white males	Lung cancer: 7 observed/3.3 expected; SMR 212 acute beryllium respiratory disease group: 6 observed/1.91 expected; SMR 314; P < 0.05 chronic beryllium respiratory disease group: 1 observed/1.38 expected	421 white males 223 198	Follow-up 1952-1975

most follow-up studies with a starting point some time in the past). The authors' analysis indicated a statistically significant excess of deaths from cancers of the trachea, bronchus and lung (ICD 162 and 163, referred to as 'lung cancer'), with 47 deaths observed and 34.29 expected ($P < 0.05$, Poisson: one-tailed test). Other statistically significant excesses were seen for non-neoplastic respiratory disease (excluding pneumonia and influenza) and heart disease. The excess of lung cancer deaths was most marked in workers who started employment in 1942-1949 and who had had a median duration of employment of 3.9 months. This excess risk of lung cancer occurred in the same group in which there was an excess of non-neoplastic respiratory disease. No dose-response relationship (as measured by duration of exposure) was noted for either disease.

Mancuso (1980a) conducted a study of lung cancer mortality among employees in the same plant examined by Wagoner et al.; but, in addition, he analysed data from a second beryllium facility in Ohio. Social Security Administration records of employee payroll listings were used. The cohorts consisted of white males employed sometime during the period 1 January 1942 - 31 December 1948. The analysis of mortality was done using the same programme as for the Wagoner et al. study. There appears to be a two-fold excess of lung cancer at the Ohio facility (25 deaths observed, 12.52 deaths expected; $P < 0.01$). This excess occurred primarily among workers with a long latent period (15 years or more) and a short duration of employment (less than 5 years).

In order to compare lung cancer mortality among beryllium-exposed workers with that of another industrial population, Mancuso (1980b) also studied viscose rayon employees. An excess of lung cancer was again noted when both beryllium cohorts were compared with the viscose rayon workers (80 deaths observed, 57.06 expected; $P < 0.01$). No dose-response relationship (as measured by duration of exposure) was noted.

A re-evaluation of the mortality patterns in the Beryllium Case Registry was undertaken by Infante et al., (1980). They studied a cohort of white males who were alive at the time of registration between 1952 and 1975. Vital status was ascertained for all but 64 of the 421 cohort members; death certificates were obtained for 124 of 139 who died. An excess risk of dying from lung cancer (ICD codes 162 and 163) was observed in the registry cohort, as compared with US white males (7 observed, 3.3 expected). The overall excess of 73 deaths in the registry population was largely a reflection of the excess mortality from non-neoplastic respiratory diseases, excluding influenza and pneumonia (52 observed, 1.62 expected). This study analysed a selected group of individuals with lung diseases, who were registered because of known exposure to beryllium; the lung disease was defined by standard diagnostic criteria; other unknown selection factors may have been involved. The two-fold excess risk of lung cancer (cell-type unspecified) in this group is not statistically significant at the 5% level. Subdivision of the group into 'acute' (nonmalignant respiratory disease) and 'chronic' (berylliosis cases) provided the possibility of further analysing the data: the 'acute' group then showed a statistically significant excess of lung cancer ($P < 0.05$) [The Working Group noted that the use of lung cancer rates for the entire US white male population may be inappropriate for comparison with a selected population].

[The Working Group noted several points. The life-table programme used by both Wagoner *et al*. (1980) and Mancuso (1980a) involves a straight-line extrapolation from 1965-1967 rates as an estimate of rates for the period 1968-1975 in calculating expected values for lung cancer; since the mortality rates for lung cancer increased during that period, this procedure underestimates expected values and thus overestimates the SMR. Two beryllium production plants in the US provide the data base for all 4 studies cited. Six of the 7 lung cancer cases studied by Infante *et al*. (1980) were employees at these production facilities. Although there is a consistent finding of excess lung cancer in the shortest exposure group (less than 5 years), the 4 studies are not totally independent. The authors of the 4 studies suggest that beryllium exhibits a carcinogenic effect after a short exposure period and a long latent period. No data on total beryllium dose are available. The Working Group was aware that of the 47 lung cancer cases described by Wagoner *et al*. (1980), 31 (66%) were employed for less than 12 months. Although this could reflect the high percentage (60%) of beryllium workers who worked for less than 1 year, it is unusual to identify a carcinogenic effect from such a short exposure].

4. Summary of Data Reported and Evaluation

4.1 Experimental data

Beryllium compounds are carcinogenic in three animal species (rat, rabbit and monkey). In particular, beryllium metal, beryllium-aluminium alloy, beryl ore, beryllium chloride, beryllium fluoride, beryllium hydroxide and beryllium sulphate (or its tetrahydrate) produced lung tumours in rats exposed by inhalation or intratracheally; beryllium oxide and beryllium sulphate produced lung tumours in monkeys following intrabronchial implantation or inhalation ; and beryllium metal, beryllium carbonate, beryllium oxide, beryllium phosphate, beryllium silicate and zinc beryllium silicate produced osteosarcomas in rabbits following intravenous and/or intraosseus administration.

On the basis of the available data from experiments in rats and hamsters involving the inhalation of bertrandite ore, in rats involving the single intratracheal instillation of beryllium-copper alloy, beryllium-nickel alloy or beryllium-copper-cobalt alloy and in rabbits involving the intraosseus injection of beryllium acetate, no evaluation of the carcinogenicity of these compounds could be made. An experiment in which mice were injected intravenously with zinc beryllium silicate or beryllium oxide was also inadequate.

Beryllium sulphate was not mutagenic in various bacterial systems. In the *rec* assay, beryllium sulphate gave positive results and beryllium chloride negative results. Positive results were obtained with beryllium chloride in DNA misincorporation tests. Beryllium chloride induced chromosomal aberrations in cultured peripheral lymphocytes from domestic pigs; beryllium sulphate induced morphological transformation in Syrian hamster embryo cells. No data on the mutagenicity of other beryllium compounds were available.

Beryllium crosses the placenta to only a small extent. No data on the embryotoxicity or teratogenicity of beryllium or beryllium compounds were available.

4.2 Human data

Commercial production of beryllium began during the 1940s. Its use in industry increased until 'early 1970' and decreased thereafter. Exposures can occur during the mining of beryl ore, the initial processing of ore into beryllium and beryllium compounds or in the use of these substances in manufacturing processes.

Beryllium and several beryllium compounds are known to cause acute and chronic lung disease, even in low doses. For this reason, the use of beryllium in fluorescent tubes was discontinued from about 1950; the risk of exposure to beryllium compounds in the general population is therefore small. Additionally, control measures aimed at reducing occupational exposure have been introduced in industries producing and using beryllium.

Four epidemiological studies carried out between 1967 and 1970 did not provide evidence of a relationship between exposure to beryllium compounds and the occurrence of human cancer. Four subsequent studies of these same populations all show an excess of lung cancer in white males who were occupationally exposed to beryllium or beryllium compounds in the only two beryllium extraction operations in the US; there is thus overlapping of the study populations. The demonstrated excess risk is small (1.4 times that of the comparison populations); the majority of the cases occurred in a subgroup of the population with very short employment in the beryllium industry. The Working Group, while considering that the data raised a suspicion of a carcinogenic effect of beryllium, could not evaluate the contribution of beryllium to the occurrence of lung cancer due to the absence of additional information on exposure to beryllium and on the contribution of confounding factors.

4.3 Evaluation

There is *sufficient evidence* that beryllium metal and several beryllium compounds are carcinogenic to three experimental animal species. The epidemiological evidence that occupational exposure to beryllium may lead to an increased lung cancer risk is limited[1]. Taken together, the experimental and human data indicate that beryllium should be considered suspect of being carcinogenic to humans.

---

[1]One member of the Working Group disassociated himself from this conclusion on the grounds that he considered the epidemiological data sufficient to conclude that beryllium is a confirmed carcinogen in humans.

5. References

Aldridge, W.N., Barnes, J.M. & Denz, F.A. (1950) Biochemical changes in acute beryllium poisoning. *Br. J. exp. Pathol., 31,* 473-484

Araki, M., Okada, S. & Fujita, M. (1954) Beryllium. Experimental studies on beryllium-induced malignant tumours of rabbits (Jpn.). *Gann, 45,* 449-451

Ballance, J., Stonehouse, A.J., Sweeney, R. & Walsh, K. (1978) *Beryllium and beryllium alloys.* In: Kirk, R.E. & Othmer, D.F., eds, *Encyclopedia of Chemical Technology,* 3rd ed., Vol. 3, New York, NY, John Wiley & Sons, pp. 803-823

Barnes, J.M. (1950) Experimental production of malignant tumours by beryllium. *Lancet, i,* 463

Barnes, J.M., Denz, F.A. & Sissons, H.A. (1950) Beryllium bone sarcoma in rabbits. *Br. J. Cancer, 4,* 212-222

Beaver, W.W. (1963) *Beryllium-base alloys.* In: *The Metallurgy of Beryllium,* London, Chapman & Hall, pp. 601-621

Boland, L.F. (1958) Beryllium. Present and potential uses. *Anal. J.,* November, 27-31

Brittain, H.G. (1978) The use of hydroxynapththol blue in the ultramicrodetermination of alkaline earth and lanthanide elements: an improved method. *Anal. chim. Acta, 96,* 165-170

Brown, R. & Taylor, H.E. (1975) *Trace Element Analysis of Normal Lung Tissue and Hilar Lymph Nodes by Spark Source Mass Spectrometry,* HEW Publication No. (NIOSH) 75-129, Springfield, VA, National Technical Information Service

Brush Wellman, Inc. (undated) *Ceramic Products, Beryllium Oxide,* Elmore, OH

Bugryshev, P.F., Moskalev, Y.I., Kuznetsov, A.A. & Nazarova, V.A. (1976) Beryllium distribution in rats (Russ.). *Farmakol. Toksikol., 39,* 615-618

Bureau of National Affairs, Inc. (1979a) Beryllium: comments on HEW consultants' report fail to end carcinogenicity controversy. *Occup. Saf. Health Rep., 95-3237,* pp. 1485-1486

Bureau of National Affairs, Inc. (1979b) Occupational safety and health standards. *Occup. Saf. Health Rep., 1910.1001,* p. 31:8304

Casto, B.C., Meyers, J. & DiPaolo, J.A. (1979) Enhancement of viral transformation for evaluation of the carcinogenic or mutagenic potential of inorganic metal salts. *Cancer Res., 39,* 193-198

Cianciara, M. & Swiatkowski, J. (1978) Examination of respiratory tract in workers occupationally exposed to beryllium (Pol.). *Med. Pracy, 29,* 153-161

Cloudman, A.M., Vining, D., Barkulis, S. & Nickson, J.J. (1949) Bone changes observed following intravenous injections of beryllium (Abstract). *Am. J. Pathol., 25,* 810-811

Constantinidis, K. (1978) Acute and chronic beryllium disease. *Br. J. clin. Pract., 32,* 127-136, 153

Copper Development Association, Inc. (1973) *Standards Handbook; Wrought Copper and Copper Alloy Mill Products,* Part 2, *Alloy Data,* New York, pp. 55-60

Coulson, D.M. & Haynes, D.L. (1972) *Survey of Manual Methods of Measurements of Asbestos, Beryllium, Lead, Cadmium, Selenium, and Mercury in Stationary Source Emissions,* US Environmental Protection Agency, Menlo Park, CA, Stanford Research Institute, pp. 9-13, BI.I-B8.1

Cowgill, U.M. (1976) The hydrogeochemistry of Linsley Pond, North Branford, Connecticut. IV. Minor constitutents by optical emission spectroscopy. *Arch. Hydrobiol., 78,* 279-309

Curtis, G.H. (1951) Cutaneous hypersensitivity due to beryllium. A study of thirteen cases. *Arch. Dermatol. Syphilol., 64,* 470-482

Dean, J.A., ed. (1973) *Lange's Handbook of Chemistry,* 11th ed., New York, NY, McGraw-Hill, p. 4-23

DeNardi, J.M., Van Ordstrand, H.S. & Carmody, M.G. (1949) Chronic pulmonary granulomatosis. Report of ten cases. *Am. J. Med., 7,* 345-355

DeNardi, J.M., Van Ordstrand, H.S. & Curtis, G.H. (1952) Berylliosis: summary and survey of all clinical types in ten-year period. *Cleveland Clin. Q., 19,* 171-193

DiPaolo, J.A. & Casto, B.C. (1979) Quantitative studies of *in vitro* morphological transformation of Syrian hamster cells by inorganic metal salts. *Cancer Res., 39,* 1008-1013

Dreher, G.B., Muchmore, C.B. & Stover, D.W. (1977) *Major, Minor, and Trace Elements of Bottom Sediments in Lake Du Quoin, Johnston City Lake, and Little Grassy Lake in Southern Illinois,* Environmental Geology Notes No. 82, Urbana, IL, Illinois State Geological Survey

Drevenkar, V., Stefanac, Z. & Brbot, A. (1976) A new selective reagent for the spectrofluorometric determination of beryllium. *Microchem. J., 21,* 402-410

Drury, J.S., Shriner, C.R., Lewis, E.G., Towill, L.E. & Hammons, A.S. (1978) *Reviews of the Environmental Effects of Pollutants: VI. Beryllium,* Report No. EPA-600/1-78-028, US Environmental Protection Agency, Cincinnati, OH, pp. 1-191

Dutra, F.R. (1951) Experimental beryllium granulomas of the skin. *Arch. ind. Hyg. occup. Med., 3,* 81-89

Dutra, F.R. & Largent, E.J. (1950) Osteosarcoma induced by beryllium oxide. *Am. J., Pathol., 26,* 197-209

Dutra, F.R., Largent, E.J.& Roth, J.L. (1951) Osteogenic sarcoma after inhalation of beryllium oxide. *Arch. Pathol., 51,* 473-479

Epstein, M.S., Rains, T.C., Brady, T.J., Moody, J.R. & Barnes, I.L. (1978) Determination of several trace metals in simulated fresh water by graphite furnace atomic emission spectrometry. *Anal. Chem., 50,* 874-880

Ermakova, N.G. & Vasilieva, E.G. (1978) Determination of the T- and B-lymphocytes populations under an occupational effect of the chemical allergen - beryllium (Russ.). *Gig. Tr. Prof. Zabol., 4,* 32-35

Farkas, M.S. (1979) Beryllium. Alloy sales bolstered by favorable economic conditions. *Eng. Min. J., 180,* 166, 171

Feldman, I., Havill, J.R. & Neuman, W.F. (1953) The state of beryllium in blood plasma. *Arch. Biochem. Biophys., 46,* 443-453

Fisher, R.P. (1978) Priority pollutants in wastewaters. The analysis for thirteen inorganic pollutants by modern atomic absorption spectrometric methods. *Tec. Assoc. Pulp Paper Ind., 61,* 63-67

Fodor, I. (1977) Histogenesis of beryllium-induced bone tumours. *Acta morphol. acad. sci. hung., 25,* 99-105

Fonda, G.R. (1952) *Luminescent materials.* In: Kirk, R.E. & Othmer, D.F., eds, *Encyclo-pedia of Chemical Technology,* 1st ed., Vol. 8, New York, NY, Interscience, pp. 545-549

Foreman, J.K., Gough, T.A. & Walker, E.A. (1970) The determination of traces of beryl-lium in human and rat urine samples by gas chromatography. *Analyst, 95,* 797-804

Frame, G.M. & Ford, R.E. (1974) Trace determination of beryllium oxide in biological sam-ples by electron-capture gas chromatography. *Anal. Chem., 46,* 534-539

Gardner, L.U. & Heslington, H.F. (1946) Osteosarcoma from intravenous beryllium com-pounds in rabbits (Abstract). *Fed. Proc., 5,* 221

Gladney, E.S. (1977) Direct determination of beryllium in NBS SRM 1632 coal by flameless atomic absorption. *At. Absorpt. Newsl., 16,* 42-43

Gosink, T.A. (1976) Gas chromatographic analysis of beryllium in the marine system. Inter-ference, efficiency, apparent biological discrimination and some results. *Mar. Sci. Commun., 2,* 183-199

Grewal, D.S. & Kearns, F.X. (1977) A simple and rapid determination of small amounts of beryllium in urine by flameless atomic absorption. *At. Absorpt. Newsl., 16,* 131-132

Griciute, L.A. (1971) *On the role of beryllium compounds in experimental lung carcino-genesis (Russ.).* In: Bramberga, V.M., ed., *Proceedings of the III Conference of Cancerologists of Estonian, Lithuanian and Latvian SSR, Riga, 1971,* Riga, Health Ministry, pp. 95-96

Griffitts, W.R., Allaway, W.H. & Groth, D.H. (1977) Beryllium. *Geochem. Environ., 2,* 7-10

Groth, D.H. (1980) Carcinogenicity of beryllium: review of the literature. *Environ. Res., 21,* 56-62

Groth, D.H., Scheel, L.D. & MacKay, G.R. (1972) Comparative pulmonary effects of beryl-lium and arsenic compounds in rats (Abstract). *Lab Invest., 26,* 477-478

Groth, D.H., Kommineni, C. & MacKay, G.R. (1980) Carcinogenicity of beryllium hydroxide and alloys. *Environ. Res., 21,* 63-84

Gusarskii, V.V., Chueva, L.A. & Artamonova, V.M. (1977) Spectral aerosol-spark determination of beryllium in technological solutions (Russ.). *Zavod. Lab., 43,* 1472-1473

Guyatt, B.L., Kay, H.D. & Branion, H.D. (1933) Beryllium 'rickets'. *J. Nutr., 6,* 313-324

Hardy, H.L. (1976) Correction on the number of presumed beryllium-induced osteosarcomas in human beings. *New Engl. J. Med., 295,* 624

Hardy, H.L & Tabershaw, I.R. (1946) Delayed chemical pneumonitis occurring in workers exposed to beryllium compounds *J. ind. Hyg. Toxicol., 28,* 197-211

Hardy, H.L. & Tepper, L.B. (1959) Beryllium disease. A review of current knowledge. *J. occup. Med., 1,* 219-224

Hardy, H.L., Rabe, E.W. & Lorch, S. (1967) United States Beryllium Case Registry (1952-1966). Review of its methods and utility. *J. occup. Med., 9,* 271-276

Havezov, I. & Tamnev, B. (1978) Atomic-absorption spectrophotometric determination of beryllium in β-Al_2O_3 ceramics. *Fresenius' Z. anal. Chem., 290,* 299-301

Higgins, G.M., Levy, B.M. & Yollick, B.L. (1964) A transplantable beryllium-induced chondrosarcoma of rabbits. *J. Bone Jt Surg., 46A,* 789-796

Hoagland, M.B., Grier, R.S. & Hood, M.B. (1950) Beryllium and growth. I. Beryllium-induced osteogenic sarcomata. *Cancer Res., 10,* 629-635

Hurlbut, J.A. (1974) *The History, Uses, Occurrences, Analytical Chemistry, and Biochemistry of Beryllium - A Review,* Albuquerque, NM, US Atomic Energy Commission

Hurlbut, J.A. (1978) Determination of beryllium in biological tissues and fluids by flameless atomic absorption spectroscopy. *At. Absorpt. Newsl., 17,* 121-124

IARC (1972) *IARC Monographs on the Evaluation of Carcinogenic Risk of Chemicals to Man,* Vol. 1, Lyon, pp. 17-28

Infante, P.F. & Wagoner, J.K. (1975) *Evidence for the carcinogenicity of beryllium.* In: Hutchinson, T.C., ed., *Proceedings of the International Conference on Heavy Metals in the Environment,* Toronto, Institute for Environmental Studies, pp. 329-338

Infante, P.F., Wagoner, J.K. & Sprince, N.L. (1980) Mortality patterns from lung cancer and nonneoplastic respiratory disease among white males in the Beryllium Case Registry. *Environ. Res., 21,* 35-43

Janes, J.M., Higgins, G.M. & Herrick, J.F. (1954) Beryllium-induced osteogenic sarcoma in rabbits. *J. Bone Jt Surg., 36B,* 543-552

Janes, J.M., McCall, J.T. & Kniseley, R.N. (1975) Osteogenic sarcoma: influence of trace metals in experimental induction. *Trace Subst. environ. Health, 9,* 433-439

Japanese Society of Industrial Hygiene (1978) Recommendations for the concentrations permitted (Jpn.). *Jpn. J. ind. Health, 20,* 290-293

Jones Williams, W. (1977) Beryllium disease - Pathology and diagnosis. *J. Soc. occup. Med., 27,* 93-96

Kada, T., Hirano, K. & Shirasu, Y. (1980) Screening of environmental chemical mutagens by the *rec*-assay system with *Bacillus subtilis. Chem. Mutagens, 6* (in press)

Kawecki, H.C. (1953) Basic beryllium acetate, *US Patent 2,641,611,* 9 June, to Beryllium Corporation (*Chem. Abstr., 47,* 10184b)

Kawecki Berylco Industries, Inc. (1968) *Product Specifications: Beryllium Chemical Compounds,* New York, NY, File 401 1-SP1

Kelly, P.J., Janes, J.M. & Peterson, L.F.A. (1961) The effect of beryllium on bone. A morphological study of the progressive changes observed in rabbit bone. *J. Bone Jt Surg., 43A,* 829-844

Komitowski, D. (1968) Experimental beryllium-induced bone tumours as a model of osteogenic sarcoma (Pol.). *Chir. Narzad. Ruchu. Ortop. Pols., 33,* 237-242

Komitowski, D. (1971) Histochemical study into histogenesis of bone tumours developing under the effect of beryllium (Russ.). *Vest. Akad. Med. Nauk. SSR, 26,* 10-11

Komitowski, D. (1974) Beryllium-induced bone sarcomas (Ger.). *Verh. dtsch. Ges. Pathol., 58,* 438-440

Kubinski, H., Zeldin, P.E. & Morin, N.R. (1977) Survey of tumor-producing agents for their ability to induce macromolecular complexes (Abstract). *Proc. Am. Assoc. Cancer Res., 18,* 16

Kuznetsov, A.V., Matveev, O.G. & Suntsov, G.D. (1974) Differences in the distribution of labelled beryllium chloride with or without carrier in rats following intratracheal administration (Russ.). *Gig. Sanit., 10,* 113-114

Lagas, P. (1978) Determination of beryllium, barium, vanadium and some other elements in water by atomic absorption spectrometry with electrothermal atomization. *Anal. chem. Acta, 98,* 261-267

Lieben, J., Dattoli, J.A. & Israel, H.L. (1964) Probable berylliosis from beryllium alloys. *Arch. environ. Health, 9,* 473-477

Litvinov, N.N., Bugryshev, P.F. & Kazenashev, V.F. (1975) Toxic properties of some soluble beryllium compounds (based on experimental morphological investigations). *Gig. Tr. Prof. Zabol., 7,* 34-37

Lloyd Davies, T.A. & Harding, H.E. (1950) Beryllium granulomata in the lungs of rats. *Br. J. ind. Med., 7,* 70-72

Lövblad, G. (1977) *Trace Element Concentrations in Some Coal Samples and Possible Emissions From Coal Combustion in Sweden,* Gothenburg, Sweden, Swedish Water and Air Pollution Research Laboratory

Luckey, T.D. & Venugopal, B. (1977) *Metal Toxicity in Mammals,* Vol. 2, New York, NY, Plenum Press, pp. 43-50

Luke, M.Z., Hamilton, L. & Hollocher, T.C. (1975) Beryllium-induced misincorporation by a DNA-polymerase: a possible factor in beryllium toxicity. *Biochem. biophys. Res. Commun., 62,* 497-501

Mancuso, T.F. (1970) Relation of duration of employment and prior respiratory illness to respiratory cancer among beryllium workers. *Environ. Res., 3,* 251-275

Mancuso, T.F. (1980a) *Occupational lung cancer among beryllium workers.* In: Lemen, R. & Dement, J., eds, *Conference on Occupational Exposures to Fibrous and Particulate Dust and their Extension into the Environment,* Washington DC, Society for Occupational and Environmental Health (in press)

Mancuso, T.F. (1980b) Mortality study of beryllium industry workers, occupational lung cancer. *Environ. Res., 21,* 48-55

Mancuso, T.F. & El-Attar, A.A. (1969) Epidemiological study of the beryllium industry. Cohort methodology and mortality studies. *J. occup. Med., 11,* 422-434

Marcotte, J. & Witschi, H.P. (1972) Synthesis of RNA and nuclear proteins in early regenerating rat livers exposed to beryllium. *Res. Commun. chem. Pathol. Pharmacol., 3,* 97-104

Matsuura, K. (1974) Experimental studies on the production of osteosarcoma by beryllium compounds, and the effects of irradiation (Jpn.). *Jpn. J. Orthop. Assoc., 48,* 403-418

Mazabraud, A. (1975) Experimental production of osteosarcomas in rabbits by single local injection of beryllium (Fr.). *Bull. Cancer, 62,* 49-58

Meehan, W.R. & Smythe, L.E. (1967) Occurrence of beryllium as a trace element in environmental materials. *Environ. Sci. Technol., 1,* 839-844

Mellor, J.W. (1946) *A Comprehensive Treatise on Inorganic and Theoretical Chemistry,* Vol. 4, London, Longmans, Green & Co., pp. 221-248

Morgareidge, K., Cox, G.E., Bailey, D.E. & Gallo, M.A. (1977) Chronic oral toxicity of beryllium in the rat (Abstract no. 175). *Toxicol. appl. Pharmacol., 41,* 204-205

Mulwani, H.R. & Sathe, R.M. (1977) Spectrophotometric determination of beryllium in air by a sensitised chrome azurol S reaction. *Analyst, 102,* 137-139

Nash, P. (1950) Experimental production of malignant tumours by beryllium. *Lancet, i,* 519

National Institute for Occupational Safety & Health (1972) *Criteria for a Recommended Standard . . . Occupational Exposure to Beryllium,* DHEW (NIOSH) Publication No. 72-10268, Washington DC, US Government Printing Office

Nishimura, M. (1966) Clinical and experimental studies on acute beryllium disease. *Nagoya J. med. Sci, 28,* 17-44

Nishioka, H. (1975) Mutagenic activies of metal compounds in bacteria. *Mutat. Res., 31,* 185-189

van Oss, J.F., ed. (1970) *Chemical Technology: an Encyclopedic Treatment,* Vol. 3, New York, Barnes & Noble, pp. 236-239

Paton, G.R. & Allison, A.C. (1972) Chromosome damage in human cell cultures induced by metal salts. *Mutat. Res., 16,* 332-336

Peterson, L.F.A., Brown, A.L. & Janes, J.M. (1964) The ultrastructure of beryllium-induced osteogenic sarcoma in the rabbit (Abstract). *J. Bone Jt Surg., 46A,* 920

Petkof, B. (1975) *Beryllium.* In: *Mineral Facts and Problems, 1975,* Washington DC, US Bureau of Mines, US Government Printing Office, pp. 137-146

Petkof, B. (1976) *Beryllium*. In: *Mineral Yearbook, 1976,* Vol. 1, Washington DC, US Bureau of Mines, US Government Printing Office, pp. 213-216

Petkof, B. (1979) *Beryllium*, Preprint from the *1977 Bureau of Mines Minerals Yearbook*, Washington DC, US Department of the Interior, pp. 1-4

Pinto, N.P. & Greenspan, J. (1968) *Beryllium*. In: Gonser, B.W., ed., *Modern Materials, Advances in Development and Applications,* Vol. 6, New York, NY, Academic Press, pp. 319-372

Policard, A. (1950) Histological studies of the effects of beryllium oxide (glucine) on animal tissues. *Br. J. ind. Med., 7,* 117-121

Pough, F.H. (1960) *A Field Guide to Rocks and Minerals,* Boston, MA, Houghton Mifflin Co., pp. 283-284

Presas-Barrosa, M.J., Bermejo-Martiniz, F. & Rodriguez-Vazquez, J.A. (1977) The ultraviolet spectrophotometric determination of beryllium, cobalt and some other metals with uramildiacetic acid. *Anal. chim. Acta, 88,* 395-398

Reeves, A.L. (1965) The absorption of beryllium from the gastrointestinal tract. *Arch. environ. Health, 11,* 209-214

Reeves, A. (1978a) *Environmental Assessment of Beryllium,* Report No. EPA-600/1-78-028, US Environmental Protection Agency, Cincinnati, OH, US Government Printing Office, pp. 192-197

Reeves, A.L. (1978b) *Beryllium carcinogenesis.* In: Schrauzer, G.N., ed., *Inorganic and Nutritional Aspects of Cancer,* New York, NY, Plenum Press, pp. 13-27

Reeves, A.L. (1979) *Beryllium*. In: Friberg, L., Nordberg, G.F. & Vouk, V.B., eds, *Handbook on the Toxicology of Metals,* Amsterdam, Elsevier, pp. 329-343

Reeves, A.L. & Vorwald, A.J. (1961) The humoral transport of beryllium. *J. occup. Med., 3,* 567-574

Reeves, A.L. & Vorwald, A.J. (1967) Beryllium carcinogenesis. II. Pulmonary deposition and clearance of inhaled beryllium sulfate in the rat. *Cancer Res., 27,* 446-451

Reeves, A.L., Deitch, D. & Vorwald, A.J. (1967) Beryllium carcinogenesis. I. Inhalation exposure of rats to beryllium sulfate aerosol. *Cancer Res., 27,* 439-445

Robinson, F.R., Brokeshoulder, S.F., Thomas, A.A. & Cholak, J. (1968) Microemission spectrochemical analysis of human lungs for beryllium. *Am. J. clin. Pathol., 49,* 821-825

Rosenkranz, H.S. & Poirier, L.A. (1979) Evaluation of the mutagenicity and DNA-modifying activity of carcinogens and noncarcinogens in microbial systems. *J. natl Cancer Inst., 62,* 873-892

Roskill Information Services (1975) *Copper: Survey of World Production, Consumption and Prices,* London

Ross, W.D., Pyle, J.L. & Sievers, R.E. (1977) Analysis for beryllium in ambient air particulates by gas chromatography. *Environ. Sci. Technol., 11,* 467-471

Safe Drinking Water Committee (1977) *Drinking Water and Health,* Advisory Center on Toxicology, Assembly of Life Sciences, National Research Council, Washington DC, National Academy of Sciences, pp. 211, 231-232

Sanders, C.L., Cannon, W.C. & Powers, G.J. (1978) Lung carcinogenesis induced by inhaled high-fired oxides of beryllium and plutonium. *Health Phys., 35,* 193-199

Saxén, L. & Pasila, M. (1978) Pulmonary berylliosis. Report of a case (Finn.). *Duodecim, 94,* 504-508

Schepers, G.W.H. (1961) Neoplasia experimentally induced by beryllium compounds. *Prog. exp. Tumor Res., 2,* 203-244

Schepers, G.W.H. (1964) Biological action of beryllium. Reaction of the monkey to inhaled aerosols. *Ind. Med. Surg., 33,* 1-16

Schepers, G.W.H., Durkan, T.M., Delehant, A.B. & Creedon, F.T. (1957) The biological action of inhaled beryllium sulfate. *Arch. ind. Health, 15,* 32-58

Schroeder, H.A. & Mitchener, M. (1975) Life-term studies in rats: effects of aluminum, barium, beryllium and tungsten. *J. Nutr., 105,* 421-427

Schulert, A.R., Glasser, S.R., Stant, E.G., Jr, Brill, A.B., Koshakji, R.P. & Mansour, M.M. (1969) Development of placental discrimination among homologous elements. *At. Energy Comm. Symp. Ser., 17,* 145-152

Schwenzfeier, C.W., Jr (1964) *Beryllium compounds.* In: Kirk, R.E. & Othmer, D.F., eds, *Encyclopedia of Chemical Technology,* 2nd ed., Vol. 3, New York, NY, John Wiley & Sons, pp. 474-480

Scott, D.R., Loseke, W.A., Holboke, L.E. & Thompson, R.J. (1976) Analysis of atmospheric particulates for trace elements by optical emission spectrometry. *Appl. Spectrosc.,* *30,* 392-405

Simmon, V.F. (1979a) *In vitro* mutagenicity assays of chemical carcinogens and related compounds with *Salmonella typhimurium. J. natl Cancer Inst., 63,* 893-899

Simmon V.F. (1979b) *In vitro* assays for recombinogenic activity of chemical carcinogens and related compounds with *Saccharomyces cerevisiae* D3. *J. natl Cancer Inst., 62,* 901-909

Simmon, V.F., Rosenkranz, H.S., Zeiger, E. & Poirier, L.A. (1979) Mutagenic activity of chemical carcinogens and related compounds in the intraperitoneal host-mediated assay. *J. natl Cancer Inst., 62,* 911-918

Sirover, M.A. & Loeb, L.A. (1976) Metal-induced infidelity during DNA synthesis. *Proc. natl Acad. Sci. USA, 73,* 2331-2335

Sissons, H.A. (1950) Bone sarcomas produced experimentally in the rabbit, using compounds of beryllium. *Acta unio int. contra cancrum, 7,* 171-172

Skilleter, D.N. & Price, R.J. (1978) The uptake and subsequent loss of beryllium by rat liver parenchymal and non-parenchymal cells after the intravenous administration of particulate and soluble forms. *Chem. -biol. Interactions, 20, 383-396*

Spencer, H.C., Jones, J.C., Sadek, S.E., Dodson, K.B. & Morgan, A.H. (1965) Toxicological studies on beryllium oxides (Abstract no. 63). *Toxicol. appl. Pharmacol., 7,* 498

Steinmetz, H. (1907) On beryllium acetate. *Z. anorg. Chem., 54,* 217-222 *[Chem. Abstr., 1,* 2672]

Stephen, H. & Stephen, T., eds (1963) *Solubilities of Inorganic and Organic Compounds,* Vol. 1, New York, NY, MacMillan, pp. 233, 759

Sterner, J.H. & Eisenbud, M. (1951) Epidemiology of beryllium intoxication. *Arch. ind. Hyg. occup. Med., 4,* 123-151

Stoeckle, J.D., Hardy, H.L. & Weber, A.L. (1969) Chronic beryllium disease. Long-term follow-up of sixty cases and selective review of the literature. *Am. J. Med., 46,* 545-561

Sunderman, F.W., Jr (1971) Metal carcinogenesis in experimental animals. *Food Cosmet. Toxicol., 9,* 105-120

Sunderman, F.W., Jr (1977) Metal carcinogenesis. *Adv. mod. Toxicol., 1,* 257-295

Talluri, M.V. & Guiggiani, V. (1967) Action of beryllium ions on primary cultures of swine cells. *Caryologia, 20,* 355-367

Tapp, E. (1966) Beryllium induced sarcomas of the rabbit tibia. *Br. J. Cancer, 20,* 778-783

Tapp, E. (1969a) Osteogenic sarcoma in rabbits following subperiosteal implantation of beryllium. *Arch. Pathol., 88,* 89-95

Tapp, E. (1969b) Changes in rabbit tibia due to direct implantation of beryllium salts. *Arch. Pathol., 88,* 521-529

Truhaut, R., Festy, B. & Le Talaer, J.-Y. (1968) Interaction of beryllium with DNA and its incidence with some enzymatic systems (Fr.). *C.R. Acad. Sci. Paris, Série D, 266,* 1192-1195

Uesugi, K. & Miyawaki, M. (1976) A highly sensitive spectrophotometric determination of beryllium with chromal blue G and cetyltrimethylammonium chloride. *Microchem. J., 21,* 438-444

US Bureau of Mines (1979a) *Minerals in the US Economy: Ten-Year Supply-Demand Profiles for Nonfuel Mineral Commodities (1968-77),* Washington DC, US Government Printing Office, p. 11

US Bureau of Mines (1979b) *Mineral Commodity Summaries 1979,* Washington DC, US Government Printing Office, pp. 20-21

US Department of Commerce (1978) *US Exports, Schedule B Commodity Groupings, Schedule B Commodity by Country,* Bureau of the Census, FT410/December 1977, Washington DC, US Government Printing Office, p. 2-228

US Department of Commerce (1979) *US General Imports,* Bureau of the Census, IM146/December 1978, Washington DC, US Government Printing Office, pp. 1348, 1628, 1740

US Environmental Protection Agency (1973) *Background Information on the Development of National Emission Standards for Hazardous Air Pollutants: Asbestos, Beryllium, and Mercury,* Publication No. APTD-1503, Washington DC, US Government Printing Office, pp. 52-56

US Environmental Protection Agency (1977) *The Determination of Antimony, Arsenic, Beryllium, Cadmium, Lead, Selenium, Silver and Tellurium in Environmental Water Samples by Flameless Atomic Absorption,* Publication No. EPA-905/4-77-002, Metals Section, Washington DC, US Government Printing Office

US Environmental Protection Agency(1978) National emission standard for beryllium. *US Code Fed. Regul., Title 40,* parts 61.30-61.32, pp. 276-277

Vacher, J. & Stoner, H.B. (1968) The transport of beryllium in rat blood. *Biochem. Pharmacol., 17,* 93-107

Vacher, J., Deraedt, R. & Benzoni, J. (1973) Compared effects of two beryllium salts (soluble and insoluble): toxicity and blockade of the reticuloendothelial system. *Toxicol. appl. Pharmacol., 24,* 497-506

Van Cleave, C.D. & Kaylor, C.T. (1955) Distribution, retention and elimination of Be^7 in the rat after intratracheal injection. *Arch. ind. Health, 11,* 375-392

Van Ordstrand, H.S., Hughes, R. & Carmody, M.G. (1943) Chemical pneumonia in workers extracting beryllium oxide. Report of three cases. *Cleveland clin. Q., 10,* 10-18

Van Orstrand, H.S., Hughes, R., DeNardi, J.M. & Carmody, M.G. (1945) Beryllium poisoning. *J. Am. med. Assoc., 129,* 1084-1090

Vorwald, A.J. (1967) *The induction of experimental pulmonary cancer in the primate* (Abstract). In: Harris, R.J., ed., *Proceedings of the IV International Cancer Congress, Tokyo, 1966,* Berlin, Springer, p. 125

Vorwald, A.J. (1968) *Use of Nonhuman Primates in Drug Evaluation,* Austin, TX, University of Texas, pp. 222-228

Vorwald, A.J., Pratt, P.C. & Urban, E.J. (1955) The production of pulmonary cancer in albino rats exposed by inhalation to an aerosol of beryllium sulfate (Abstract). *Acta unio int. contra cancrum, 11,* 735

Vorwald, A.J., Reeves, A.L. & Urban, E.C.J. (1966) *Experimental beryllium toxicology.* In: Stokinger, H.E., ed., *Beryllium: Its Industrial Hygiene Aspects,* New York, NY, Academic Press, pp. 201-234

Wagner, W.D., Groth, D.H., Holtz, J.L., Madden, G.E. & Stokinger, H.E. (1969) Comparative chronic inhalation toxicity of beryllium ores, bertrandite and beryl, with production of pulmonary tumors by beryl. *Toxicol. appl. Pharmacol., 15,* 10-29

Wagoner, J.K., Infante, P.F. & Bayliss, D.L. (1980) Beryllium: an etiologic agent in the induction of lung cancer, nonneoplastic respiratory disease and heart disease among industrially exposed workers. *Environ. Res., 21,* 15-34

Walsh, K. & Rees, G.H. (1978) *Beryllium compounds.* In: Kirk, R.E. & Othmer, D.F., eds, *Encyclopedia of Chemical Technology,* 3rd ed., Vol. 3, New York, NY, John Wiley & Sons, pp. 824-829

Weast, R.C., ed. (1977) *CRC Handbook of Chemistry and Physics,* 58th ed., Cleveland, OH, The Chemical Rubber Company, p. B-94

Wicks, S.A. & Burke, R.W. (1977) *Determination of beryllium by fluorescence spectrometry.* In: Mavrodineanu, R., ed., *Procedures Used at the National Bureau of Standards to Determine Selected Trace Elements in Biological and Botanical Materials,* NBS Special Publication 492, US Department of Commerce, Washington DC, US Government Printing Office, pp. 85-89

Windholz, M., ed. (1976) *The Merck Index,* 9th ed., Rahway, NJ, Merck & Co., pp. 153-155

Winell, M.A. (1975) An international comparison of hygienic standards for chemicals in the work environment. *Ambio, 4,* 34-36

Witschi, H.P. (1968) Inhibition of deoxyribonucleic acid synthesis in regenerating rat liver by beryllium. *Lab. Invest., 19,* 67-70

Witschi, H.P. (1970) Effects of beryllium on deoxyribonucleic acid-synthesizing enzymes in regenerating rat liver. *Biochem. J., 120,* 623-634

Yamaguchi, S. (1963) Study of beryllium-induced osteogenic sarcoma (Jpn.). *Nagasaki Iggakai Zasshi, 38,* 127-142

Zdrojewski, A., Dubois, L. & Quickert, N. (1976) Reference method for the determination of beryllium in airborne particulates. *Sci. total Environ., 6,* 165-173

CHROMIUM and CHROMIUM COMPOUNDS

Chromium and chromium compounds were first considered by an IARC Working Group in 1972 (IARC, 1973). Since that time new data have become available, and these are included in the present monograph and have been taken into consideration in the evaluation.

1. Chemical and Physical Data

1.1 Synonyms, trade names and molecular formulae

Table 1. Synonyms (Chemical Abstracts Services names are given in bold), trade names and atomic or molecular formulae of chromium and chromium compounds

Chemical name	Chem. Abstr. Reg. Serial No.	Synonyms and trade names	Formula	Oxidation state
Chromite ore	1308-31-2	Chrome ore; chromite; **chromite mineral [Cr$_2$FeO$_4$]**; iron chromite	Cr$_2$O$_3$.FeO	+3
Chromium	7440-47-3	Chrome	Cr	0
Barium chromate	10294-40-3	Barium chromate [VI]; barium chromate (1:1); barium chromate oxide; **chromic acid [H$_2$CrO$_4$], barium salt (1:1)**; C.I. 77103; C.I. pigment yellow 31 Baryta Yellow; Lemon Chrome; Lemon Yellow; Permanent Yellow; Steinbühl Yellow; Ultramarine Yellow	BaCrO$_4$	+6
Basic chromic sulphate	12336-95-7	Basic chromium sulphate; **chromium hydroxide sulfate [Cr(OH)(SO$_4$)]**; chromium sulphate; mono-basic chromium sulphate; sulphuric acid, chromium salt, basic	CrOHSO$_4$	+3

Table 1 (contd)

Chemical name	Chem. Abstr. Reg. Serial No.	Synonyms and trade names	Formula	Oxidation state
Calcium chromate	13765-19-0	**Chromic acid [H$_2$CrO$_4$], calcium salt (1:1)**; C.I. 77223; C.I. pigment yellow 33 Calcium Chrome Yellow; Gelbin; Yellow Ultramarine	CaCrO$_4$	+6
Chromic acetate	1066-30-4	**Acetic acid, chromium (3+) salt**; chromium acetate; chromium [III] acetate; chromium triacetate	Cr(OOCCH$_3$)$_3$	+3
Chromic chloride	10025-73-7	**Chromium chloride [CrCl$_3$]**; chromium [III] chloride; chromium trichloride; C.I. 77295 Puratronic® chromium chloride	CrCl$_3$	+3
Chromic oxide	1308-38-9	Chrome oxide; chromia; **chromium oxide [Cr$_2$O$_3$]**; chromium sesquioxide; chromium (3+) trioxide; C.I. 77288; C.I. pigment green 17; dichromium trioxide Anadonis Green; Casalis Green; Chrome Green; Chrome Ochre; Chrome Oxide Green; Chrome Oxide Pigment; Chrome Oxide X1134; Chromium III Oxide; Chromium Oxide Green; 11661 Green; Green Chrome Oxide; Green Chromic Oxide; Green Chromium Oxide; Green Cinnabar; Green Oxide of Chromium; Green Oxide of Chromium OC-31; Green Rouge; Guignet's Green; Leaf Green; Levanox Green GA (hydrated chromic oxide); Oil Green; Oxide of Chromium; Pure Chromium Oxide Green 59; Ultramarine Green	Cr$_2$O$_3$	+3

Table 1 (contd)

Chemical name	Chem. Abstr. Reg. Serial No.	Synonyms and trade names	Formula	Oxidation state
Chromic phosphate	7789-04-0	Chromium phosphate; chromium *ortho*phosphate; **phosphoric acid, chromium (3+) salt (1:1)**; phosphoric acid chromium [III] salt Arnaudon's Green (hemiheptahydrate); Plessy's Green (hemiheptahydrate)	$CrPO_4$	+3
Chromium carbonyl	13007-92-6	**Chromium carbonyl [Cr(CO)$_6$]**; chromium hexacarbonyl; hexacarbonyl chromium	$Cr(CO)_6$	0
Chromium potassium sulphate	10141-00-1	Chrome alum (dodecahydrate); chromic potassium sulphate; potassium chromic sulphate; potassium chromium alum; potassium chromium sulphate; potassium disulphatochromate [III]; **sulfuric acid, chromium (3+) potassium salt (2:1:1)** 0% Basicity chrome alum; Crystal chrome alum	$CrK(SO_4)_2$	+3
Chromium sulphate	10101-53-8	Chromic sulphate; chromium sulphate (2:3); dichromium sulphate; dichromium trisulphate; **sulfuric acid, chromium (3+) salt (3:2)** Koreon	$Cr_2(SO_4)_3$	+3
Chromium trioxide	1333-82-0	Chromic acid; chromic [VI] acid; chromic acid, solid; chromic anhydride; chromic trioxide; **chromium oxide [CrO$_3$]**; chromium [VI] oxide; chromium (6+) trioxide; monochromium oxide Puratronic® chromium trioxide	CrO_3	+6

Table 1 (contd)

Chemical name	Chem. Abstr. Reg. Serial No.	Synonyms and trade names	Formula	Oxidation state
Cobalt-chromium alloy	11114-92-4	**Cobalt alloy, Co, Cr**		0
		DIN 2.4964; DIN 2.4602; EP-375; HEV-4; HS 21; HS 25; Hastelloy C; Haynes 25; Haynes alloy number 25; Haynes stellite 21; Kh15N55M16; Kh15N55M16V; S 816; Stellite 8; Stellite 21; Stellite 23; Stellite 25; Stellite 27; Stellite 30; Stellite 31; Stellite 36; Stellite 8A; Stellite C; Vitallium; Zimalloy		
Ferrochromium	11114-46-8	Carbon ferrochromium; chrome ferroalloy; **chromium alloy, Cr, C, Fe, N, Si**; ferrochrome		0
Lead chromate	7758-97-6	**Chromic acid [H_2CrO_4], lead (2+) salt (1:1)**; C.I. 77600; crocoite; pigment green 15; plumbous chromate	$PbCrO_4$	+6
		Canary Chrome Yellow 40-2250; Chrome Green; Chrome Green UC61; Chrome Green UC74; Chrome Green UC76; Chrome Lemon; Chrome Yellow 5G; Chrome Yellow GF; Chrome Yellow LF; Chrome Yellow Light 1066; Chrome Yellow Light 1075; Chrome Yellow Medium 1074; Chrome Yellow Medium 1085; Chrome Yellow Medium 1295; Chrome Yellow Medium 1298; Chrome Yellow Primrose 1010; Chrome Yellow Primrose 1015; Cologne Yellow; Dainichi Chrome Yellow G; Leipzig Yellow; Paris Yellow; Pure Lemon Chrome L3GS		

Table 1 (contd)

Chemical name	Chem. Abstr. Reg. Serial No.	Synonyms and trade names	Formula	Oxidation state
Lead chromate oxide	1344-38-3	Basic lead chromate; C.I. 77601; **C.I. pigment orange 21**; C.I. pigment red; red lead chromate Arancio Cromo; Austrian Cinnabar; Chinese Red; Chrome Orange; Chrome Orange 54; Chrome Orange 56; Chrome Orange 57; Chrome Orange 58; Chrome Orange G; Chrome Orange R; Chrome Orange 5R; Chrome Orange Dark; Chrome Orange NC-22; Chrome Orange RF; Chrome Orange XL; Chrome Red; C.P. Chrome Orange Dark 2030; C.P. Chrome Orange Extra Dark 2040; C.P. Chrome Orange Light 2010; C.P. Chrome Orange Medium 2020; Dainichi Chrome Orange R; Dainichi Chrome Orange 5R; Genuine Acetate Orange Chrome; Genuine Orange Chrome; Indian Red; International Orange 2221; Irgachrome Orange OS; Light Orange Chrome; No. 156 Orange Chrome; Orange Chrome; Orange Nitrate Chrome; Pale Orange Chrome; Persian Red; Pure Orange Chrome M; Pure Orange Chrome Y; Vynamon Orange CR	$PbO.PbCrO_4$	+6
Potassium chromate	7789-00-6	Bipotassium chromate; **chromic acid** $[H_2CrO_4]$, **dipotassium salt**; dipotassium chromate; dipotassium monochromate; neutral potassium chromate; potassium chromate [VI]	K_2CrO_4	+6

Table 1 (contd)

Chemical name	Chem. Abstr. Reg. Serial No.	Synonyms and trade names	Formula	Oxidation state
Potassium di-chromate	7778-50-9	**Chromic acid [$H_2Cr_2O_7$], dipotassium salt**; dichromic acid dipotassium salt; dipotassium dichromate; lopezite; potassium bichromate; potassium dichromate [VI]	$K_2Cr_2O_7$	+6
Sodium chromate	7775-11-3	**Chromic acid [H_2CrO_4], disodium salt**; chromium disodium oxide; disodium chromate; neutral sodium chromate	Na_2CrO_4	+6
Sodium dichromate	10588-01-9	Bichromate of soda; **chromic acid [$H_2Cr_2O_7$], disodium salt**; chromium sodium oxide; disodium dichromate; dichromic acid, disodium salt; sodium bichromate; sodium chromate; sodium dichromate [VI]	$Na_2Cr_2O_7$	+6
Strontium chromate	7789-06-2	**Chromic acid [H_2CrO_4], strontium salt (1:1)**; C.I. pigment yellow 32; strontium chromate [VI]; strontium chromate (1:1) Deep Lemon Yellow; Strontium Chromate 12170; Strontium Chromate A; Strontium Chromate X-2396; Strontium Yellow	$SrCrO_4$	+6
Zinc chromate [a,b]	13530-65-9	**Chromic acid [H_2CrO_4], zinc salt (1:1)**; zinc yellow	$ZnCrO_4$	+6

Table 1 (contd)

Chemical name	Chem. Abstr. Reg. Serial No.	Synonyms and trade names	Formula	Oxidation state
Zinc chromate hydroxide	15930-94-6	**Chromic acid [H$_2$CrO$_4$], zinc salt (1:2);** zinc chromate hydroxide; zinc chromate [VI] hydroxide; zinc hydroxychromate **Buttercup Yellow**	Zn$_2$CrO$_4$(OH)$_2$	+6
Zinc potassium chromate	11103-86-9	**Chromic acid [H$_2$CrO$_4$], potassium zinc salt (2:2:1);** potassium zinc chromate; zinc chrome; zinc yellow **Buttercup Yellow; Citron Yellow**	KZn$_2$(CrO$_4$)$_2$(OH)	+6
Zinc yellow[a]	37300-23-5	Basic zinc chromate; C.I. 77955; **C.I. pigment yellow 36;** zinc chromate pigment; zinc chrome; zinc potassium chromate; zinkgelb **Buttercup Yellow; Citron Yellow**	Approximately: 4ZnO.K$_2$O. 4CrO$_3$.3H$_2$O	+6

[a]The names 'zinc chromate' and 'zinc yellow' are often used interchangeably, even though they are distinct chemically.

[b]A form of zinc chromate, basic zinc chromate, has the empirical formula, Zn$_5$CrO$_{12}$H$_8$ (Lalor, 1973).

1.2 Chemical and physical properties of the pure substances

Physical properties of the chromium compounds considered in this monograph are given, when available, in Table 2. Information on solubility, from Weast (1977), unless otherwise specified, is given below. In the following text, the terms 'soluble' and 'insoluble' refer to the aqueous solubility of chromium compounds.

Chromite ore - no information available

Chromium - insoluble in water; reacts with dilute hydrochloric acid and sulphuric acid

Barium chromate - practically insoluble in water (4.4 mg/l at 28°C); reacts with mineral acids

Basic chromic sulphate - no information available

Calcium chromate - soluble in water (163 g/l at 20°C and 182 g/l at 45°C); reacts with acids and ethanol

Chromic acetate - soluble in cold water, insoluble in ethanol (Weast 1977); soluble in acetone (2 g/l at 15°C) and methanol (45.4 g/l at 15°C)

Chromic chloride - anhydrous form is insoluble in cold water and slightly soluble in hot water; in its hydrated forms it is very soluble in water (585 g/l) and insoluble in methanol, ethanol, acetone and diethyl ether

Chromic oxide - insoluble in water; does not react with ethanol or alkali

Chromic phosphate - slightly soluble in cold water; reacts with most acids and alkali but not with acetic acid

Chromium carbonyl - insoluble in water, ethanol, diethyl ether and acetic acid; slightly soluble in carbon tetrachloride and iodoform

Chromium potassium sulphate - soluble in water (243.9 g/l at 25°C); reacts with dilute acids; insoluble in ethanol

Chromium sulphate - the heptahydrate is soluble in water (124 g/l at 0°C); the anhydrous salt is slightly soluble in ethanol; does not react with acids

Chromium trioxide - soluble in water (625.3 g/l at 20°C)

Cobalt-chromium alloy - no information available

Ferrochromium - no information available

Table 2. Physical properties of chromium and chromium compounds[a]

Chemical name	Atomic/molecular weight	Melting-point (°C)	Boiling-point (°C)	Density (g/cm³)	Crystal system
Chromite ore	—	—	—	4.6 (specific gravity)[b]	—
Chromium	51.996	1857±20	2672	7.2 (28°C)	cubic
Barium chromate	253.33	—	—	4.498 (15°C)	rhombic
Calcium chromate (dihydrate)	192.09	200	—	—	monoclinic prism
Chromic acetate (hydrate)	247.15	—	—	—	powder or pasty mass
Chromic chloride	158.15	1150	1300 (sublimes)	2.76 (15°C)	trigonal
Chromic oxide	151.99	2435	4000	5.21	hexagonal
Chromic phosphate (dihydrate)	183.00	—	—	2.42 (32.5°C)	crystal
Chromium carbonyl	220.06	110 (decomposes)	210 (explodes)	1.77	orthorhombic
Chromium potassium sulphate (dodecahydrate)	499.41	89	400	1.826 (25°C)	cubic, octahedral
Chromium sulphate					
$CrSO_4.7H_2O$	274.17	—	—	—	crystal
$Cr_2(SO_4)_3$	392.18	—	—	3.012	powder
Chromium trioxide	99.99	196	decomposes	2.70	rhombic
Ferrochromium					
low-carbon	—	1710	—	—	—
2% carbon	—	1240	—	—	—
high-carbon	—	1532	—	—	—
Lead chromate	323.18	844	decomposes	6.12 (15°C)	monoclinic
Lead chromate oxide	546.37	—	—	6.63	powder
Potassium chromate	194.20	968.3	decomposes[c]	2.732 (18°C)	rhombic
Potassium dichromate	294.19	398	500 (decomposes)	2.676 (25°C)	monoclinic or triclinic
Sodium chromate	161.97	792[c]	decomposes[c]	2.710-2.736	rhombic bipyramidal

Table 2 (contd)

Chemical name	Atomic/molecular weight	Melting-point (°C)	Boiling-point (°C)	Density (g/cm³)	Crystal system
Sodium dichromate	262.00	356.7	400 (decomposes)	2.52 (13°C)	monoclinic prisms
Strontium chromate	203.61	(decomposes)[d]	—	3.895 (15°C)	monoclinic
Zinc chromate					
$ZnCrO_4$	181.36	—	—	3.40	powder
$Zn_5CrO_{12}H_8$	578.96	—	—	3.87-3.97[g]	powder
Zinc chromate hydroxide	280.74[e]	—	—	—	powder[e]
Zinc potassium chromate	418.76	—	—	—[f]	—
Zinc yellow	873.81[g]	—	—	3.47[f]	triclinic plates[f]

[a]From Weast (1977), unless otherwise specified

[b]Hawley (1977)

[c]Udy, M.C. (1956)

[d]Hartford (1979)

[e]Windholz (1976)

[f]Hartford & Copson (1964)

[g]Lalor (1973); molecular weight is for formula shown in Table 1.

Lead chromate - practically insoluble in water (580 μg/l at 25°C); reacts with most acids and alkali but not with acetic acid or ammonia

Lead chromate oxide - insoluble in water; reacts with acids and alkali

Potassium chromate - soluble in water (629 g/l at 20°C and 792 g/l at 100°C); insoluble in ethanol

Potassium dichromate - soluble in water (49 g/l at 0°C and 1020 g/l at 100°C); insoluble in ethanol

Sodium chromate - soluble in water (873 g/l at 30°C) and methanol (3.44 g/l at 25°C)

Sodium dichromate - soluble in water (2380 g/l at 0°C) and methanol (513.2 g/l at 19.4°C)

Strontium chromate - slightly soluble in water (1.2 g/l at 15°C); reacts with hydrochloric, nitric and acetic acids and ammonium salts

Zinc chromate - soluble in acids and liquid ammonia; insoluble in cold water and acetone; decomposes in hot water

Zinc chromate hydroxide - slightly soluble in water; reacts with dilute acids, including acetic acid (Windhlz, 1976)

Zinc potassium chromate - no information available

Zinc yellow - partially soluble in water (Hawley, 1977).

1.3 Technical products and impurities

Chromite ore consists of varying percentages of chromium, iron, aluminium and magnesium oxides, as the major components. Chromite ore has been classified into three general grades associated with their use: metallurgical, chemical and refractory grades (Morning, 1976a). During the past decade, technological advances have allowed considerable interchangeability among the various grades, particularly for the so-called chemical grade, which can be utilized by all three industries. A stricter classification is: (1) 'high-chromium' chromite ore, containing 46% min. chromic oxide and a chromium:iron content ratio greater than 2:1; (2) 'high-iron' chromite, with 40-46% chromic oxide and a chromium: iron ratio of 1.5:1 to 2:1; and (3) 'high-aluminium' chromite, containing 20% min. aluminium oxide and 60% min. aluminium oxide plus chromic oxide.

The most common minor elements in chromite ores are titanium, manganese, nickel, vanadium and carbon (Thayer, 1956).

Typical analysis of chromite ore imported into Japan from India is as follows: chromium (as Cr_2O_3), 55.47%; iron (as FeO), 14.74%; aluminium (as Al_2O_3), 10.07%; magnesium (as MgO), 10.84%, silicon (as SiO_2), 3.26%; and calcium (as CaO), 0.18%.

Chromium metal is available in the US as electrolytic chromium (99.5% Cr), alumino-thermic chromium (98.5% Cr) and ductile chromium (99.9% Cr). Electrolytic chromium and aluminothermic chromium typically contain traces of silicon, carbon, sulphur, oxygen and iron (Bacon, 1964). The purity of chromium metal available in Japan is usually over 99.2%.

Barium chromate available in the US has the following specifications: purity, 98.5% min; granulation, 100.0% through USS Sieve No. 325; apparent density, 0.33-0.50; chlorides (as Cl), 0.05% max; water-soluble matter, 0.05%, max; and volatile matter, 0.10% max (Barium & Chemicals, Inc., 1978a). The specifications for barium chromate available in Japan are: purity, 98.4% min; chlorides, 0.1% max; sulphate, 0.005% max; water, 0.05% max; water-soluble matter, 0.05% max; and average particle diameter, 1.4 μm.

Basic chromic sulphate is available from one company in the US in three grades containing 24%, 24.5% and 25% Cr (calculated as chromic oxide), respectively. All grades dissolve readily to give clear solutions substantially free from iron, vanadium and silica (Allied Chemical, 1960). Similar grades are available in Japan.

One technical grade of *calcium chromate* available in the US typically contains the following: calcium carbonate and calcium hydroxide, 4.0%; aluminium (as Al_2O_3), 0.5%; sodium (as Na_2O), 0.5%; silicon, 0.2%; sulphur, 0.1%; and chlorides (as Cl), 0.01% (Barium & Chemicals, Inc., 1978b).

Chromic acetate is available commercially from one US company in the form of a 50% aqueous solution (McGean Chemical Co., Inc., 1978). In Japan, it is available as a 55-57% aqueous solution.

Chromic chloride is available in the US as an aqueous solution containing 62% of the pure substance (McGean Chemical Co., Inc., 1978). Two technical grades in crystalline form are available in Japan, each containing 18-19% chromium. Two grades available from one company in western Europe contain 20 and 100 mg/kg max. of metallic impurities.

Typical composition of *chromic oxide* available from one US company is as follows: purity, 98.5%; water-soluble materials, 0.2%; moisture, 0.3%; iron, 0.05%; sulphur, 0.2%; and inert materials, 0.75% (Hercules Inc., 1978). Chromic oxide available in Japan has minimum purities of 99.3% (for use in pigments and abrasives) and 98.0% (for production of refractory materials).

Chromic phosphate is believed to be produced by one company in the US and on a laboratory scale for reagent use in Japan; however no data on specifications were available.

Chromium carbonyl is produced by two companies in the US, but no data on specifications were available.

Two grades of *chromium potassium sulphate*, varying in degree of hydration, are available from one US producer; these are identified as 'Crystal' (crystals) and '0% Basicity' (powder) (McGean Chemical Co., Inc., 1978). Two crystalline forms, with purities greater than 99.9 and 99%, respectively, are available in Japan.

US government specifications for *chromium trioxide* are as follows: purity, 99.5% min; chloride, 0.10% max; sulphate, 0.20% max; water-insoluble materials, 0.10% max; particle size, 10% min. passes through -30 mesh ($<$590 μm US sieve) (Hartford, 1979). Two grades available from one company in Europe contain 20 and 100 mg/kg max. metallic impurities. Chromium trioxide is available in Japan in flake form (99.7% purity) and as a 60% solution.

Cobalt-chromium alloys are available commercially in the US as master alloys, stellites, superalloys and as Vitallium.

Master cobalt-chromium alloys typically contain 3.77% cobalt, 13.6% chromium and approximately 80% iron. They are usually combined with small amounts of vanadium, nickel or titanium for use in specific applications (Roskill Information Services, 1974).

Haynes stellites are available in several grades, with the following ranges of composition: cobalt, 35-55%; chromium 25-34%; tungsten, 3-20%; carbon, 0.5-2%; and up to 13% other elements. Other stellites have the following compositions (% by weight): carbon, 0.15-0.60; chromium, 17.5-30.0; nickel, 1.5-58.4; molybdenum, 3.5-7.0; tungsten, 3.5-16; cobalt, 30.0-68.8; and other elements, 0.01-4.0 (Cross, 1956).

Chromium-cobalt superalloys are available in several grades, with the following ranges of composition: cobalt, 36-68%; carbon, 0.1-0.85%; chromium, 3-29.5%; nickel, 0.28%; molybdenum, 0-5%; tungsten, 0-25%; tantalum, 0-9%; titanium, 0-4%; boron, 0-0.4%; zirconium, 0-2.25%; iron, 0-21%; and other elements, 0-4.3%.

Vitallium is available containing: 67.5% cobalt, 27% chromium, 5% molybdenum and 0.5% carbon (Sullivan *et al.*, 1970).

Ferrochromium is available in the US in several grades with the following compositions (% by weight) (Morning, 1976b):

Grade	Cr	Si	C	S	P
High-carbon	65-70	1-2	5-6.5	0.04	0.03
Charge chromium:					
50-55 percent chromium	50-55	3-6	6-8	0.04	0.03
66-70 percent chromium	66-70	3	5-6.5	0.04	0.03
Low-carbon					
0.025 percent carbon	67-75	1	0.025	0.025	0.03
0.05 percent carbon	67-75	1	0.05	0.025	0.03
Ferrochromium-silicon					
36/40 grade	35-37	39-41	0.05	—	—
40/43 grade	39-41	42-45	0.05	—	—

All single values are maximums. The difference between the sum of percentage shown and 100% is chiefly iron content.

The American Society for Testing and Materials' specifications for the *lead chromate* content of pigments containing it are: primrose chrome yellow, 50% min; lemon chrome yellow, 65% min; medium chrome yellow, 87% min; and chrome orange, 55% min (Hartford, 1979). Lead chromate is produced in Japan by two companies, with the following specifications: purity, 87 and 99.12% min; water, 1 and 0.04% max; chloride, no specification and 0.008% max; iron, no specification and 0.005% max; and water-soluble matter, 1 and 0.04% max.

No data on *lead chromate oxide* were available.

The following partial specifications were reported in 1956 (Copson, 1956) for the various grades of *potassium chromate* available in the US:

	Technical granular (%)	Chemically pure granular (%)	Chemically pure crystalline (%)
K_2CrO_4	99.8	99.9	99.3
Chloride (as Cl)	0.06	0.005	0.005
Sulphate (as SO_4)	0.1	0.05	0.05

In Japan, two grades are available, with 99.0 and 99.9% min. purity.

Technical *potassium dichromate* is available in the US in granular and powder forms, with the following typical analyses (Allied Chemical, 1973a):

	Granular	Powder
% Purity	99.9	99.9
% Chloride (as Cl)	0.03	0.03
% Sulphate (as SO_4)	0.006	0.006
% Insoluble material	0.007	0.01

Potassium dichromate available in Japan has a purity of 99.7%.

Technical-grade anhydrous *sodium chromate* available from one US company has the following typical analysis: purity, 99.5%; sulphates (as Na_2SO_4), 0.41%; chlorides (as NaCl), 0.02%; vanadium (as V), <0.001%; and water-insoluble materials, <0.01% (PPG Industries, 1978). Sodium chromate was also available as a chemically pure grade, as the tetrahydrate and in solutions (Copson, 1956). It is available in Japan in two grades, with 99.0 and 99.9% purity.

Technical-grade *sodium dichromate* is available in the US in crystalline form and as an aqueous solution, with the following typical analyses (Allied Chemical, 1973b):

	Granular	Solution
% Sodium dichromate dihydrate	100.5	69.1
% Chloride (as Cl)	0.02	0.20
% Sulphate (as SO_4)	0.05	0.17
% Vanadium (as V)	0.0015	0.013
mg/kg insoluble material	—	10

In Japan, technical-grade sodium dichromate is available in crystalline form as the dihydrate (99.5% purity) and as an aqueous solution containing $66 \pm 0.5\%$, calculated as the dihydrate.

A typical analysis of *strontium chromate* as produced by one company in the US is as follows: purity, 97.0%; moisture, 0.36%; chlorides (as Cl), 0.005%; iron (as Fe), 0.0025%; and barium (as Ba), 0.10% (Barium & Chemicals, Inc., 1978c). Strontium chromate available in Japan has the following specifications: chromium (as CrO_3), 44.0% min; strontium (as SrO), 47.0% min; moisture, 1% max; and water-soluble material, 4-7%.

Zinc chromate is available commercially in the US only in the form of basic zinc chromate. A typical analysis of basic zinc chromate is ZnO, 71.0% by weight; CrO_3, 17.0%; combined water, 10.0%; moisture, 1.5%; and total water-soluble salts, 0.2% (Lalor, 1973).

Technical *zinc chromate hydroxide* available in Japan has the following specifications: chromium (as CrO_3), 16-19%; zinc (as ZnO), 68-71%; moisture, 1% max; and water-soluble material, 0.2-0.6%.

Zinc potassium chromate available in Japan has the following specifications: chromium (as CrO_3), 43-46%; zinc (as ZnO), 37-40%; moisture, 1% max; water-soluble material, 5.5-7.5%.

Zinc yellow is available in the US in two grades which differ in their soluble salt contents (% by weight) (Lalor, 1973): Type I: ZnO, 3.60; CrO_3, 45.0; K_2O, 10.0; SO_3, <0.05; Cl, <0.05; and Type II: ZnO, 38.0; CrO_3, 44.0; K_2O, 10.0; SO_3, 1.0; Cl, 0.1. Both contain 6.0% water (combined) and 0.5% moisute and 0.1% acetic acid-insolubles.

2. Production, Use, Occurrence and Analysis

The early history of chromium compounds, including synthetic methods used in their preparation, was reviewed (Mellor, 1931).

2.1 Production and use

CHROMITE ORE

(a) Production

Mining of chromite ore started in the US in 1827, and the US produced most of the world's supply until 1860, when production in other countries became significant (Udy, M. J., 1956). World mine production of chromite ore in 1974 was about 7459 million kg, and preliminary figures for 1976 showed it to be about 8611 million kg (Morning, 1978). Table 3 gives the world production by country in 1976.

Table 3. World mine production of chromite ore by country[a]

Country[b]	Million kg
Albania	794
Brazil	172
Cuba	32
Cyprus	9
Egypt	1
Finland	414
Greece	27
India	401
Iran	160
Japan	22
Malagasy Republic	221
New Caledonia	10
Pakistan	11
Philippines	427
Rhodesia, Southern	608
South Africa, Republic of	2409
Sudan	22
Turkey	740
USSR	2120
Vietnam	9
Yugoslavia	2
Total	8611

[a] From Morning (1978)

[b] In addition to the countries listed, Argentina, Bulgaria, Colombia, North Korea and Thailand may also have produced chromite ore, but available information was inadequate for reliable estimates of production to be made.

In addition to the 22 million kg of chromite ore mined in Japan in 1976, 132 million kg were imported from India. The rate of production in Japan has been relatively constant since 1972, but quantitites imported have risen by about 3% per year.

Production in the US ceased in 1961 but was started again in 1976 (Morning, 1976a). However, current US production is believed to be negligible. In 1978, imports of chromite ore, containing a minimum of 46% chromic oxide, amounted to 8093 million kg; exports of chromite ore in that year totalled 20.9 million kg (US Department of Commerce, 1979).

No information was available on whether it is produced elsewhere as well.

(b)   Use

Use of chromite ore in the US decreased from 1315 million kg in 1974 to 912 million kg in 1976, when utilization by the three consuming industries was as follows: metallurgical, 59.3%; refractory, 20.1%; and chemical, 20.6% (Morning, 1978).

The metallurgical grade is used primarily to produce ferrochromium alloys, which are used as additives in the production of stainless and other special steels (Bacon, 1964). The major use of chromite refractory materials is in iron and steel processing, nonferrous alloy refining, glass-making and cement processing (Morning, 1975). Chemical-grade chromite ore is converted (by a series of operations involving roasting with soda ash and/or lime and leaching, with appropriate control of acidity) to sodium dichromate, used as such and in the production of many other chromium chemicals (Copson, 1956).

The major use of chromite ore in Japan is in the production of ferrochromium (90%), the balance being used in the manufacture of refractory materials (6%), chromium compounds (3%) and chromium metal (1%).

CHROMIUM

(a)   Production

Chromium is made commercially in the US by two processes: (1) an electrolytic method in which a chromium-containing electrolyte, prepared by dissolving a high-carbon ferrochromium in a solution of sulphuric acid and chromium potassium sulphate, is subjected to electrolysis; and (2) an aluminothermic reduction method in which chromic oxide is reduced with finely divided aluminium.

In 1970, US production of chromium metal and metal alloys, other than ferrochromium alloys, was 14 million kg; about 75% was made by the electrolytic method. This included production of chromium briquets, exothermic chromium additives and miscellaneous chromium alloys, in addition to chromium metal. By 1976, US production had increased to 18 million kg (Morning, 1978). In 1977, combined US imports of chromium metal from the UK, Japan and France were 2.2 million kg (US Department of Commerce, 1978). In 1978, US exports of chromium (including unwrought, wrought and scrap) were 1.02 million kg (US Department of Commerce, 1979).

Chromium metal has been produced in Japan since 1956. It is manufactured by electrolysis of an ammonium chromic sulphate solution. About 9 million kg were produced in 1977; there were no exports or imports.

No information was available on whether it is produced elsewhere as well.

(b)   Use

Chromium metal and metal alloys are used primarily in stainless and heat-resisting steel and alloy steel. They are used in alloys to impart strength, hardness and resistance to corrosion, oxidation, wear and heat.

In 1976, 70% (264 million kg) of all US chromium alloys were used in stainless steel. Of the total of chromium metal and alloys used in the production of commercial alloys, about 60% was in high-carbon ferrochromium, 25% in low-carbon ferrochromium, 16% in ferrochromium-silicon, 3% in other alloys and 1% in chromium metal (Morning, 1978).

The only current use for chromium in Japan is in the production of alloys, but future use is expected to include chromium-plating.

BARIUM CHROMATE

(a)   Production

Barium chromate is produced commercially by the reaction of barium chloride with sodium chromate (Copson, 1956). Five companies in the US produce this chemical, but no data were available. Barium chromate is produced by one company in Japan; production in 1977 is estimated to have been less than 50 thousand kg; there were no exports or imports. Available information indicated that barium chromate is also produced by one company in Spain, two companies in Belgium, three companies in France and by four companies in each of the Federal Republic of Germany, Italy and the UK, although it may be produced elsewhere as well.

(b)   Use

Barium chromate is used in pyrotechnics and in high-temperature batteries (Hartford, 1979). In Japan, the principal use is believed to be in explosive fuses.

BASIC CHROMIC SULPHATE (see CHROMIUM SULPHATE, below)

CALCIUM CHROMATE

(a)   Production

Calcium chromate is produced commercially by the reaction of calcium chloride with sodium chromate. Hydrated forms can be made, but the anhydrous salt is the only product of commercial significance.

Four companies in the US produce this chemical, but no data were available. Calcium chromate was formerly produced in Japan at an annual rate of about 100 thousand kg, but during the last few years it has been produced in only small amounts for reagent use. Available information indicated that it is also produced by one company in the UK, although it may be produced elsewhere as well.

(b)   Use

Calcium chromate is largely used as a corrosion inhibitor and as a depolarizer in batteries. Its use in protective coatings for steel and light metals is sometimes reported as a pigment use, but its primary function in these products is that of a corrosion inhibitor. The use of calcium chromate as a pigment was discontinued in Japan several years ago.

CHROMIC ACETATE

(a)   Production

Solutions of chromic acetate are produced by dissolving freshly-prepared hydrous chromic oxide in acetic acid. Commercial mixtures of chromic acetate with sodium acetate are prepared by reduction of sodium dichromate with glucose or corn sugar in the presence of acetic acid (Copson, 1956).

Five companies in the US produce this chemical, but no data on production levels were available. Annual production in Japan is about 30 thousand kg. Available information indicated that chromic acetate is also produced by one company in the Federal Republic of Germany, two in Italy, three in France and four in the UK, although it may be produced elsewhere as well.

(b) Use

Chromic acetate is used in printing and dyeing textiles (Howarth, 1956). Most of the chromic acetate produced in Japan is used in dyeing processes.

CHROMIC CHLORIDE

(a) Production

Chromic chloride hexahydrate is prepared by dissolving freshly-made hydrous chromic oxide in hydrochloric acid. Anhydrous chromic chloride can be produced by passing chlorine over a mixture of chromic oxide and carbon (Hawley, 1977).

Two companies in the US produce this chemical, but no data on production levels were available. In Japan, chromic chloride is produced from chromic sulphate by conversion to purified chromic carbonate, which is treated with hydrochloric acid. About 100 thousand kg of the chemical were produced by one Japanese company in 1977; there were no imports or exports. Available information indicated that chromic chloride is also produced by one company in the Federal Republic of Germany, two in Italy and four in the UK, although it may be produced elsewhere as well.

(b) Use

Chromic chloride is used for the production of commercial solutions of the basic chlorides [$Cr(OH)Cl_2$, $Cr(OH)_2Cl$] by reaction with sodium hydroxide. In 1956, these solutions were reported to have minor special applications, such as use as a mordant for alizarin dyes on cotton yarn and certain cyamine dyes on silk. They are also used in Japan for decorative chromium plating.

Anhydrous chromic chloride is used as a catalyst for polymerizing olefins, for chromium plating (including vapour plating) and for preparing sponge chromium (Hawley, 1977).

CHROMIC OXIDE

(a) Production

The anhydrous material is produced industrially by heating chromic hydroxide, by heating dry ammonium dichromate, or by heating sodium dichromate with sulphur and washing out the sodium sulphate. The hydrated material is made commercially by calcining sodium dichromate with boric acid and hydrolysing the resulting chromic borate.

Six companies in the US produce this chemical. US production of the most important type of chromic oxide, chromic oxide green, was reported to be about 6 million kg in 1971, about 3.7 million kg in 1976 and 2.7 million kg in 1977 (Hartford, 1979). US imports of chromic oxide green in 1977 were about 948 thousand kg, primarily from the UK, Japan, Poland and the Federal Republic of Germany (US Department of Commerce, 1978).

Chromic oxide is produced in Japan by two companies, either by heating hydrous chromic oxide or chromium trioxide or by reducing sodium dichromate with carbon. An estimated 2.7 million kg were produced in 1977 (only a slight increase over 1974 production). Imports, consisting of chromic oxide and hydrated chromic oxide, amounted to 3.1 million kg in 1977, compared with 1.6 million kg in 1974; exports increased from 3.3 million in 1974 to 5.3 million kg in 1977.

Available information indicated that it is also produced by approximately 30 companies in western Europe, although it may be produced elsewhere as well.

(b) Use

The major portion of chromic oxide (anhydrous and hydrated) is used as a pigment. A substantial portion is also used in metallurgy and, to a lesser extent, as a catalyst, in refractory brick, and as a chemical intermediate.

Anhydrous chromic oxide is the most stable green pigment known and is used in applications requiring heat-, light- and chemical-resistance (e.g., in glass and ceramics). It is used in dyeing polymers, and its resistance to alkali makes it a valuable colourant for latex paints. It has special use in colouring Portland cement, granules for asphalt roofing and in camouflage paints. Metallurgical-grade anhydrous chromic oxide is used in the manufacture of chromium metal and aluminium-chromium master alloys. It is used as a catalyst in the preparation of methanol, butadiene and high-density polyethylene. Chromic oxide is used in refractory brick as a minor component to improve performance. When used as a mild abrasive for polishing jewellery and fine metal parts, it is known as 'green rouge'.

Hydrated chromic oxide is also used as a green pigment, especially for automotive finishes.

In Japan, chromic oxide is used for the production of refractory materials (36%), pigments (35%), abrasives (15%), and other uses such as glaze for glass (14%).

CHROMIC PHOSPHATE

(a) Production

A violet hexahydrate form of chromic phosphate is formed by mixing cold solutions of potassium chromium sulphate (chrome alum) with disodium phosphate. A green crystalline dihydrate is obtained by boiling the violet hexahydrate with acetic anhydride or by heating it in dry air (Udy, M.C., 1956).

Chromic phosphate is made by one company in the US; it is not produced commercially in Japan. Available information indicated that it is also produced by one comany in each of The Netherlands, Spain and the UK, two companies in France and three companies in the Federal Republic of Germany, although it may be produced elsewhere as well.

(b) Use

Chromic phosphate is used in pigments, phosphate coatings and wash primers (Hartford, 1979).

CHROMIUM CARBONYL

(a) Production

Chromium carbonyl is produced by the reaction of carbon monoxide with chromic chloride and aluminium metal. Two companies in the US produce this chemical, but no data on production levels were available. No information was available on whether chromium carbonyl is produced elsewhere as well.

(b) Use

There is no known commercial use for chromium carbonyl, but it is reported to be useful for the synthesis of 'sandwich' compounds from aromatic hydrocarbons (such as dibenzene chromium from benzene). Some of these compounds have been investigated as possible sources of vapour-deposited chromium and for the production of carbides (Hartford, 1979).

CHROMIUM POTASSIUM SULPHATE

(a) Production

Chromium potassium sulphate is produced commercially by the reduction of potassium dichromate with sulphur dioxide (Copson, 1956).

Two companies produce this chemical in the US, but no data on production levels were available. Chromium potassium sulphate was first produced commercially in Japan before 1940. Production reached a level of about 20-30 thousand kg in 1970; subsequently, the annual quantity produced decreased rapidly, and only about 1000 kg were produced in 1977.

Available information indicated that it is also produced by one company in France, two companies in each of the Federal Republic of Germany, Italy and Spain and four companies in the UK, although it may be produced elsewhere as well.

(b)   Use

Chromium potassium sulphate was reported in 1956 to be used as a mordant for wool prior to application of mordant dyes. It is also used to treat cotton which has been dyed with certain direct cotton dyes and sulphur dyes, rendering the dyed textile faster to washing. Another important application is in the preparation of hydrous chromic oxide which, in turn, is used to make many of the trivalent chromium mordants (Howarth, 1956).

This chemical is also used for hardening photographic emulsions (Hartford, 1979).

CHROMIUM SULPHATE

(a)   Production

Solutions of mixed hydrated chromic sulphates are obtained by dissolving hydrous chromic oxide in concentrated sulphuric acid and allowing it to stand until crystals of the hydrated chromic sulphate separate. The anhydrous form is produced by heating any of the hydrates to 400°C in air or to 280°C in a stream of carbon dioxide.

Mixtures of basic chromic sulphates [containing mainly $Cr(OH)SO_4$] with sodium sulphate are produced commercially by the organic reduction (with such substances as molasses) of a solution of sodium dichromate in the presence of sulphuric acid or by reduction of dichromate solutions with sulphur dioxide (Copson, 1956).

Three companies in the US produce chromium sulphate in research quantities, and one produces basic chromic sulphate, but no data were available.

Both chromium sulphate and basic chromic sulphate have been produced in Japan since about 1950. The process involves reduction of sodium dichromate with glucose. The combined production of the two producers of basic chromic sulphate in Japan was about 2 million kg in 1977. The combined production of the two producers of chromium sulphate was about 120 thousand kg in 1977.

Available information indicated that chromium sulphate is also produced by about 30 companies in western Europe, although it may be produced elsewhere as well.

(b) Use

Chromium sulphate is used as a mordant for textile dyeing. The basic chromic sulphates are the principal chemicals used in chrome tanning of leather (Darrin, 1956).

CHROMIUM TRIOXIDE

(a) Production

Chromium trioxide is produced commercially by the reaction of sodium dichromate with concentrated sulphuric acid.

In 1978, there were two US producers of chromium trioxide, each with a capacity to produce 18 million kg per year (Anon., 1978). The annual US production rate in 1973, 1976 and 1977 was in the range of 26 million kg (Hartford, 1979). US exports in 1977 were 4 million kg, and imports were 224 thousand kg, mostly from the Federal Republic of Germany (US Department of Commerce, 1978).

Commercial production in Japan was started before 1940. It is produced there by the reaction of sodium dichromate with sulphuric acid. In 1977, three companies produced a total of 8.3 million kg, of which 1.2 million kg were exported; there were no imports.

Available information indicated that chromium trioxide is also produced by about 15 companies in western Europe, although it may be produced elsewhere as well.

(b) Use

Use of chromium trioxide in the US amounted to 31 million kg in 1977 and 31.5 million in 1978; it is projected to reach 34 million kg in 1982 (Anon., 1978).

The major use of chromium trioxide is in chromium plating, particularly in the production of automobiles. Additional uses in other metal-finishing operations include aluminium anodizing, which has been used extensively on military aircraft assemblies; chemical conversion coatings, which provide both decoration and corrosion protection; and the production of phosphate films on galvanized iron or steel. Important non-plating uses of chromium trioxide include use as a corrosion inhibitor for ferrous alloys in recirculating water systems, as an oxidant in organic synthesis and in catalyst manufacture. Small amounts are used to modify the properties of basic magnesite refractories.

The pattern of use in the US in 1978 is estimated to have been as follows: metal treating and plating, 80%; wood treatment, 10%; chemical manufacturing, 5%; and other, 5% (Anon., 1978).

In Japan, the major use of chromium trioxide is in chromium plating (90%); 3% is used in pigments and 7% in other uses such as abrasives. The total used in Japan dropped from 11.8 million kg in 1972 to 8.3 million kg in 1977.

COBALT-CHROMIUM ALLOY

(a) Production

Cobalt-chromium alloys were first made in 1907 by fusion of cobalt with 10-60% chromium (Haynes, 1907; Sibley, 1976). Commercial production began shortly thereafter, and since 1920 more than 75% of the cobalt used in the US has been for the manufacture of alloys with chromium (Sibley, 1976).

Eight US companies produced chromium alloys in 1975 (the last year for which information is available), but no separate data on the quantity of cobalt-chromium alloys produced were available (Morning, 1976). Stellite has been produced by one company in the UK (Roskill Information Service, 1974). These alloys may be produced elsewhere as well.

(b) Use

Cobalt-chromium alloys were originally developed for use in cutting tools. Subsequently, because of their corrosion resistance, they have also been used for equipment in contact with acids and other chemicals. They are used for facing valves and seats in internal combustion engines; wearing surfaces or cutting edges of hot shears, trimming dies, cam gauges, punches and turbine blades; pipeline linings; and pumps for corrosive liquids. Stellite alloys are used in mirrors. The superalloys are used for turbine discs and blades and nozzle vanes in jet engines; grates and quenching baskets in furnaces; and high-temperaure springs and fasteners (Roskill Information Services, 1974). Vitallium alloy is most commonly used as a denture alloy (Sullivan *et al.*, 1970).

FERROCHROMIUM

(a)   Production

Ferroalloys were produced in the mid-1890s by the addition of ferrosilicon to steel to achieve complete deoxidation (Matthews, 1976). High-carbon ferrochromium is produced by reducing chromite with coke in submerged-arc furnaces. Medium-carbon ferrochromium is produced from the high-carbon material, usually by refining in an open-arc furnace with chromite and adding lime, silicon and fluorospar, or by blowing with oxygen in a Bessemer converter.

In one process, low-carbon ferrochromium is made in two stages: (1) production of high-silicon ferrochromium in a submerged-arc furnace, either by direct smelting of chromite, quartz and coke or by smelting high-carbon ferrochromium with quartz and coke; and (2) either crushing and mixing the high-silicon ferrochromium with ore, lime and fluorospar with subsequent open-arc furnace refining using sodium nitrate as an oxidant, or reacting the high-silicon ferrochromium with a molten mixture of ore and lime with subsequent refining. In another process for low-carbon ferrochromium, high-carbon ferrochromium is crushed and briquetted with an oxidant, and the briquettes are heated in a vacuum at a programmed rate (Roskill Information Services, 1974).

Ferroalloys were being produced commercially in the US by 1900 (Matthews, 1976), but no specific information on ferrochromium was found. Five US companies produce it: US production in 1976 was 25.6 million kg of low-carbon ferrochromium and 151.7 million kg high-carbon ferrochromium. In 1976, US imports were 162.6 million kg 3% min carbon ferrochromium and 58 million kg of 3% max carbon ferrochromium. Total US exports of ferrochromium in 1976 were 12 million kg (Jones, 1978).

Data on world production of ferrochromium alloys in electric furnaces in 1976 is summarized in Table 4.

(b)   Use

Ferrochromium is used primarily in the production of stainless and heat-resisting steels. These are used mostly in corrosive environments (such as petrochemical processing), high-temperature environments (such as turbines and furnace parts) and in consumer goods (such as cutlery and decorative trims). Ferrochromium is also used as a constituent of iron coatings, steels and superalloys. Because of their resistance to oxidation and corrosion at high temperatures, the superalloys are used in jet engines, gas turbines and chemical processing equipment.(Johnson, 1974).

Table 4. World production of ferrochromium alloys in electric furnaces in 1976 by country[a]

Country	Production (million kg)	Number of producers
Australia[b]	3.6	1
Brazil	65.5	1
Finland	40.0	1
France[c]	101.8	1
Germany, Federal Republic of	—	1
India	14.5	2
Italy	45.5	2
Japan	464.5	7
Norway	27.3	1
Philippines		1
Rhodesia, Southern		3
South Africa, Republic of	239.1	5
Spain	19.1	1
Sweden	120.0	3
Turkey	9.1	1
USSR	210.0	—
US	177.3	5
Yugoslavia	55.5	—
TOTAL[d]	1.8 billion kg	

[a]From Jones (1978) and Morning (1977)
[b]1975 data
[c]Includes ferrochromium-silicon
[d]Totals may not add up due to rounding off

The US consumption pattern for ferrochromium in 1976 was as follows: stainless and heat-resisting steel, 68%; steel alloys, 20%; cast iron, 3%; superalloys, 3%; alloys (except steels and superalloys), 2%; carbon steel, 1%; tool steel, 1%; and miscellaneous uses, 1% (Jones, 1978).

LEAD CHROMATE

(a) Production

Lead chromate can be produced by reacting sodium chromate with lead nitrate, or by reacting lead monoxide with chromic acid solution. Details of the various commercial processes for the manufacture of lead chromates are not generally revealed by the producers. By varying the proportion of reactants, either lead chromate ($PbCrO_4$) or lead chromate oxide ($PbO.PbCrO_4$) can be produced. High-lead chromate content is associated with the yellow pigments; increasing the lead chromate oxide content gives orange colours; and mixing with lead molybdate gives red pigments (Chalupski, 1956).

US production data for lead chromate are not available; however, the combined production of chrome yellow and chrome orange amounted to 29.4 million kg in 1970 and 28.2 million kg in 1977 (Hartford, 1979). Assuming an average of 70% lead chromate in these pigments, about 20 million kg of lead chromate were produced in the US or imported for use in these pigments in 1977. US imports of chrome yellow amounted to 2.6 million kg in 1977, mostly from Canada but also from the Federal Republic of Germany and Japan (US Department of Commerce, 1978).

Commercial production in Japan was started in about 1910, and there are now three major producers and one minor producer. Production in 1977 was 10.8 million kg, and exports were 1.8 million kg. This represents a substantial decrease in production, from 17 million kg in 1973 (when exports were also greater).

Available information indicated that lead chromate is produced by about 30 companies in western Europe, although it may be produced elsewhere as well.

(b) Use

Lead chromate is used to make pigments for paints for both wood and metal. Chrome yellows (containing 52-98% lead chromate) are considered to be the most versatile of the inorganic pigments and are therefore found in many formulations designed for a wide spectrum of uses. The largest use of chrome yellows in the early 1970s was in paint for automotive finishes, farm machinery, architectural and air-dried finishes, and water-thinned coatings for exterior and interior use. Medium chrome yellow paints make up about 30% of the paint used for traffic control. Chrome yellows are also used as colourants in vinyls, rubber and paper. The second largest use of chrome yellows is in printing inks (Schiek, 1973).

The major use for lead chromate in Japan is in production of pigments for paint and inks (85%); other uses include application as a colourant for synthetic resins (14%) and in miscellaneous uses (1%).

LEAD CHROMATE OXIDE

(a) Production

Lead chromate oxide is produced by the reaction of lead oxide with sodium dichromate in the presence of acetic acid or by the reaction of lead nitrate with sodium chromate in the presence of sodium carbonate (Chalupski, 1956).

US production data for lead chromate oxide are not available; however, the combined production of chrome yellow and chrome orange, containing varying proportions of lead chromate oxide, amounted to 29.4 million kg in 1970 and 28.2 million kg in 1977 (Hartford, 1979).

Lead chromate oxide is formed during the production of lead chromate in Japan, but no data on production levels were available.

Available information indicated that lead chromate oxide is also produced by one company in Belgium, two in Italy and four in the Federal Republic of Germany, although it may be produced elsewhere as well.

(b) Use

Chrome orange pigments, consisting largely of lead chromate oxide, have been widely used in paints, metal protective primers and linoleum (Chalupski, 1956). In the early 1970s, use of chrome oranges in the US was decreasing, although they were still being used in tints and rust-inhibiting paints (Schiek, 1973). The lead chromate oxide produced in Japan is used primarily as a pigment.

POTASSIUM CHROMATE

(a) Production

Potassium chromate is produced by the reaction of potassium dichromate with potassium hydroxide or potassium carbonate. Combined US production of potassium dichromate and potassium chromate in 1966 was estimated at 2.6-3.8 million kg, with the potassium dichromate believed to be the more important industrially.

There is one US producer, but no data were available. Combined US imports of potassium chromate and potassium dichromate amounted to 2.7 thousand kg in 1977 (US Department of Commerce, 1978). The two Japanese producers made about 1000 kg in 1977 for reagent uses; there were no exports or imports. Available information indicated that potassium chromate is also produced by one company in each of the Federal Republic of Germany, Italy and Switzerland and by 5 companies in the UK, although it may be produced elsewhere as well.

(b) Use

Because of the higher cost of potassium chromate, compared with sodium chromate, its application in the textile industry is limited to special cases in which a potassium rather than a sodium salt is essential, or in which differences in solubility or other physical properties make its use desirable (Howarth, 1956). Among these uses are as a mordant for wool, in dyeing nylon and wool with mordant acid dyes, in oxidizing vat dyes and indigosol dyes on wool, in dyeing with chromate colours, in treating direct dyes and some sulphur dyes on cotton to render them faster to washing, in oxidizing aniline black, and in stripping dyed wool.

POTASSIUM DICHROMATE

(a) Production

Potassium dichromate is produced industrially by roasting chrome ore with potassium carbonate, or, preferably, by reacting sodium dichromate with potassium chloride. Combined US production of potassium dichromate and potassium chromate in 1966 was estimated to be 2.6-3.8 million kg, with the potassium dichromate believed to be the more important industrially.

Two companies in the US are believed to produce a reagent grade, and one produces a technical grade, but no production data were available. Combined US imports of potassium chromate and dichromate amounted to 2.7 thousand kg in 1977 (US Department of Commerce, 1978).

It was first produced commercially in Japan before 1940. Production by two companies in 1978 amounted to about 1 million kg, well below the 3.2 million kg level of 1972 and below the 1977 level of 1.4 million kg. Exports are believed to be minor.

Available information indicated that potassium dichromate is also produced by about 15 companies in western Europe, although it may be produced elsewhere as well.

(b)   Use

Potassium dichromate was once the most important chromium compound, but it has been largely replaced in many applications by sodium dichromate. It is used in a large number of small volume applications; probably the largest uses are photomechanical processing, chrome-pigment production and wool preservative formulations.

The major use for potassium dichromate in Japan is pigment production (54%); dye manufacture consumes an estimated 22%, with the remaining 24% used as an oxidizing agent in miscellaneous uses (as a catalyst and in other applications).

SODIUM CHROMATE

(a)   Production

Sodium chromate is produced commercially by roasting chromite ore (a chromium iron oxide) with sodium carbonate, or with sodium carbonate and calcium oxide and leaching to dissolve the sodium chromate. After treatment to remove hydrated alumina, the sodium chromate solution is either marketed directly or evaporated to produced hydrated or anhydrous crystals (Hartford & Copson, 1964). Sodium chromate may also be produced from sodium dichromate by treatment with sodium hydroxide.

Two companies produce sodium chromate in the US. In 1978, the estimated combined US production of sodium chromate and sodium dichromate was 159 million kg. Combined exports in 1977 were 14 million kg; combined imports were 102 thousand kg (US Department of Commerce, 1978).

Commercial production in Japan started before 1940. Production in 1977 by the two producing companies was less than 10 thousand kg.

Available information indicated that sodium chromate is also produced by one company in each of Italy and Spain, two companies in the Federal Republic of Germany and four companies in the UK; although it may be produced elsewhere as well.

(b)   Use

Sodium chromate is used in leather tanning, wood preservation, corrosion inhibition, pigment manufacture, and as a raw material for production of other chromium compounds (Hawley, 1977). In Japan, its principal use is as a mordant in dyeing operations.

SODIUM DICHROMATE

(a) Production

Sodium dichromate is produced industrially by the reaction of sulphuric acid with sodium chromate.

Three companies produce sodium dichromate in the US. The combined US production of sodium chromate and sodium dichromate increased from 123 million kg in 1967 to 142-144 million kg in 1973, 1976 and 1977 (Hartford, 1979). In 1977, combined US exports of sodium chromate and sodium dichromate amounted to 14 million kg, and combined imports were 102 thousand kg (US Department of Commerce, 1978).

It was first produced commercially in Japan in about 1908. In 1978, the combined production of two companies was estimated to be 20.7 million kg, slightly below the 1977 level of 21 million kg.

Available information indicated that sodium dichromate is also produced by about 15 companies in western Europe, although it may be produced elsewhere as well.

(b) Use

Use of sodium dichromate in the US amounted to 146 million kg in 1978 and 147 million kg in 1979 and is projected to reach 153 million kg in 1983. The pattern of use in the US in 1978 was as follows: manufacture of chromic acid, 28%; manufacture of pigments, 24%; leather tanning, 17%; corrosion control, 7%; metal treatment, drilling muds and textiles, 8%; and miscellaneous uses (chemical manufacture, catalysts, wood preservatives and other), 16% (Anon., 1979).

The major use for sodium dichromate (57% of the total) in Japan is in chrome tanning; other uses include pigment manufacture, 31%; dye manufacture, 48%; and other uses (including use as an oxidizing agent in chemical manufacture, and as a catalyst), 8%.

STRONTIUM CHROMATE

(a) Production

Strontium chromate is prepared from strontium chloride and sodium chromate (Hartford & Copson, 1964).

Three US companies manufacture it; 1970 production was estimated to be 680 thousand kg and rising at the rate of 5% per year (Lalor, 1973). US imports in 1977 amounted to 242 thousand kg, essentially all from Canada (US Department of Commerce, 1978).

Production in Japan began after 1940. The combined production of three companies in 1977 was about 600 thousand kg, comparable with that of the previous seven years. No exports or imports were reported.

Available information indicated that strontium chromate is also produced by about 15 companies in western Europe, although it may be produced elsewhere as well.

(b) Use

Strontium chromate was first used commercially (near the end of the nineteenth century) as a colourant in artists' paints under the name 'citron yellow'. It was replaced for this use by organic pigments in 1936, at which time it was also being used for corrosion resistance on aluminium and magnesium alloys. Later, it was used in chemical-resistant coatings because of its low reactivity, and in epoxy-polyamide vehicles and vinyl sheeting because of its heat-resistant properties.

In 1973, some strontium chromate was still used in vinyl sheeting and chemical-resistant coatings and in primer coatings for water tanks, but most of it was used, either alone or in combination with basic zinc chromate, in wash primers or in aluminium flake coatings (Lalor, 1973).

Strontium chromate has also been used as an additive to control the sulphate content of solutions in electrochemical processes (Hartford & Copson, 1964).

In Japan, the only known use is as a corrosion inhibitor.

ZINC CHROMATE

(a) Production

Basic zinc chromate was first developed as a commercial product in 1940 (Lalor, 1973). It is prepared by adding a solution of chromic acid to a slurry of zinc oxide or zinc hydroxide.

In 1979, there were three producers of basic zinc chromate in the US. It is believed that many of the western European producers of zinc yellow also produce basic zinc chromate; it may be produced elsewhere as well.

No quantitative data on production, imports or exports were available to the Working Group.

(b) Use

All of the basic zinc chromate produced is used in surface coatings as a corrosion-resistant primer coating or in metal conditioners (wash primers) applied before priming (Lalor, 1973).

ZINC CHROMATE HYDROXIDE

(a) Production

Zinc chromate hydroxide is produced by the reaction of zinc oxide and chromium trioxide in aqueous solution. Estimated US production in 1970 was 450 thousand kg and was rising at a rate of about 5% per year (Lalor, 1973). More recent data are not available.

Zinc chromate hydroxide was first produced in Japan in about 1950. In 1977, three companies produced a combined total of about 900 thousand kg, compared with about 1.3 million kg in 1973. No information was available on whether it is produced elsewhere as well.

(b) Use

Zinc chromate hydroxide is used as a pigment in paints, varnishes, oil colours, linoleum and rubber (Windholz, 1976). It is an ingredient, along with phosphoric acid and polyvinyl butyral, of a wash primer designated WP #1, developed in the US during World War II (Wash primers are used to pretreat metals before the application of a conventional primer) (Lalor, 1973).

The only known use of zinc chromate hydroxide in Japan is in the manufacture of corrosion-inhibiting pigments.

ZINC POTASSIUM CHROMATE

(a) Production

Zinc potassium chromate is produced by the reaction of potassium dichromate with zinc oxide and sulphuric or hydrochloric acids (Chalupski, 1956).

Two US companies produce this chemical. During World War II, the annual US production rate for zinc yellow, a pigment based on zinc potassium chromate, was 11 million kg, a level not reached since that period (Hartford, 1979). US production of zinc chromate pigment in 1970 was about 8 million kg (Lalor, 1973).

Zinc potassium chromate was first produced in Japan in about 1950. It is manufactured there by the reaction of zinc oxide with potassium dichromate and chromium trioxide. The combined production of three Japanese companies in 1977 was about 900 thousand kg, down from about 1.3 million kg in 1973. There were no exports or imports.

Available information indicated that zinc potassium chromate is also produced by about 15 companies in western Europe, although it may be produced elsewhere as well.

(b) Use

Zinc potassium chromate is used in corrosion inhibiting paints and artists' colours (Hawley, 1977). It is reported to be the best corrosion-inhibiting pigment for primers on aircraft parts fabricated from aluminium or magnesium and is specified by the US Navy for use in many applications. It is used in structural steel priming, as well as in combination with ferric oxide pigments, and is also an ingredient of dips for automotive bodies (Hartford & Copson, 1964).

In Japan, the only known use for zinc potassium chromate is in the manufacture of corrosion-inhibiting pigments.

ZINC YELLOW

(a) Production

Zinc yellow has been known since the early 1800s and was first suggested for paint use in 1829. Zinc yellow (Type I) is prepared by the addition of a sodium dichromate solution to a slurry of zinc oxide immediately after potassium chloride has been added (Lalor, 1973). The relative proportions of the coreactants determine the colour, tinting characteristics and other properties of the pigment.

Commercial production of zinc yellow in the US probably began during or just before World War II, when demand for anti-corrosion marine paints was high (Lalor, 1973): production during that period reached 11 million kg annually. Currently, there are believed to be three major producers of zinc yellow in the US. Production levels of Types I and II in 1976 and 1977 were 2.5 million kg and 1.7 million kg, respectively (Hartford, 1979). US imports amounted to 1.5 million kg in 1977, mainly from Norway, Canada, Poland and France (US Department of Commerce, 1978); imports in 1979 were also approximately 1.5 million kg; separate data on exports were not available.

Available information indicated that zinc yellow is also produced by three companies in each of France and the Federal Republic of Germany; two each in Spain and Belgium; and one each in Portugal, The Netherlands and the UK; although it may be produced elsewhere as well.

(b) Use

The major use of zinc yellow is as an anti-corrosion pigment in primers for metal surfaces. It is also used as a colouring agent in linoleum, rubber, artists' oil paints and plastics (acrylics, cellulosics and general-purpose polystyrene).

2.2 Regulatory status (see also preamble, p. 21)

The 1970 WHO European and 1978 Japanese standard for Cr[VI] in drinking-water (Ministry of Health & Welfare, 1978; WHO, 1970) and the European standard for chromium in surface water intended for the abstraction of drinking-water (EEC, 1975) is 0.05 mg/l. The US Environmental Protection Agency has established a maximim contaminant level for chromium in drinking-water, also of 0.05 mg/l (US Environmental Protection Agency, 1978). This is the maximum permissible level in water delivered to any user of a public water system.

The US Environmental Protection Agency has also established pretreatment standards that establish the concentration of chromium which may be introduced into a publicly owned waste-treatment works by leather tanning and finishing plants. The maximum total chromium permitted for existing sources in any one day is 6 mg/l, and the average daily values for 10 consecutive days shall not exceed 3 mg/l (US Environmental Protection Agency, 1979).

According to the US Occupational Safety & Health Administration's (1978) health standards for air contaminants, an employee's exposure to chromium in the form of soluble chromic or chromous salts should not exceed an 8-hour time-weighted average of 0.5 mg/m^3 (as Cr); in the form of chromium metal or insoluble salts it should not exceed an 8-hour time-weighted average of 1 mg/m^3 in the workplace air in any 8-hour work shift of a 40-hour work week. The time-weighted average allowable concentrations for chromic acid and chromates (as Cr) in Sweden and Czechoslovakia are 0.05 mg/m^3; the ceiling concentration in the USSR is 0.01 mg/m^3 (Winell, 1975).

In Japan, 'tolerance concentrations' have been established for occupational exposure to chromium chemicals as follows: 0.1 mg/m^3 (as CrO_3) for barium chromate, calcium chromate, lead chromate, potassium chromate, potassium dichromate, sodium chromate, sodium dichromate and strontium chromate; 0.5 mg/m^3 (as CrO_3) for chromic chloride; 1.0 mg/m^3 for chromium sulphate; and 5 mg/m^3 (as CrO_3) for zinc chromate hydroxide and zinc potassium chromate.

2.3 Occurrence

(a) Natural environment

Chromium is widely distributed in the earth's crust but is concentrated in the extremely basic rocks. At an overall crust concentration of 125 mg/kg Cr, it is the twentieth most abundant element (Hartford, 1979), ranking with vanadium, zinc, copper and tungsten. Only the trivalent and hexavalent compounds are detected in the environment in significant quantities (Fishbein, 1976). Chromium is found in nature only in the combined state and not as the free metal. It exists mainly as chromite, which has the idealized composition $FeO.Cr_2O_3$, although this composition has been found in nature only in meteorites. Chromite usually has the formula $(Fe, Mg) (Cr, Al, Fe)_2O_4$ (Hartford, 1963) and as such is found in considerable quantities in Rhodesia, the USSR, South Africa, New Caledonia and the Philippines; it contains 40-50% chromium (Bidstrup & Case, 1956).

Of the chromium chemicals (other than chromite ore) included in this monograph, only two are known to occur in nature in mineral form: lead chromate as crocoite and potassium dichromate as lopezite (Hartford, 1963). Cobalt-chromium alloys and ferrochromium are not known to occur in nature.

(b) Air

Falk (1970) found a chromium content (as metal) of 15 ng/m³ in the particulates of air samples taken in the US in 1964 and 1965. Generally, the concentration in air is between 0.002-0.02 $\mu g/m^3$. Current data on chromium concentrations in the ambient air of major urban areas in the US are apparently inadequate to depict trends accurately, although there appears to be a slight downward trend since 1960 in 20 of the larger industrialized areas. In 1966, only 7/58 cities in the National Air Sampling Network had annual average chromium levels of 0.01 $\mu g/m^3$ or more, and only 16 had maximum single values above that level. Approximately 200 urban stations in the US during 1960-1969 had annual mean concentrations of 0.01-0.03 $\mu g/m^3$ (The minimum level detectable was 0.01 $\mu g/m^3$). In nonurban areas, the level of chromium was less than 0.01 $\mu g/m^3$. Levels of 0.9-21.5 $\mu g/m^3$ were reported in 23 localities in northern England and Wales in 1956-1958 . Analysis of chromium in the air of cities has failed to reveal seasonal variations (Fishbein, 1976).

In the period 1957-1974 the amount of chromium contained in the atmospheric aerosol at a rural site in the UK declined at an average yearly rate of 11.3% (Salmon et al., 1977).

During the period May 1972-April 1975, the range of average levels of chromium determined at 15 stations in Belgium was 0.01-0.04 $\mu g/m^3$. The data are reported to reflect background pollution and the levels that are representative of the air inhaled by the majority of the population. Sampling station locations were selected to avoid, as much as possible, the direct influence of local sources (Kretzschmar et al., 1977).

Coal from many sources can contain as much chromium as soils and rocks, or approximately 60 mg/kg; consequently, the burning of coal can contribute to chromium levels in air and is probably responsible for much of it in cities. Particulates emitted from coal-fired power plants contained 2.3-31 mg/kg chromium, depending on the type of boiler firing; the emitted gases contained 0.22-2.2 mg/m^3. These concentrations were reduced by fly-ash collection to 0.19-6.6 mg/kg and 0.018-0.5 mg/m^3, respectively (Fishbein, 1976).

Mean concentration in the air of 6 US cities with metallurgical chromium producers was 0.016 μg/m^3; in 3 cities where chromium chemicals were made it was 0.012 μg/m^3; and in 8 cities with refractories, it was 0.016 μg/m^3. All were higher than the US national average. Cement-producing plants are probably an additional source of chromium in the air: Portland cement contains 41.2 mg/kg chromium (range 27.5-60), as might be expected from the presence of chromium in limestone. Soluble chromium in cement averaged 4.1 mg/kg (range 1.6-8.8), of which 2.9 mg/kg (range 0.03-7.8) were hexavalent chromium. When chromate chemicals are used as rust inhibitors in cooling towers, they are dissolved in re-circulating water systems, which continually discharge about 1% of their flow to waste. Additionally, chromate and water are lost to the atmosphere. Another important source of chromium in the atmosphere is asbestos, which contains approximately 1500 mg/kg chromium. The wearing of brake linings thus represents a source of chromium, since asbestos particles are emitted in this way (Fishbein, 1976).

A potential source of chromium to the atmosphere (particularly the urban atmosphere) is represented by the increased use of catalytic emission control systems on passenger cars in the US (beginning with the 1975 model year). Reduction catalysts, such as copper chromite (the composition is variable), have been found to emit high concentrations ($>10^{12}$/m^3 metal-containing condensation nuclei) under a broad range of controlled conditions (Fishbein, 1976).

(c)   Occupational exposure

The National Institute for Occupational Safety & Health (1975) estimated that there are 175,000 persons in the US who are potentially exposed occupationally to hexavalent chromium and listed 104 occupations in which such exposure could occur. In 1973, it was estimated that 15,000 persons in the US were potentially exposed occupationally to chromium[VI] trioxide mist (National Institute for Occupational Safety & Health, 1973).

Chromium and its compounds are found in three main types of industrial activity: (i) most chromium derivatives are used in the metallurgical industry, particularly in relation to the production and use of ferrochromium alloys and stainless steel; (ii) chromium compounds are also an important component of refractory materials, such as bricks, glass, ceramics and certain ferrous metals; and (iii) many of the highly coloured chromate salts of various metals are used in the pigment, paint, tanning and dyeing industries.

Potential occupational exposures in the manufacture of chromium products to chromium compounds are, briefly, as follows:

Occupation	Chromium compounds
Chromium extraction and ferro-alloy production	Chromite[III] ore, sodium chromate[VI], sodium dichromate[VI], chromium[VI] trioxide
Electroplating	Chromium[VI] trioxide, sodium and potassium dichromates[VI]
Refractory materials	Chromic[III] oxide, chrome-magnesium alloys
Pigment production	Sodium dichromate[VI], potassium chromate[VI], chromates[VI] of ammonium, barium, calcium, lead, molybdenum and zinc

Chromite ore processing: Water-soluble hexavalent chromium compounds do not occur as such in ore but comprise almost the entire Cr content of roast and residue materials. The types of chromium to which there is occupational exposure in the course of processing chromium-barium ores are chromates[VI], chromate[VI]-chromite[III] complex and chromic[III] oxide in process residues, and calcium chromate[VI], chromic chromate and chromium[VI] trioxide (Kuschner & Laskin, 1971).

In 1953, the US Public Health Service (Gafafer, 1953) investigated the hazards associated with the chromate-producing industry in the US. It was considered probable that throughout the industry most chromium [VI] exposures were to sodium chromate and dichromate, since these are the principal intermediate and end-products, respectively, of the usual alkaline roasting operations. The range of time-weighted exposures for the occupational groups was 5-170 $\mu g/m^3$ (mean, 68 $\mu g/m^3$) of water-soluble chromium [VI] (National Institute for Occupational Safety & Health, 1975).

Airborne concentrations of 'chromates' in 4 plants in the US over the period 1930-1947 were 0.01-4.6 mg/m^3 in kilns and mills, 0.20-21.0 mg/m^3 in packing areas and 0.003-2.17 mg/m^3 in other parts of the factories (Machle & Gregorius, 1948).

Concentrations of Cr[III], Cr[VI] and total Cr during various operations in chromite ore processing were reported by Bourne & Yee (1950), for a plant in Ohio which produced sodium chromate and dichromate, and by Buckell & Harvey (1951), for a chromate-producing plant in the UK, as follows:

Operation	Cr[III] (mg/m^3)		Cr[VI] (mg/m^3)		Total Cr (mg/m^3)	
	US	UK	US	UK	US	UK
Chromite and lime mixing	1.52	2.14	0.03	0.005	1.55	2.145
Roasting	0.39	0.17	0.26	0.029	0.65	0.199
Filtering	0.08	0.037	0.12	0.52	0.2	0.557
Shipping	0.30	0.0053	0.2	0.88	0.5	0.8853

Levels of 0.11-0.15 mg/m^3 Cr[VI] were reported over a 3-year period during which workers were exposed to alkaline chromate in an Italian factory (Vigliani & Zurlo, 1955).

The many uses of chromium and chromium compounds may involve alterations in the original material. Four examples are given below.

Chromium plating: In a study of the different chromium exposures of workers, Guillemin & Berode (1978) found that exposure was higher during 'hard' than during 'bright' chromium plating; techniques used to minimize mist formation were discussed. Gresh (1944) reported that concentrations of Cr[VI] in the vicinity of anodizing tanks were 210-600 µg/m^3. Under these conditions, persons working up to 200 feet (60 m) from the tanks would have been affected by aerosols of Cr[VI]. When better ventilation was installed, levels decreased to 45-50 µg/m^3.

In a chromium-plating establishment in the US, the chromium- and nickel-plating line used a solution of technical-grade chromic [III] oxide at a concentration of approximately 300 g/l at 118-120°F (47.8-48.9°C). In the chromium- and nickel-plating area, airborne Cr[VI] concentrations ranged from <0.71-9.12 µg/m^3 (mean 3.24 µg/m^3) (National Institute for Occupational Safety & Health, 1975).

In a study in Finland of 33 chromium platers, the highest airborne chromium concentration found, reported as chromic [III] oxide, was 3 µg/m^3 (Lumbio, 1953).

Airborne concentrations to which chromium plating workers were exposed from the solution and airborne mist emanating from tanks of acidic Cr[VI] were 180-1400 µg/m^3; after installation of local exhaust ventilation, 3-9 µg/m^3 were detected (Kleinfeld & Rosso, 1965).

In a study of electroplaters in the state of Sao Paulo, Brazil, the concentrations of airborne chromium [VI] trioxide in electroplating operations in 2/8 hard-chrome plants using solutions of Cr[VI] were less than 0.1 mg/m^3; in 3 they were between 0.1-0.2 mg/m^3, in 2 between 0.3-0.4 mg/m^3 and in 1 greater than 1 mg/m^3. Of 73 brilliant-chrome electroplating industries surveyed, 33 had environmental levels of Cr[VI] of less than 0.1 mg/m^3, while the others had higher levels (Gomes, 1972).

Welding: Welders of stainless steel and, to a lesser extent, welders of aluminium alloys are exposed to fumes which contain chromium of several oxidation states, in a wide range of levels and proportions which depend to a great extent on the process and working conditions. Typical particle concentrations of fumes in stainless-steel welding shops are of the order of 1-4 mg/m³ (Stern, 1977). The composition of these fumes is extremely varied, but, on average, manual arc-welding fumes contain 2-4% Cr[VI] (most of which is water-soluble) and 0.2-2% insoluble Cr[III] (and chromium metal). Inert gas welding fumes contain 3.5-14% insoluble Cr[III] (and chromium metal) and less than 1% soluble and insoluble Cr[VI] (Stern, 1980).

Chromium pigment industries: Chromium pigment workers are exposed primarily to lead chromate[VI], although in the past they were also exposed to zinc chromate[VI] and to its raw material, sodium dichromate[VI]. The total mean amount of dust in a zinc chromate-producing plant ranged from 1.2-9.8 mg/m³, with a maximum of 13.6 mg/m³ for workers filling sacks; lower exposure was found for workers mixing raw materials (2.9-6 mg/m³) and for foremen (1.9-3.8 mg/m³). The concentration of chromate (as Cr) in the air varied from 0.01-1.35 mg/m³ (Langård & Norseth, 1975).

Leather tanning: Mineral leather tanners are exposed primarily to basic chromium [III] sulphate, although they may also be exposed to aluminium (used in the most ancient method) or to zirconium (used for heavy white leathers). In one-bath chrome tanning, now the most commonly employed method, chrome liquors consisting of a colloidal solution of basic chromium [III] sulphate are loaded into the tanning drums directly from outer storage tanks. Chromic [III] sulphite or chromium [III] potassium sulphate may be used instead.

The two-bath tannage system, initially the only chrome-tanning method, is now seldom used in industrialized countries, except for the production of special leathers, such as that for kid gloves. However, it was still common in tanneries in the US and in Italy in the 1950s and 1960s and may be used currently elsewhere in the world. With this method, the hide is immersed in a bath of hexavalent chromium salts (potassium or sodium dichromate[VI]), sodium chloride and sulphuric acid, and then removed, manually, and placed in a reduction bath that reduces the dichromate to tanning trivalent chromium sulphate.

Reduction of hexavalent dichromates to basic chromium [III] sulphate is now usually carried out in separate chemical factories, although it may be carried out in a separate part of a tannery. A highly exothermic reaction takes place between sulphuric acid, dichromates and a reducing agent (such as glucose, starch, dextrin, sulphur dioxide) in a lead-sheathed vat, exposing workers to hexavalent chromium.

Tannery workers may be exposed to trivalent chromium salts when the salts are being weighed and introduced into the tanning drums and when the tanning baths are emptied. Levels of 0.02-0.05 mg/m³ Cr[III] were measured in the air in a room where drums were emptied (Laboratorio Provinciale di Igiene e Profilatti, 1975).

(d)   Water and sediments

In rivers, concentrations of chromium have been found to range between 1 and 10 μg/l. Chromium (both hexavalent and trivalent) is generally less concentrated in seawater than in rivers and wells, with concentrations well below 1 μg/l. It has been estimated that 6.7 million kg of chromium are added to the oceans every year. As a result, much of the chromium lost from the land by erosion and mining is eventually deposited on the ocean floor (Fishbein, 1976).

Of 1500 samples of US surface waters taken between 1960 and about 1968, 24.5% contained chromium detectable spectrographically. The maximum and mean levels observed were 112 and 9.7 μg/l, respectively (Kroner, 1973). A survey of chromium content of 15 North American rivers showed levels of 0.7-84 μg/l, with most in the range of 1-10 μg/l. Levels in public water supplies ranged from no detectable content to 36 μg/l of chromium, with the median 0.43 μg/l (Hartford, 1979). Naturally occurring hexavalent chromium was found in groundwater in Arizona in concentrations greater than 0.05 mg/l (Robertson, 1975).

The mean concentration of dissolved chromium compounds in the Rhine River during 1975 was 6.5±1.76 μg/l with a range of 3.7-11.4 μg/l (Nissing, 1975). The concentration of chromium compounds in Austrian medicinal and table waters was determined as 1.2-4.2 μg/l (Sontag *et al*., 1977). The average levels of chromium compounds in three tributaries of the Han River in Korea were found to be 0.096, 0.106 and 0.065 mg/l (Min, 1976).

The vertical distribution of chromium compounds in dated sediments of four sedimentary profiles from the central part of Lake Constance was examined: between 1900 and about 1960-1970, an increase of 2-3-fold occurred (Mueller, 1977).

(e)   Soil and plants

Chromium is present in the soil at levels which vary from traces to 250 mg/kg (as chromic [III] oxide) and is particularly prevalent in soil derived from basalt or serpentine.

The chromium content of mosses and liverworts collected in 1951 in a remote rural area in Denmark was compared with that in the same plants collected in 1975: an increase of about 62% was observed, which coincided with the increase in industrial activity and fossil-fuel combustion (Rasmussen, 1977).

The chromium content of cigarette tobacco from different sources has been reported as follows: Iraq, 8.6-14.6 mg/kg (two varieties); Iran, 4.3-6.2 mg/kg (two brands); and the US, 0.24-6.3 mg/kg (Al-Badri *et al.*, 1977).

With the exception of cotton seeds, every plant tissue analysed prior to 1956 contained a trace of chromium. Vegetables from 25 botanical families were found to contain chromium in amounts varying from 10-1000 μg/kg of dry matter, with most samples in the range of 100-500 μg/kg (Davis, 1956).

(f)   Food

The chromium content of most foods is considered to be extremely low; small amounts were found in vegetables (20-50 μg/kg), fruits (20 μg/kg) and grains and cereals (excluding fats, 40 μg/kg). The mean daily intakes of chromium from food, water and air have been estimated to be 280, 4 and 0.28 μg, respectively (Fishbein, 1976). Hartford (1979) indicated that nearly all foodstuffs contain chromium in the range of 20-590 μg/kg, resulting in a daily intake for humans of 10-400 μg, with an average of about 80 μg.

(g)   Marine organisms

Samples of 119 fish caught in 1974 in Austria contained 0.02-0.21 mg/kg chromium (Teherani et al., 1977).

(h)   Human tissues and secretions

The normal concentration of chromium in human tissues ranges from 0.020 to several hundred μg/g and decreases from birth to the age of 10. Later in life the concentration in lung increases, probably as a result of deposition from inhaled air, but the concentration in other organs falls continuously (Schroeder et al., 1962). The ranges of concentration of chromium found in normal human body tissues and in those from workers in the chromate-producing industry are given in Table 5.

In a recent study (Versieck et al., 1978) in which neutron activation analysis was applied to the determination of chromium in the sera of 20 apparently healthy individuals, a mean value of 0.160 μg/l, a standard deviation of 0.083 μg/l and a range of 0.0382-0.351 μg/l were found. These levels were markedly lower than those reported by earlier workers. The mean value of chromium in the sera of 8 men, as determined by atomic absorption spectrometry, was 0.14 μg/l (Kayne et al., 1978).

Concentrations of chromium in blood and urine from persons with varying degrees of exposure to chromium compounds are given in Table 6.

Table 5. Concentrations of chromium compounds, calculated as chromium, in body tissues of persons without and with known exposure to chromium[a]

Tissue	Normal tissues (μg/kg wet tissue)	Tissues from chromate workers (μg/kg wet tissue)
Lung	0-330	1300-98,870
Lung tumour		0-16,580
Metastatic tumour		20-1000
Tracheobronchial lymph node	0-10	120-75,900
Bronchus		950-3860
Trachea		0-320
Nasal septum		2870
Larynx		210
Kidney	0-96	0-2110
Liver	10-110	0-1590
Spleen	0-980	0-910
Abdominal lymph node	10	40-800
Stomach	0-50	40-110
Intestine	100	40-50
Bladder	—	30-2260
Heart	—	0-200
Muscle	0-80	0-190
Pancreas	210	80-360
Thyroid	430	240-530
Adrenal	0-410	50-760
Brain	0-40	0-50
Bone	50	0-2920
Cartilage	—	60
Bile	—	10
Hair	—	310
Skin	—	50
Aorta	—	30

[a] From Baetjer (1956)

Table 6. Concentrations of chromium in blood and urine from persons with varying degrees of exposure to chromium[a]

Degree of exposure to chromium	Blood concentration ($\mu g/l$)	Urine concentration ($\mu g/l$)
No exposure	0-200	0-160
Slight exposure	–	0-180
Chromate workers	0-5800	0-780
Chromium platers	–	0-2800
Chromite workers	0-20	0

[a]From various literature sources, as reported by Baetjer (1956)

(i)   Other

Cr[III] has been found in ribonucleic acid (RNA) from all sources examined. It is possible that chromium helps to stabilize the structure of RNA (Wacker & Vallee, 1959).

2.4   Analysis (see also preamble, p. 21)

Methods for sampling chromium-containing materials and for the analytical separation of chromium, and methods for their detection, identification and determination have been reviewed (Gahler, 1962; Hartford, 1963). Sampling and analytical methods used to monitor air, water and soil near industrial sites have been summarized (US Environmental Protection Agency, 1977). The application of neutron activation techniques for the measurement of trace metals such as chromium in the marine environment has also been reviewed (Robertson & Carpenter, 1972), as have selected methods for the determination of chromium in natural fresh water (Whitney & Risby, 1975).

Typical methods of analysis for determining levels of chromium in environmental samples are summarized in Table 7. Abbreviations are: AAS/EA, atomic absorption spectrometry/electrothermal atomization; FAAS, flameless atomic absorption spectrometry; GC, gas chromatography; IDMS, isotope dilution mass spectrometry; NAA, neutron activation analysis; X-REA, X-ray emission analysis.

Table 7. Analytical methods for chromium and chromium compounds

Sample matrix	Sample preparation	Assay procedure	Sensitivity or limit of detection	Reference
Formulations				
Tanning liquors (trivalent chromium)	Oxidize to hexavalent chromium (dichromate) with ammonium persulphate (oxidant) and cupric sulphate-cobaltous nitrate mixture (catalyst)	Iodometric titration		Makarov-Zemlyanskii et al. (1978)
Catalysts (chromium metal)	Extract chromium with 2,4-pentanedione (forming a volatile chelate)	Gas chromatography	1 μg	Astapova et al. (1978)
Pigments	Dissolve in hydrofluoric acid	AAS/EA	0.1 mg/kg	Kolihova et al. (1978)
Air	Extract collection filter with hot mixture of hydrochloric and nitric acids; concentrate extract on liquid; hold overnight; dilute	AAS		Smith et al. (1976)
	Collect particulate sample on acetate fibre superfilter; use filter as thin target sample and bombard in a proton beam for 10 min	X-REA	0.1 μg	Li et al. (1979)
Water				
Waste waters (hexavalent and total chromium)	—	Pulse polarography	0.04 mg/l (total); 0.01 mg/l (hexavalent)	Heigl (1978)

Table 7 (contd)

Sample matrix	Sample preparation	Assay procedure	Sensitivity or limit of detection	Reference
River water	Separate suspended particles by centrifugation; add diethyldithiocarbamate; filter through acetate superfilter; use filter as thin target sample and bombard in a proton beam for 10 min	X-REA		Li *et al.* (1979)
Seawater (hexavalent and total chromium)	Extract with ammonium pyrrolidine dithiocarbamate into chloroform at pH 2	IDMS	0.001 µg/l	Osaki *et al.* (1976)
Seawater (hexavalent and trivalent chromium, selective)	Extract hexavalent chromium with Aliquat-336 (a mixture of methyl tri-*n*-alkyl ammonium chlorides) at pH 2; extract trivalent chromium by adding thiocyanate to at least one molar concentration; adjust pH to 6-8	FAAS	0.01 µg/l (hexavalent) 0.03 µg/l (trivalent)	de Jong & Brinkman (1978)
Sediments	Activate with neutrons for 6 hrs	NAA	1.5 mg/kg	Ackermann (1977)
Food				
Tinned foods	Oxidize to hexavalent chromium with hydrogen peroxide; treat with diphenylcarbazide	Colorimetry	0.05 mg/kg	Il'inykh (1977)
Biological samples				
SRM 1569 brewers' yeast; SRM 1577 bovine liver; SRM 1570 spinach; human hair and nails	Chemical procedures were developed for digestion of biological matrices and separation of chromium without large analytical blanks or significant losses by volatilization	IDMS	1 µg	Dunstan & Garner (1977)

Table 7 (contd)

Sample matrix	Sample preparation	Assay procedure	Sensitivity or limit of detection	Reference
Whole human blood	Heat about 1 ml in a quartz crucible in an oven to about 400°C for a few hrs; grind residual ash gently; press powder onto a thin Mylar film; irradiate	X-ray fluorescence	0.15 mg/l	Paradellis (1977)
Blood serum	Dilute 1:1 with deionized water before direct injection into air-acetylene flame	AAS	0.02 mg/l	Arpadzhyan & Kachov (1978)
	Oxidize with permanganate to dichromate; destroy excess permanganate with azide; add diphenylcarbazide	Long-path photometry		Yarbro & Flaschka (1976)
Serum	—	NAA		Versieck *et al.* (1978)
Human urine (trivalent chromium)	React a buffered (pH 5.8-6.2) sample of reconstituted lyophilized urine with doubly distilled trifluoroacetylacetone in sealed tubes	GC	0.1 pg	Ryan & Vogt (1977)
Plant materials	Dry in an oven at 120°C for 2-4 hrs; ash in a muffle furnace at 500°C for 6 hrs	Emission spectrography	2 mg/kg	Dixit *et al.* (1976)
Other				
Welding fumes; complex matrices with redox systems (insoluble and total hexavalent chromium)	Add sodium carbonate; warm; remove precipitate by filtration	AAS	1 μg/m^3	Thomsen & Stern (1979)

3. Biological Data Relevant to the Evaluation
of Carcinogenic Risk to Humans

3.1 Carcinogenicity studies in animals

(A summary of these studies is given in Table 8, on pp. 264-273.)

(a)   Oral administration

Mouse: Groups of 54 male and 54 female Swiss mice that received 5 mg/l *chromic [III] acetate* in drinking-water for life developed no more tumours than did control mice. No difference was found in the survival of treated females compared with controls, but treated males died 100 days earlier than control males (831 *versus* 957 days): only 60% of the males survived 18 months (Schroeder *et al.*, 1964) [The Working Group noted the low dose used].

Rat: Chromic *[III] acetate* was given in drinking-water at a level of 5 mg/l to 46 male and 50 female Long Evans rats for lifespan.   There was no significant increase in the incidence of tumours at various sites in rats of either sex as compared with the controls.   The total numbers of tumour-bearing animals among rats autopsied were: 16/39 treated males, 18/35 treated females, 9/35 male controls and 15/35 female controls.   At least 70% of the animals survived for up to two years.   Treated females lived as long as control females, but treated males lived up to 100 days longer than control males (Schroeder *et al.*, 1965) [The Working Group noted the low dose used].

Chromic [III] oxide obtained by the reduction of chromate at 600°C was incorporated and baked in bread with other nutrients at levels of 1, 2 and 5%, and the bread was fed to groups of 60 male and female inbred BD rats on 5 days per week for 2 years. Average survival times were 860-880 days.   Mammary fibroadenomas were found in 3 rats given 1%, in 1 given 2% and in 3 given 5%.   In the controls, 1 mammary carcinoma and 2 fibroadenomas were detected (Ivankovic & Preussmann, 1975).

(b)   Inhalation and/or intratracheal administration

Mouse: Groups of mice were exposed in dust chambers for 4 hours per day on 5 days per week to a *mixed chromate [VI] dust*[1] containing 1-2 mg/m³ soluble chromium (as chromium [VI] trioxide) until they died or were killed (total dose of chromium trioxide inhaled, 272-1330 mg-hours): 127 Swiss females were exposed for up to 58 weeks, 10 Swiss

---

[1] In the publications by Baetjer *et al.*, the mixed chromium dust used was prepared by grinding to a fine powder the roast which is produced when chromite [III] ore is heated at a high temperature with sodium carbonate and calcium hydroxide. The mixture contained approximately 12% chromium, which consisted of water-soluble hexavalent sodium chromate, water-insoluble but acid-soluble chromium chemicals which were partly trivalent and partly hexavalent and some unchanged chromite [III] ore.

males and 11 Swiss females for up to 39 weeks, 34 strain A females for 16 weeks, 45 strain A females for 24 weeks, 110 strain A females for 38 weeks, 52 strain A males for 46 weeks and 50 C57BL males for 42 weeks and 61 C57BL females for 41 weeks. No lung carcinomas were observed, and the incidence of lung adenomas did not significantly exceed that in control mice in any strain. The experiment lasted for up to 101 weeks (Baetjer *et al.*, 1959b).

Groups of 136 C57BL/6 mice of each sex were exposed by inhalation to *calcium chromate [VI]* dust at a level of 13 mg/m³ for 5 hours per day on 5 days per week over their lifespan. No evidence was found of excess induction of lung adenomas: 6 adenomas appeared in treated males and 8 in females, compared with 3 and 2 in the 136 respective controls. No carcinomas were seen (Nettesheim *et al.*, 1971).

Five to six intratracheal instillations of a *mixed chromate dust*[1], equivalent to 0.04 mg chromium [VI] trioxide per instillation, were given either to 14 and 20 Swiss males, which were then observed for 26 and 32 weeks, respectively; to 45 and 110 Swiss females observed for up to 32 and 48 weeks, respectively; to 28, 52, 77 and 48 strain A females observed for up to 31, 37, 43 and 52 weeks, respectively; to 17 strain A males observed for up to 52 weeks; or to 48 C57BL males and 47 C57BL females observed for up to 32 weeks. Treated animals developed no more lung tumours than did untreated control animals (Baetjer *et al.*, 1959b).

Six intratracheal injections of 0.03 ml of a 0.2% saline suspension of *zinc yellow [VI]* were given at 6-week intervals to 62 strain A mice, which were observed until their death. No pulmonary carcinomas were found; pulmonary adenomas occurred in 31/62 exposed, in 7/18 untreated control and in 0/2 zinc carbonate-treated control animals (Steffee & Baetjer, 1965).

Rat: A group of 78 Wistar rats were exposed by inhalation to a *mixed chromate dust*[1] for 4-5 hours/day on 4 days a week over their lifespan, to give an average *chromic [III] oxide* concentration of 3-4 mg/m³. A group of 38 Sherman rats received 16 monthly intratracheal injections of 0.1 ml of a suspension consisting of 0.5% *mixed chromate dust* plus 0.6% *potassium dichromate [VI]*, equivalent to 0.07 mg chromium/dose. No significant difference in tumour incidence was observed between experimental and control groups. Rats survived for 16 or more months (Steffee & Baetjer, 1965).

---

[1] See footnote on p. 254.

Random-bred and Wistar rats were given single intratracheal applications of 50 or 20 mg *chromic [III] oxide,* respectively. Malignant lung tumours developed in 7/34 and 6/18 animals; and 4 and 5 of these, respectively, were lung sarcomas which appeared between 11 and 22 months after the injection of chromium (Dvizhkov & Fedorova, 1967) [The Working Group noted that no controls were reported].

A 50:50 mixture of *calcium chromate [VI]* with a cholesterol binder was implanted in a stainless-steel pellet (1 x 5 mm) into a segmental bronchus of 100 rats (strain and sex unspecified). Six squamous-cell carcinomas and 2 adenocarcinomas of the lung were found in animals observed up to 136 weeks. The median time of appearance of tumours was 540 days. In parallel tests, *chromate process residue* (see section 2) yielded 1 squamous-cell carcinoma, while *chromic [III] oxide* and *chromium [VI] trioxide* produced no such tumours in similar groups of 98 and 100 animals observed up to 136 weeks. No lung tumours occurred in 24 cholesterol binder-treated controls (Laskin *et al.*, 1970).

It was reported in an abstract that stainless-steel pellets loaded with various chromium compounds (with cholesterol as a carrier) were implanted into the left bronchiolus of rats (strain unspecified). Two pure, medium-soluble, hexavalent chromium salts, *calcium chromate [VI]* and *zinc potassium chromate [VI]*, induced squamous-cell carcinomas of the bronchus similar to those produced by 3-methylcholanthrene. Highly-soluble chromates, presumably *sodium* and *potassium chromate [VI]* and *dichromate [VI]*, and *Cr [III]* compounds were inactive (Levy & Venitt, 1975) [The Working Group noted the incomplete reporting of this experiment].

Groups of 35-62 female rats were given one intratracheal intubation of 10 mg powdered *chromium* alone or in combination with 1 or 5 mg methylcholanthrene (MC) and killed at various intervals up to 12 weeks. Squamous-cell carcinomas of the lung developed 12 weeks after intubation in 7/12 rats given 5 mg MC + Cr, in 3/12 given 1 mg MC + Cr, in 3/7 given 5 mg MC, in 1/8 given 1 mg MC and in 0/12 given Cr alone (Mukubo, 1978) [The Working Group noted that the chromium could have been acting as a carrier of the 3-methylcholanthrene].

Rats (number and strain unspecified) were exposed by inhalation to 2 mg/m³ *calcium chromate [VI]* in air during 589 exposures over a period of 891 days. One squamous-cell carcinoma of the lung and one of the larynx and one malignant 'peritruncal tumour' were reported (Laskin, 1972) [The Working Group noted the incomplete reporting of the experiment].

Hamster: Hamsters (number, sex and strain unspecified) were exposed by inhalation to 2 mg/m³ *calcium chromate [VI]* in air during 589 exposures for 891 days. One squamous-cell carcinoma and one papilloma of the larynx were observed (Laskin, 1972) [The Working Group noted the incomplete reporting of the experiment].

Guinea-pig: Of guinea-pigs exposed by inhalation to a combination of *mixed chromate dust*[1], aerosols of *potassium dichromate [VI]* and *sodium chromate [VI]* and 'pulverized residue dust' (roast material from which soluble chromates had been leached) for 4-5 hours/day on 4 days/week for lifespan (average dose, 3-4 mg/m^3 *chromic [III] oxide*), 3/50 developed pulmonary adenomas. Pulmonary adenomas also occurred in 0/19 guinea-pigs that were given 6 intratracheal instillations at 3-monthly intervals of 0.3 ml of a 1% suspension in saline of a *mixed chromate dust*[1]; in 0/19 that were similarly exposed to the pulverized residue dust; in 1/21 that were similarly exposed to *zinc yellow [VI]*; and in 0/13 that were similarly exposed to *lead chromate [VI]*. The animals were observed until they died. No pulmonary carcinomas developed in any experimental group. No pulmonary adenomas occurred in 44 controls in the inhalation experiment or 18 vehicle controls in the intratracheal experiment (Steffee & Baetjer, 1965).

Rabbit: Eight rabbits were exposed by inhalation for 4-5 hours/day on 4 days/week for up to 50 months to a combination of *mixed chromate dust*[1], aerosols of *potassium dichromate [VI]* and *sodium chromate [VI]* and 'pulverized residue dust' (roast material from which soluble chromates had been leached), according to a complex dosage schedule (average dose, 3-4 mg/m^3 *chromic [III] oxide*); other groups were exposed at 3-monthly intervals by 3-5 intratracheal injections of 1 ml of 1% suspensions in saline of *mixed chromate dust*[1] (10 rabbits), *zinc yellow [VI]* (7 rabbits), *lead chromate [VI]* (7 rabbits) or the 'pulverized residue dust' (7 rabbits). These studies all gave negative results (Steffee & Baetjer, 1965).

(c)   Subcutaneous and/or intramuscular administration

Mouse: Groups of 26 female and 26 male C57BL mice received *calcium chromate [VI]* or *sintered calcium chromate [VI]*[2] by i.m. implantation of 10 mg of the chromium compound mixed with 20 mg of sheep fat; the mice were observed for a total of 14 months. Nine implantation-site sarcomas were observed among 46 mice given sintered calcium chromate that lived longer than 6 months; 2 sarcomas were observed in 50 mice given calcium chromate; and no sarcomas were found among 50 control mice that lived 6 months or more. The same compounds as well as *sintered chromium [VI] trioxide* were also injected subcutaneously into 26 female and 26 male C57BL mice at a dose of 10 mg of the chromium compound in tricaprylin, and the animals were observed for 18-25 months. One sarcoma was observed in 13 mice treated with calcium chromate [VI] that lived longer than 6 months, but none were seen at the injection site in the other treated groups or in vehicle controls. Histologically, the tumours were spindle-cell sarcomas or fibrosarcomas (Payne, 1960a).

---

[1]
See footnote on p. 254.

[2]
The sintered compound was prepared by heating calcium chromate [VI] with less than 1% impurities to about 1100°C for about 1 hour.

Four monthly i.m. injections of 3 mg *lead chromate [VI]* in trioctanoin were given to 25 female NIH-Swiss mice. Two lymphomas were seen within 16 months and 3 lung adeno-carcinomas within 24 months among 17 mice necropsied. Similar incidences occurred in vehicle-injected and untreated control mice (Furst *et al*., 1976).

None of 52 C57BL mice given i.m. implantations of 10 mg *roasted chromite [III] ore* (equivalent to 0.79 mg chromium) developed tumours at the implantation site. Details of survival are not given (Payne, 1960b).

Rat: A single s.c. injection of 30 mg *lead chromate [VI]* or *lead chromate [VI] oxide* in water to groups of 40 Sprague-Dawley rats gave rise to 26/40 and 27/40 sarcomas, respectively, at the site of injection within 117-150 weeks. No local sarcomas occurred in 60 vehicle-treated control rats; 1 local sarcoma occurred in 80 control rats that received comparable s.c. injections of unspecified iron pigments (Maltoni, 1974, 1976a).

When 39 Bethesda Black rats (20 males, 19 females) were given 16 i.m. injections of 2 mg *sodium dichromate [VI]* in gelatin at monthly intervals and observed for 2 years (17 alive at 18 months), no tumours appeared at the injection site. After i.m. implantation of 12.5 mg *calcium chromate [VI]* in a gelatin capsule to 8 rats, 4 malignant tumours deve-loped at the implantation site in animals observed for 2 years. A group of 35 Bethesda Black rats received an i.m. implantation of 25 mg *chromic [III] acetate* in a gelatin capsule; and a further 7 i.m. implantations were made over a period of 24 months, at which time the rats were sacrificed. One spindle-cell sarcoma was observed at the site of implantation (Hueper & Payne, 1962).

Tumours were observed after 17 months in 14/74 female Strangeways rats at the site of i.m. injection of 28 mg of wear particles from prostheses made from a *cobalt-chromium alloy* (26.9% chromium, 65.3% cobalt, 6.11% molybdenum and 0.36% manganese) sus-pended in horse serum. All 7 histologically observed tumours were fibrosarcomas. No con-trols were reported (Heath *et al*., 1971).

A group of 24 CB stock rats were given once-weekly injections for 20 weeks of *calcium chromate [VI]* in arachis oil (total dose, 19 mg); 18 developed spindle-cell and pleo-morphic-cell sarcomas at the injection site, none of which metastasized. The mean time to tumour appearance was 323 days (duration of experiment, 440 days). No tumours deve-loped in a control group given arachis oil only (Roe & Carter, 1969) [It was not clear from the article whether the test material was injected intramuscularly or subcutaneously].

Groups of 25 male and 25 female Fischer-344 rats received monthly i.m. injections of 8 mg *lead chromate [VI]* suspended in trioctanoin for 9 months or 4 mg *calcium chromate [VI]* suspended in trioctanoin for 12 months. Calcium chromate produced 3 fibrosarcomas and 2 rhabdomyosarcomas at the injection site in 5/45 rats, whereas lead chromate induced 14 fibrosarcomas and 17 rhabdomyosarcomas at the site of injection in 31/47 rats. In addition, 3/24 lead chromate-treated rats had renal carcinomas. No such tumours appeared in a similar group of 22 controls injected with the vehicle (Furst *et al.*, 1976).

Single i.m. injections of 2 mg powdered *chromium* metal in 0.5 ml oily penicillin G-procaine suspension given to 24 male Fischer rats resulted in no local tumours in 22 survivors at 24 months (Sunderman *et al.*, 1974).

Small cubes composed of 25 mg *roasted chromite [III] ore* suspended in 75 mg sheep fat were implanted intramuscularly into 31 female Bethesda Black rats. Three fibrosarcomas were found at the site of implantation after 24 months. No implantation-site tumours occurred in vehicle-treated controls (Hueper, 1958). Sarcomas (spindle-cell sarcomas and fibrosarcomas) at the implantation site were also seen after 1 year in 8/35 rats implanted intramuscularly with pellets of 25 mg *calcium chromate [VI]*, in 8/35 rats implanted with pellets of 25 mg *sintered calcium chromate [VI]* and in 15/35 rats implanted with pellets of 25 mg *sintered chromium [VI] trioxide*, all in 50 mg sheep fat. No implantation-site tumours were obtained in 35 rats given the insoluble *barium chromate [VI]* (25 mg in 75 mg sheep fat) or in 35 controls (Hueper & Payne, 1959).

In groups of 22-34 rats that received i.m. implantations of various chromium compounds, the following incidences of implantation-site tumours (type unspecified) were observed after 27 months: *calcium chromate [VI]*, 9/32 (22 alive at 1 year); *strontium chromate [VI]*, 15/33 (20 alive at 1 year); *barium chromate [VI]*, 0/34 (30 alive at 1 year); *lead chromate [VI]*, 1/33 (28 alive at 1 year); *sodium dichromate [VI]*, 0/33 (25 alive at 1 year); *zinc yellow [VI]* [1], 16/34 (22 alive at 1 year); *chromite [III] roast residue*, 1/34 (32 alive at 1 year); *chromic [III] acetate*, 1/34 (30 alive at 1 year); and *sintered calcium chromate [VI]*, 12/34 (22 alive at 1 year). None of 32 control rats given implants of sheep fat alone developed local tumours (30 alive at 1 year) (Hueper, 1961).

---

[1] It was not specified whether this compound was zinc chromate, zinc potassium chromate or zinc yellow.

(d)   Intraperitoneal administration

Mouse: Fifty male C57BL mice, approximately 6 weeks old, were given weekly i.p. injections for 4 consecutive weeks of 0.2 ml of a 0.005% suspension of *chromium* powder in a 2.5% gelatin-saline solution; 40 mice survived from 6-21 months. One mouse developed myeloid leukaemia; no other tumours were noted (Hueper, 1955).

Three groups of 10 male and 10 female strain A/Strong mice were given thrice-weekly i.p. injections of *chromium [III] sulphate* suspended in tricaprylin for 8 weeks (total doses, 480, 1200 and 2400 mg/kg bw). Animals were killed 30 weeks after the first injection. No significant increases in the incidences of pulmonary adenomas over those in 20 vehicle-treated or 20 untreated control mice of each sex were observed (Stoner *et al.*, 1976).

Rat: In experiments with Wistar and random-bred rats, 4/20 animals developed lung sarcomas 16-19 months after a single i.p. injection of 20 mg *chromic [III] oxide*. No controls were reported (Dvizhkov & Fedorova, 1967).

A group of 25 male Wistar rats, 3-4 months old, were given weekly i.p. injections for 6 consecutive weeks of 0.1 ml of a 0.05% suspension of *chromium* powder in a 2.5% gelatin-saline solution.   One rat developed a scirrhous carcinoma, two rats developed round-cell sarcomas, 1 rat had both a round-cell sarcoma and an insulinoma of the pancreas, and 1 rat had an insulinoma.   No vehicle-treated controls were reported.   The author stated that although round-cell sarcomas also occurred in controls, insulinomas were found only in treated rats (Hueper, 1955).

(e)   Intravenous administration

Mouse: A group of 25 C57BL mice (sex unspecified) received 6 weekly injections of 0.05 ml of a 0.005% suspension of *chromium* powder in gelatin-saline solution. Six animals lived up to 12 months, but none to 18 months. No tumours were observed (Hueper, 1955).

Rat: Of 25 male Wistar rats given 6 weekly injections of 0.18 ml of a 0.05% suspension of *chromium* powder in gelatin-saline solution, 15 lived to 1 year. Round-cell sarcomas were observed in 4 rats; 1 rat had a haemangioma; and 2 rats had papillary adenomas of the lungs, one of which showed extensive squamous-cell carcinomatous changes. No vehicle-treated controls were reported. The author stated that although round-cell sarcomas also occurred in controls, lung adenomas were found only in treated rats (Hueper, 1955).

Rabbit: Eight rabbits received 6 weekly i.v. injections of 0.5 ml/kg bw of a 5% sus-pension of *chromium* powder in gelatin-saline solution in the ear vein; the same course of treatment was given 4 months later; and 3 years after the first injection, a third series of in-jections were given to 3 surviving rabbits.   Four rabbits given i.v. injections of the vehicle alone served as controls.   One of 3 rabbits that lived 6 months after the last injection develo-ped a tumour (apparently an immature carcinoma) involving a lymph node, but no tumours occurred in controls.   In a further experiment, 6 female rabbits received 6 weekly i.v. injec-tions of 5 ml of a 5% suspension of *chromite [III] ore* in gelatin-saline solution; and the treatment was repeated in 4 of the 6 rabbits 9 months later. The 6 rabbits died or were killed at 13, 20, 22, 22, 48 and 48 months. No tumours were observed during these periods in test animals (Hueper, 1955).

(f)   Intrapleural administration

Mouse: No tumours were observed after 14 months in 50 C57BL male mice that received 6 intrapleural injections of 0.2 ml of a 0.005% suspension of *chromium* powder in gelatin-saline solution every other week; 32 mice lived for 7-14 months (Hueper, 1955).

Groups of 30 male and 25 female A mice were given 4 intrapleural injections of 0.05 ml of a 2 or 4% suspension of *mixed chromium dust*[1] in olive oil at 4-6 week intervals. No more lung tumours were seen during an observation period of 38 weeks than in a control group of 23 males and 18 females observed for 101 weeks (Baetjer *et al.*, 1959b).

Only granulomas were produced when *chromite [III]* dust [FeO(CrAl)$_2$O$_3$] particles (average diameter, 1 μm; range, 0.1-5 μm) were injected intrapleurally at a level of 10 mg in 0.5 ml distilled water into Balb/C mice. Animals were killed at intervals from 2 weeks to 18 months after the injection (Davis, 1972).

Rat: Groups of 17 female and 8 male Osborne-Mendel rats were given 6 monthly intrapleural injections of 0.05 ml of a 33.6% (by weight) suspension of *chromium* powder in lanolin; and 25 male Wistar rats received 6 weekly intrapleural injections of 0.1 ml of a 0.5% suspension of *chromium* powder in a gelatin-saline solution. Six Osborne-Mendel rats sur-vived up to 19-24 months and 12 Wistar rats up to 25-30 months. Three haemangiomas (in a female Osborne-Mendel rat) and 1 angiosarcoma were observed at different sites in the treated animals. Round-cell sarcomas were observed in 1 treated animal (group unspecified) and in 3/12 male Wistar vehicle-treated controls that lived for 18 months (Hueper, 1955).

---

[1] See footnote on page p. 254.

Groups of 20 male and 19 female Bethesda Black rats received 16 monthly intrapleural injections of 2 mg *sodium dichromate [VI]* in gelatin and were observed for up to 2 years. One adenocarcinoma of the lung was observed; no tumours at the injection site were observed in 60 control rats treated with gelatin solution. After intrapleural implantation of 12.5 mg *calcium chromate [VI]* in a gelatin capsule to 14 rats, 8 developed malignant tumours (unspecified) at the site of implantation after 2 years; no tumours occurred after 2 years at the site of 8 intrapleural implantations over 13 months of 25 mg *chromic [III] acetate* in gelatin capsules to 42 rats (Hueper & Payne, 1962).

Other chromium compounds tested in rats in experiments lasting 27 months gave the following numbers of tumours at the site of their intrapleural implantation (details of dose and tumour type not given): *calcium chromate [VI]*, 20/ 32 (0 alive at 1 year); *sintered calcium chromate [VI]*, 17/33 (9 alive at 1 year); *strontium chromate [VI]*, 17/28 (9 alive at 1 year); *barium chromate [VI]*, 1/31 (30 alive at 1 year); *lead chromate [VI]*, 3/34 (32 alive at 1 year); *sodium dichromate [VI]*, 0/26 (20 alive at 1 year); *chromite [III] roast residue*, 5/32 (28 alive at 1 year); *zinc yellow [VI]* [1], 22/33 (11 alive at 1 year); and *chromic [III] acetate*, 1/34 (18 alive at 15 months). None of 34 control rats had tumours (30 alive at 1 year) (Hueper, 1961).

Of 14 male and 11 female Osborne-Mendel rats that received 6 monthly intrapleural injections of 0.05 ml of a 73.4% (by weight) suspension of *unroasted chromite [III] ore* in lanolin, 13 survived 1 year; all animals were dead at 24 months. One thoracic tumour (fibrosarcoma) was found (Hueper, 1955).

Sheep-fat cubes containing 25 mg *roasted chromite [III] ore* [2] were implanted in the pleural cavity of 25 male Bethesda Black rats. Squamous-cell carcinomas of the lungs were observed in 2/4 rats that survived 19-24 months. Only 4/15 female controls given an implant of sheep fat survived this period, and 1 lung adenoma was observed (Hueper, 1958).

In a similar experiment, 25 mg *roasted chromite [III] ore* in 50 mg sheep fat (equivalent to 2 mg Cr) were implanted intrapleurally into 15 male and 20 female Bethesda Black rats. Implantation-site tumours (unspecified) occurred in 3 rats over 17 months. No tumours were seen in 35 rats injected intrapleurally with the sheep-fat vehicle only (Payne, 1960b).

---

[1] It was not specified whether this compound was zinc chromate, zinc potassium chromate or zinc yellow.

[2] The roasted chromite ore tested by Hueper (1958) was a process-derived material which contained unspeciated chromium compounds formed during oxidative heating of a chromium ore that had been subjected to alkaline leaching. Hueper sometimes referred to this material as 'chromate' and sometimes as 'chromite'.

Reticulum-cell sarcomas of the lung were induced in 3/17 random-bred Wistar rats after 2 intrapleural injections of 5 mg *chromic [III] oxide* (Dvizhkov & Fedorova, 1967) [The Working Group noted that no vehicle-treated or untreated controls were reported].

(g)   Other experimental systems

Intramedullary administration into the femur: A group of 25 male Wistar *rats* received an injection into the femur of 0.2 ml of a 50% (by weight) suspension of *chromium* powder (45 mg) in gelatin-saline and were observed for 24 months; 19 survived over 1 year. No tumours developed at the injection site. Of 25 male Osborne-Mendel rats injected in the femur with the same dose of *chromium* powder in lanolin and observed for 24 months, 14 survived for 1 year; 1 rat developed a fibroma at the injection site. Of 15 male and 10 female Osborne-Mendel rats injected in the femur with 0.05 ml of a 73.4% (by weight) suspension containing 58 mg   *chromite [III] ore* in lanolin, 15 survived one year; no tumours developed at the injection site (Hueper, 1955).

Injections into subcutaneously implanted tracheal rings: Seventy-two tracheal rings excised from female Wistar-Lewis *rats* were implanted subcutaneously into the backs of 13 rats of the same strain. Two weeks later, the grafts were filled by injection with 0.05 ml of an agar suspension of 2.5 mg *chromium carbonyl* with or without 2.5 mg benzo[a] pyrene. Biopsies were performed at intervals. Ten squamous-cell carcinomas developed in 24 trachea that received the mixture, and 2 carcinomas developed in 22 trachea treated with chromium carbonyl alone. Three of the tracheal carcinomas produced by the mixture met-astasized within 9 months. No tumours occurred in the 4 trachea that received the vehicle only (Lane & Mass, 1977).

Table 8. Summary of carcinogenicity studies of chromium and chromium compounds in animals

Compound	Species	Route and dosage	Findings	Reference
Chromium powder	Mouse	4 i.p. injections of 0.2 ml of a 0.005% solution	1 myeloid leukaemia in 50 treated animals	Hueper, 1955
	Mouse	6 i.v. injections of 0.05 ml of a 0.005% solution	No tumours	Hueper, 1955
	Mouse	6 intrapleural injections of 0.2 ml of a 0.005% suspension	No tumours in 50 treated mice	Hueper, 1955
	Rat	1 intratracheal injection of 10 mg	No squamous-cell carcinomas of the lung in 12 treated rats	Mukubo, 1978
	Rat	1 i.m. injection of 2 mg	No local tumours in 22 surviving treated animals	Sunderman et al., 1974
	Rat	6 i.p. injections of 0.1 ml of a 0.05% suspension	No increase in round-cell sarcoma incidence compared with controls; 2 insulinomas in treated animals, none in controls	Hueper, 1955
	Rat	6 i.v. injections of 0.18 ml of a 0.05% suspension	2 rats with pulmonary adenomas; no increase in sarcomas compared with controls	Hueper, 1955
	Rat	6 intrapleural injections of 0.05 ml of a 33.6% (by weight) suspension or 6 intrapleural injections of 0.1 ml of a 0.5% suspension	2 haemangiomas and 1 angiosarcoma in 50 treated animals and 0/25 controls	Hueper, 1955
	Rat	Intramedullary injection into the femur of 46 mg	No injection-site tumours in 25 treated animals	Hueper, 1955

Table 8 (contd)

Compound	Species	Route and dosage	Findings	Reference
Chromium powder (contd)	Rabbit	18 i.v. injections of 0.5 ml/kg bw of a 5% suspension	1 carcinoma of lymph node in 3 treated survivors and 0/4 controls	Hueper, 1955
Unroasted chromite [III] ore	Mouse	Intrapleural injection of 10 mg in 0.5 ml distilled water	Granulomas	Davis, 1972
	Rat	6 intrapleural injections of 0.05 ml of a 73.4% (by weight) suspension	Injection-site sarcoma in 1/25 treated animals	Hueper, 1955
	Rat	Intramedullary injection into the femur of 58 mg	No injection-site tumours in 25 treated rats	Hueper, 1955
	Rabbit	12 i.v. injections of 5 ml of a 5% suspension	No tumours	Hueper, 1955
Roasted chromite [III] ore	Mouse	I.m. implantation of 10 mg (equivalent to 0.79 mg chromium)	No implantation-site tumours	Payne, 1960b
	Rat	I.m. implantation of 25 mg	Sarcomas at implantation site in 3/31 treated animals and 0 vehicle controls	Hueper, 1958
	Rat	I.m. implantation	Tumours (type unspecified) at implantation site in 1/34 treated animals and 0/32 vehicle controls	Hueper, 1961
	Rat	Intrapleural implantation	Tumours (type unspecified) at implantation site in 5/32 treated animals and 0/34 controls	Hueper, 1961

Table 8 (contd)

Compound	Species	Route and dosage	Findings	Reference
Roasted chromite [III] ore (contd)	Rat	Intrapleural implantation of 25 mg	Lung squamous-cell carcinomas in 2/4 treated survivors and 1 lung adenoma in 1/4 controls	Hueper, 1958
	Rat	Intrapleural implantation of 25 mg (equivalent to 2 mg chromium)	Implantation-site tumours (type unspecified) in 3/35 treated rats and 0/35 controls	Payne, 1960b
Mixed chromate [VI] dust[a]	Mouse	Inhalation, 4 hrs/day, 5 days/wk for 16-58 wks (total dose chromium inhaled: 480-1205 mg-hrs)	No lung carcinomas; no significant increase in lung adenomas in 500 treated animals compared with controls	Baetjer et al., 1959b
	Mouse	5-6 intratracheal instillations of dust (equivalent to 0.04 mg chromium trioxide)	No more lung tumours in 506 treated mice than in controls	Baetjer et al., 1959b
	Mouse	4 intrapleural injections of 0.05 ml of a 2 or 4% suspension	No increase in lung tumour incidence in 55 treated animals compared with 41 controls	Baetjer et al., 1959b
	Rat	Inhalation, 4-5 hrs/day, 4 days/wk for lifespan (chromic oxide concentration of 3-4 mg/m^3)	No significant increase in tumour incidence in 78 treated rats compared with controls	Steffee & Baetjer, 1965

Table 8 (contd)

Compound	Species	Route and dosage	Findings	Reference
Mixed chromate dust + potassium di-chromate [VI]	Rat	16 intratracheal injections of 0.1 ml of suspension of 0.5% roasted chromate + 0.6% potassium dichromate (equivalent to 0.07 mg chromium/dose)	No significant increase in tumour incidence compared with controls	Steffee & Baetjer, 1965
Mixed chromate [VI] dust + potassium dichromate [VI] + sodium chromate [VI] + pulverized residue dust	Rabbit	Inhalation, 4 days/wk for 50 months	No increase in tumour incidence compared with controls	Steffee & Baetjer, 1965
	Guinea-pig	Inhalation, 4 days/wk for lifespan	Pulmonary carcinomas in 3/50 treated animals	Steffee & Baetjer, 1965
Barium chromate [VI]	Rat	I.m. implantation of 25 mg	No implantation-site tumours in 35 rats	Hueper & Payne, 1959
	Rat	I.m. implantation	No implantation-site tumours in 34 rats	Hueper, 1961
	Rat	Intrapleural implantation	Implantation-site tumours in 1/31 treated rats and 0/34 controls	Hueper, 1961
Calcium chromate [VI]	Mouse	Inhalation, 13 mg/m^3 5 hrs/day, 5 days/wk for lifespan	Lung adenomas in 14/136 treated animals and 5/136 controls	Nettesheim et al., 1971
	Mouse	I.m. implantation of 10 mg	Implantation-site sarcomas in 2/50 and in 0/50 controls	Payne, 1960a
	Mouse	1 s.c. injection of 10 mg	Injection-site sarcomas in 1/13 and in 0/52 controls	Payne, 1960a

Table 8 (contd)

Compound	Species	Route and dosage	Findings	Reference
Calcium chromate [VI] (contd)	Rat	Bronchial implantation	6 squamous-cell carcinomas and 2 adeno-carcinomas of the lung in 100 treated rats; 0/24 controls	Laskin et al., 1970
	Rat	Bronchial implantation	Increased incidence of bronchial squamous-cell carcinomas	Levy & Venitt, 1975
	Rat	Inhalation, 2 mg/m³, 589 exposures of 5 hrs over 891 days	1 squamous-cell carcinoma of lung, 1 of larynx, 1 'peritruncal tumour' (no. of treated animals unspecified)	Laskin, 1972
	Rat	I.m. implantation of 12.5 mg	Malignant tumours at implantation site in 4/8 treated animals	Hueper & Payne, 1962
	Rat	20 injections, total dose 19 mg	Injection-site sarcomas in 18/24 and 0 in vehicle controls	Roe & Carter, 1969
	Rat	12 injections of 4 mg	Injection-site sarcomas in 5/45 and 0/22 in vehicle controls	Furst et al., 1976
	Rat	I.m. implantation of 25 mg	Injection-site sarcomas in 8/35 treated animals and 0/32 controls	Hueper & Payne, 1959
	Rat	I.m. implantation	Tumours (type unspecified) at implantation site in 9/32 treated animals and 0/32 controls	Hueper, 1961
	Rat	Intrapleural implantation of 12.5 mg	Malignant tumours (unspecified) at implantation site in 8/14 treated animals	Hueper & Payne, 1962
	Rat	Intrapleural implantation	Tumours (type unspecified) at implantation site in 20/32 treated animals and 0/34 controls	Hueper, 1961
	Hamster	Inhalation, 2 mg/m³, 589 exposures	1 squamous-cell carcinoma and 1 papilloma of larynx (no. of treated animals unspecified)	Laskin et al., 1972

Table 8 (contd)

Compound	Species	Route and dosage	Findings	Reference
Sintered calcium chromate [VI]	Mouse	I.m. implantation of 10 mg	Implantation-site sarcomas in 9/46 treated animals and 0/50 controls	Payne, 1960a
	Mouse	S.c. injection of 10 mg	No injection-site sarcomas	Payne, 1960a
	Rat	I.m. implantation of 25 mg	Implantation-site sarcomas in 8/35 treated animals and 0 controls	Hueper & Payne, 1959
	Rat	I.m. implantation	Tumours (type unspecified) at implantation site in 12/34 treated animals and 0/32 controls	Hueper, 1961
	Rat	Intrapleural implantation	Tumours (type unspecified) at implantation site in 17/33 treated rats and 0/34 controls	Hueper, 1961
Chromic [III] acetate	Mouse	P.o., 5 mg/l drinking-water for life	No increase in tumour incidence	Schroeder et al., 1964
	Rat	P.o., 5 mg/l drinking-water for life	No increase in tumour incidence	Schroeder et al., 1965
	Rat	8 i.m. implantations of 25 mg each, over 24 months	Implantation-site sarcoma in 1/35 treated animals	Hueper & Payne, 1962
	Rat	I.m. implantation	Implantation-site tumour (type unspecified) in 1/34 and in 0/32 controls	Hueper, 1961
	Rat	8 intrapleural implantations of 25 mg each over 13 months	No implantation-site tumours after 2 years in 42 treated animals	Hueper & Payne, 1962

Table 8 (contd)

Compound	Species	Route and dosage	Findings	Reference
Chromic [III] acetate (contd)	Rat	Intrapleural implantation	Implantation-site tumour (type unspecified) in 1/34 and in 0/34 controls	Hueper, 1961
Chromic [III] oxide	Rat	P.o., 1, 2 and 5% in bread on 5 days/wk for 2 years	1% dose: 3/60 mammary fibroadenomas 2% dose: 1/60 " " 5% dose: 3/60 " " controls: 1/60 mammary carcinoma; 2/60 fibroadenomas	Ivankovic & Preussmann, 1975
	Rat	Single intratracheal application of 50 or 20 mg	50 mg dose: 7/34 with tumours (4 with lung sarcomas) 20 mg dose: 6/18 with tumours (5 with lung sarcomas) no controls	Dvizhkov & Fedorova, 1967
	Rat	Bronchial implantation	No lung tumours in 98 animals	Laskin et al., 1970
	Rat	1 i.p. injection of 20 mg	Lung sarcomas in 4/20; no controls	Dvizhkov & Fedorova, 1967
	Rat	2 intrapleural injections of 5 mg	Reticulum-cell sarcomas of lung in 3/17 treated animals; no controls	Dvizhkov & Fedorova, 1967
Chromium carbonyl	Rat	Injection of 2.5 mg into subcutaneously implanted tracheal rings	Squamous-cell carcinomas in 2/22 animals; none in 4 vehicle controls	Lane & Mass, 1977
Chromium [III] sulphate	Mouse	24 i.p. injections (total doses: 480, 1200 and 2400 mg/kg bw)	No significant increase of pulmonary adenoma incidence in 60 treated rats compared with 40 vehicle and untreated controls	Stoner et al., 1976
Chromium [VI] trioxide	Rat	Bronchial implantation	No increase in lung tumour incidence in 100 treated rats compared with 24 controls	Laskin et al., 1970

Table 8 (contd)

Compound	Species	Route and dosage	Findings	Reference
Sintered chromium [VI] trioxide	Mouse	1 s.c. injection of 10 mg	No injection-site tumours in 52 treated animals	Payne, 1960a
	Rat	I.m. implantation of 25 mg	Implantation-site sarcomas in 15/35 treated animals and 0/35 controls	Hueper & Payne, 1959
Cobalt-chromium alloy	Rat	I.m. injection of 28 mg	Injection-site sarcomas in 7/74 treated rats; other tumours in 7/74	Heath et al., 1971
Lead chromate [VI]	Mouse	4 i.m. injections of 3 mg	2 lymphomas and 3 lung adenocarcinomas in 17 mice necropsied; similar incidences in controls	Furst et al., 1976
	Rat	1 s.c. injection of 30 mg	Injection-site sarcomas in 26/40 treated animals and 0/60 vehicle controls	Maltoni, 1974, 1976a
	Rat	9 i.m. injections of 8 mg	Injection-site sarcomas in 31/47 treated rats; 3 renal carcinomas; 0/22 in vehicle controls	Furst et al., 1976
	Rat	I.m. implantation	Tumour (type unspecified) at implantation site in 1/33 treated rats and 0/32 controls	Hueper, 1961
	Rat	Intrapleural implantation	Tumours (type unspecified) at injection site in 3/34 treated rats and 0/34 controls	Hueper, 1961
Lead chromate [VI] oxide	Rat	1 s.c. injection of 30 mg	Injection-site sarcomas in 27/40 treated rats and 0/60 vehicle controls	Maltoni, 1974, 1976a

Table 8 (contd)

Compound	Species	Route and dosage	Findings	Reference
Potassium chromate [VI]	Rat	Bronchial implantation	No increased incidence of lung tumours	Levy & Venitt, 1975
Potassium dichromate [VI]	Rat	Bronchial implantation	No increased incidence of lung tumours	Levy & Venitt, 1975
Sodium chromate [VI]	Rat	Bronchial implantation	No increased incidence of lung tumours	Levy & Venitt, 1975
Sodium dichromate [VI]	Rat	16 i.m. injections of 2 mg	No injection-site tumours	Hueper & Payne, 1962
	Rat	I.m. implantation	No implantation-site tumours	Hueper, 1961
	Rat	16 intrapleural injections of 2 mg	1 lung adenocarcinoma in 39 treated animals; no injection-site tumours in 60 vehicle controls	Hueper & Payne, 1962
	Rat	Intrapleural implantation	No injection-site tumours in 26 treated animals	Hueper, 1961
	Rat	Bronchial implantation	No increase in lung tumours	Levy & Venitt, 1975
Strontium chromate [VI]	Rat	I.m. implantation	Implantation-site tumours in 15/33 treated animals and 0/32 controls	Hueper, 1961
Zinc potassium chromate [VI]	Rat	Bronchial implantation	Increased incidence of bronchial squamous-cell carcinomas	Levy & Venitt, 1975
Zinc yellow	Mouse	6 intratracheal injections of 0.03 ml of a 0.2% suspension	No pulmonary carcinomas; pulmonary adenomas in 31/62 treated animals and 7/18 untreated controls	Steffee & Baetjer, 1965

Table 8 (contd)

Compound	Species	Route and dosage	Findings	Reference
Zinc yellow (contd)	Rat	I.m. implantation	Tumours (type unspecified) at implantation site in 16/34 treated animals and 0/32 controls	Hueper, 1961[b]
	Rat	Intrapleural implantation	Tumours (type unspecified) at implantation site in 22/33 treated animals and 0/34 controls	Hueper, 1961[b]

[a]See footnote on p. 254.

[b]It was not specified whether this compound was zinc chromate, zinc potassium chromate or zinc yellow.

3.2 Other relevant biological data

Chromium [III] is considered to be an essential element in nutrition and for the main-tenance of normal glucose tolerance in experimental animals and man. The exact chemical structure of this factor is not known (Mertz, 1975).

The toxicology and metabolism of chromium compounds have been reviewed by the National Academy of Sciences (1974), Langård & Norseth (1979) and Langård (1980), and only a few aspects will be given in the following section.

When discussing biological effects of chromium and its compounds, it is important to distinguish between the different oxidation states, because of their greatly different abilities to penetrate cellular membranes and associated differences in distribution and effects in biological systems. Evaluation of experimental studies in animals and in *in vitro* test systems for carcinogenicity and mutagenicity is sometimes difficult because of lack of in-formation about the purity of the chemical compounds used and in particular about the oxi-dation state of chromium salts. It is known, for example, that not only industrial Cr[III] compounds (Petrilli & DeFlora, 1978a) but even reagent-grade Cr[III] compounds (Levis & Majone, 1979) may be contaminated by Cr[VI].

Cr[III] is the most stable oxidation state of chromium and is always present as a coordination complex, which, in aqueous media and at physiological pH, has a strong tendency to hydrolyse and to chelate (Mertz, 1969). In biological systems, Cr[III] exists in solution when complexed with biological molecules. The rate of liquid formation is ex-tremely slow, and such complexes are therefore extremely stable.

Cr[VI] is almost always linked with oxygen to form ions such as chromate and di-chromate, which are strong oxidizing agents and are reduced to Cr[III] in acidic solution. No complexes are known in which Cr[VI] is stabilized against reduction by organic matter (National Academy of Sciences, 1974).

Biological membranes are readily permeable to Cr[VI] but not to Cr[III] (National Academy of Sciences, 1974). The reduction of Cr[VI] to Cr[III] outside the cell or at other than target molecules therefore gives rise to stable Cr[III] complexes, and the metal is then unable to react with other molecules.

(a) Experimental systems

Toxic effects

The LD_{50} of chromium carbonyl by i.v. injection in mice is 30 mg/kg bw. The mean i.v. lethal dose in mice is 85 mg/kg bw for chromium [III] sulphate, 400-800 mg/kg bw for chromium [III] chloride and 2290 mg/kg bw for chromic [III] acetate (National Academy of Sciences, 1974).

Parenchymatous changes in liver and kidney with destruction of renal tubule cells were reported in various laboratory animals by Mosinger & Fiorentini (1954) after administration of potassium chromate [VI] by different routes.

Renal lesions in animals are confined to the proximal convoluted tubules (reviews: National Academy of Sciences, 1974; Langård, 1980). Franchini et al. (1978) exposed rats to a single s.c. dose (15 mg/kg bw) of potassium dichromate [VI] and observed increases in urinary β-glucuronidase, lysozyme, glucose and protein as well as morphological changes in renal tubules. The glomerular filtration rate was unchanged. In another experimental group, s.c. injections of 3 mg/kg bw potassium dichromate [VI] were given to rats every other day for 8 weeks. No clear pattern of renal accumulation of chromium was found. Urinary elimination increased continuously during the experiment in correlation with the accumulation of chromium in the renal cortex.

Oral intake of 1.9-5.5 mg/kg bw chromium in the form of monochromates or dichromates daily for 29-685 days produced no observable harmful effects in dogs, cats or rabbits (National Academy of Sciences, 1974).

Exposure of cats by inhalation to 11-23 mg/m^3 Cr[VI] as dichromate for 2-3 hours/day during 5 days caused bronchitis and pneumonia. In rabbits exposed similarly, no effects were observed. Mixed dusts containing chromates (7 mg/m^3 as chromium [VI] trioxide) were fatal to mice when inhaled for 37 hours over 10 days; whereas no marked effects were noted in rabbits or guinea-pigs that inhaled 5 mg/m^3 (as chromium [VI] trioxide) for 4 hours/day on 5 days/week for one year (National Academy of Sciences, 1974).

Increased subepithelial connective tissue and flattened epithelium in the large bronchi were observed in mice exposed to chromate (Nettesheim et al., 1971). Rats exposed by inhalation in air to 42 mg/m^3 chromic [III] oxide or to 43 mg/m^3 chromic [III] phosphate for 5 hours/day on 5 days/week for 4 months developed chronic irritation of the bronchus and lung parenchyma and dystrophic changes in the liver and kidney (Blokin & Trop, 1977).

Continuous exposure for over 32 days of the fish Rutilus rutilus to 0.1, 1.0 or 10 ppm potassium [VI] dichromate resulted in hypertrophy and hyperplasia of the gill epithelium, severe necrosis of kidney tubules, intestinal haemorrhages and lysis of intestinal epithelium (Strik et al., 1975).

As a general rule, Cr[VI] is much more toxic than Cr[III] when administered to animals (reviews: Langård, 1980; Langård & Norseth, 1979; Mertz, 1969); and very marked differences in the cytotoxicity of compounds of the two oxidation states have been observed in mammalian cells in vitro (Kaneko, 1976; Raffetto et al., 1977; Whiting et al., 1979). Potassium dichromate [VI] induced a rapid blockage of DNA replication in Syrian hamster fibroblasts (BHK line), whereas RNA and protein syntheses were inhibited secondarily (Levis *et al.,* 1978a). It also reduced the colony-forming ability of BHK cells at doses (10^{-4}-10^{-7} M) that were about 1000 times lower than those at which chromic [III] chloride (10^{-2}-10^{-5} M) was active and was 100 times more effective in inhibiting DNA synthesis (Levis *et al.,* 1978b). A large difference in cytotoxic activity between Cr[VI] and Cr[III] was also noticed when the effects of 11 water-soluble chromium compounds on BHK cells were compared; among Cr[III] compounds only chromic nitrate was really cytotoxic, since it was contaminated with about 2 parts per thousand Cr[VI] (Levis & Majone, 1979). Potassium dichromate [VI] but not chromic [III] chloride affected the passive and facilitated uptake of ribo- and deoxy-ribonucleosides (Bianchi *et al.,* 1979; Levis *et al.,* 1978b), and these two compounds also acted differentially on plasma membrane Mg^{2+}-ATPase activity of BHK cells (Luciani *et al.,* 1979). Both Cr[VI] and Cr[III] induced karyological alterations in mammalian cells (Majone, 1977; Majone & Rensi, 1979); however, these effects were observed after exposure to concentrations of Cr[VI] that were more than 100 times lower than those of Cr[III] (Levis & Majone, 1979; Majone & Rensi, 1979).

Cr[III] has been found in ribonucleic acids from all sources examined. It is possible that chromium helps stabilize the structure of RNA (Wacker & Vallee, 1959).

White *et al.* (1979) have shown that water-soluble Cr[VI] is cytotoxic in the established human cell line NHIK 3025, producing a 50% reduction in the number of cells with a concentration of 5×10^{-7} mol/l. They also showed that the observed cytotoxicity of stainless-steel welding fumes is due entirely to their water-soluble Cr[VI] content.

Effects on reproduction and prenatal toxicity

Golden hamsters received chromium [VI] trioxide intravenously on day 8 of pregnancy as single i.v. injections of either 5, 7.5, 10 or 15 mg/kg bw. The dose of 15 mg/kg bw proved to be lethal to 3/4 mother animals; with 5 mg/kg bw (173 living fetuses), no clear-cut increase in the rate of resorptions was observed, but 4% of the fetuses showed external abnormalities (oedema, exencephaly) and 34% showed cleft palate (controls, 2%). The rate of resorptions increased with the higher doses (29% with 7.5 mg/kg bw; 41% with 10 mg/kg bw; 2% in controls), as did the rate of malformations (cleft palate, 85% at 7.5 and 10 mg/kg bw). With the higher doses, 31% (7.5 mg/kg bw) and 49% (10 mg/kg bw) of the fetuses were retarded (Gale, 1974, 1978).

Placental transfer and embryotoxicity of chromic [III] chloride were studied in ICR mice. When 9.8 or 19.5 mg/kg bw (as Cr) were injected subcutaneously every other day from day 0 to day 16 of pregnancy (9 doses), a dose-dependent increase in the chromium concentration could be measured in several maternal organs (blood, liver, kidney, spleen); values exceeded those in controls by up to 20 times. There was also a slight increase in the chromium content of the placenta, although the concentration in the fetus was hardly changed under these conditions. The fetuses examined were retarded, but the resorption rates were similar in controls and treated groups. A slight increase in the rate of malformations was observed.

In another experimental series, chromic [III] chloride was given intraperitoneally on day 8 of pregnancy at doses of 9.8-24.4 mg/kg bw (as Cr). No data on placental transfer were reported. Again, no increased resorption rate was observed, except in the highest dose group, but fetal growth retardation was noticed in all dose groups. There was apparently a dose-dependent increase in malformations (especially in the frequency of exencephaly and anencephaly) and an increase in the occurrence of rib fusion (Iijima *et al.*, 1975; Matsumoto *et al.*, 1976).

Absorption, distribution and excretion

The metabolism of chromium compounds has been reviewed by the National Academy of Sciences (1974), by Langård & Norseth (1979) and by Langård (1980). Less than 1% Cr [III] is absorbed from the gastrointestinal tract of animals, whereas chromates [VI] are absorbed at a rate of 3-6% in rats. These absorption values are based on urinary excretion values and may be underestimations, since the gastrointestinal tract also takes part in chromium excretion (Mertz, 1969).

Potassium dichromate [VI] administered intratracheally to guinea-pigs is absorbed rapidly and found in the red blood cells (20% of the injected dose), in the lungs (15%) and in the spleen, liver and kidney (5% altogether) 10 minutes after the injection. Trivalent chromium binds to lung tissue more readily than does hexavalent chromium: when chromic [III] chloride was injected intratracheally, 69% of the dose was recovered from the lungs of animals killed 10 minutes after injection (Baetjer *et al.*, 1959a). In rats, brain and muscle appear to have little affinity for injected chromium as chromic [III] chloride, but there is a considerable uptake by liver, spleen and bone marrow (Visek *et al.*, 1953).

Following a single s.c. injection of 15 mg/kg bw potassium dichromate [VI], the concentration of chromium in red blood cells of rats was highest after 12 hours. After 48 hours, the highest concentrations were found in the renal cortex, liver and spleen (Mutti *et al.*, 1979a).

Water-soluble chromates disappear rapidly from the lungs into the circulation and other organs after intratracheal administration, whereas trivalent chromic chloride does not. Thirty days after injection, 30% of the trivalent chromium but only 2.4% of the hexavalent chromium was still present in the lung tissue (Baetjer *et al.*, 1959a). When injected intravenously into rats, sodium chromate [VI] accumulates in the kidneys and later in the spleen (Kovalchuk, 1966).

Zinc chromate [VI] was absorbed quickly in rats exposed to known atmospheric concentrations (6.3-10.7 mg/m^3, equivalent to 1.3-2.2 mg/m^3 chromium) in an inhalation chamber: a 5-fold increase in the blood chromium level was observed after 100 min of inhalation exposure, and this level increased at a similar rate during the next 150 min. Elimination from blood was slow: the blood chromium level fell by less than 50% during the first 3 days after exposure; and after 18 and 37 days, respectively, 20% and 9% of the initial concentration remained. Excretion occurred mainly *via* the urine (Langård *et al.,* 1978).

Trivalent chromium is transported in rat serum bound to siderophilin, albumin, γ-globulin and two α-proteins (Jett *et al.,* 1968). Onkelinx (1977) studied the metabolism of Cr[III] in rats by i.v. injection: it disappeared exponentially from plasma, and excretion took place mainly *via* the urine, with a small proportion in the faeces. Chromium accumulates in bone, kidney, spleen and liver.

Hexavalent chromium is transported (as chromate ion) through the cell membrane very effectively (Lilien *et al.,* 1970; Sanderson, 1976; Vallee, 1969), whereas trivalent chromium transport seems to be limited if not completely absent (Mertz, 1969; Polak *et al.,* 1973).

Inorganic chromium compounds, regardless of oxidation state or mode of administration, are not transferred transplacentally to any significant extent (National Academy of Sciences, 1974; Visek *et al.,* 1953). Iijima *et al.* (1975) and Matsumoto *et al.* (1976) reported similar findings for non-radioactive Cr[VI] (see section on embryotoxicity for experimental details). However, when ^{51}Cr was synthesized into the glucose tolerance factor by brewers' yeast, considerable amounts were transferred across the placenta (Mertz *et al.,* 1969).

Mutagenicity and other short-term tests

Chromium compounds of various oxidation states and solubilities were used in the experiments described below. The oxidation states for chromium given by the authors may sometimes be incorrect; this may lead to certain inconsistencies in the results cited. Cr[III] compounds, e.g., chromic [III] chloride, are extremely unstable, are frequently used as reducing agents, and may contribute only a small amount of Cr[III] to the system to which they are added. Cr[III] is known occasionally to be contaminated with Cr[VI], which may be the active agent. Water-soluble Cr[VI] is easily reduced at physiological pH, especially when autoredox systems are present (Levis & Majone, 1979; Petrilli & De Flora, 1978a).

Chromium interacted with nucleic acids in tissues treated with Cr[VI] after it had been reduced to Cr[III] by tissue components (Herrmann & Speck, 1954; Levis *et al.,* 1978b). Treatment of purified RNA (Huff *et al.,* 1964) and DNA (Kubinski *et al.,* 1977; Tamino, 1977) with Cr[III] *in vitro* induced physicochemical changes which were consistent with ligand bond formation.

Chromium [VI] trioxide decreased the fidelity and rate of DNA synthesis in an *in vitro* system containing avian myeloblastosis virus DNA polymerase, a synthetic template primer and complementary and noncomplementary nucleoside triphosphates (Sirover & Loeb, 1976).

Results with chromium compounds in bacterial tests for mutagenicity and allied effects are summarized in Table 9. In general, hexavalent chromium is convincingly mutagenic in at least three different bacterial mutation systems, whereas trivalent chromium is weakly mutagenic only in one and only at a much higher dose range. Similarly, hexavalent chromium is very much more effective than trivalent chromium in tests where the induction of DNA damage is inferred from differences in survival after treatment of DNA repair-proficient and DNA repair-deficient strains of bacteria.

That only Cr[VI] compounds are mutagenic in bacteria is supported by several further observations summarized in Table 9. The mutagenicity of Cr[VI] is decreased or abolished by chemical and biological reducing agents (such as the microsomal fraction from rat liver, erythrocyte lysate and human gastric juice, but not the microsomal fractions from rat lung or muscle) (De Flora *et al.*, 1979; Löfroth, 1978; Petrilli & De Flora, 1978b). Inactive Cr[III] compounds are converted to mutagens only by treatment with strong oxidizing agents and not with biological systems (Petrilli & De Flora, 1978a).

Stern (1980) summarized the mutagenic effects of various welding-fume matrices (containing Fe, Ni, Cr[III], Cr[VI], Al, etc.) and showed that the revertant rate observed in *Salmonella typhimurium* TA100 ($his^- \rightarrow his^+$) is due uniquely to the presence of water-soluble Cr[VI], independent of the nature of the fume matrix.

Potassium dichromate [VI] induced gene conversion in *Schizosaccharomyces pombe* (Bonatti *et al.*, 1976). Lead chromate [VI] induced mitotic recombination in *Saccharomyces cerevisiae*; rat-liver supernatant reduced this activity (Nestmann *et al.*, 1979).

Hexavalent chromium (potassium dichromate [VI] and zinc chromate [VI]) induced forward mutations to 8-azaguanine resistance in Chinese hamster V79/4 cells. Lead chromate [VI] (an insoluble salt) and chromic [III] acetate (a soluble salt) were inactive at 10 times and 200 times, respectively, the maximum dose at which cell survival was measurable after treatment with potassium dichromate [VI] (Newbold *et al.*, 1979). It was reported in an abstract that forward mutations to 6-thioguanine-resistance were induced by potassium dichromate [VI] in Chinese hamster V79 cells (Rainaldi *et al.*, 1979).

Several studies (summarized in Table 10) have shown that hexavalent chromium induces chromosomal aberrations in a variety of cultured mammalian cells; trivalent chromium, on the other hand, begins to show chromosome-damaging capacity only when tested at doses greater by 1-2 orders of magnitude. This difference in chromosome-damaging effect is paralleled by equally dramatic differences in cytotoxicity between hexavalent and trivalent chromium.

Table 9. Summary of bacterial tests for mutagenicity and allied effects of chromium compounds

Bacterial assay system	Trivalent chromium[a] Test compound(s)	Result	Hexavalent chromium Test compound(s)	Result	Reference
Reverse mutation: E. coli WP2 trp⁻ → trp⁺	none tested	–	Na_2CrO_4; $CaCrO_4$; K_2CrO_4;	+	Venitt & Levy (1974)
	none tested		$K_2Cr_2O_7$	+	Nishioka (1975)
	none tested		K_2CrO_4	+	Green et al. (1976)
Fluctuation test	none tested		$PbCrO_4$; CrO_3	+	Nestmann et al. (1979)
Plate test	none tested		$PbCrO_4$; CrO_3	–	
Reverse mutation: E. coli Hs30R arg⁻ → arg⁺	$Cr(OOCCH_3)_3$ (high dose)	+	$K_2Cr_2O_7$; K_2CrO_4	+	Nakamuro et al. (1978)
Reverse mutation: S. typhimurium (various strains)	$CrCl_3$	–	$K_2Cr_2O_7$; K_2CrO_4	+	Tamaro et al. (1975)
his⁻ → his⁺	$CrK(SO_4)_2$; $CrCl_3$	–	$Na_2Cr_2O_7$; CrO_3; $CaCrO_4$; K_2CrO_4	+	Petrilli & De Flora (1977)
	$CrK(SO_4)_2$; $CrCl_3$	–*	none tested		Petrilli & De Flora (1978a)
	$Cr_2O_3.FeO$ (also contained Cr[VI]) (*addition of oxidizing agent made these trivalent compounds mutagenic)	+			

Table 9 (contd)

Bacterial assay system	Trivalent chromium[a] Test compound(s)	Result	Hexavalent chromium Test compound(s)	Result	Reference
	none tested		$Na_2Cr_2O_7$; CrO_3; K_2CrO_4; $Zn_2CrO_4(OH)_2$; $PbO.PbCrO_4$ (*mutagenicity suppressed by addition of rat liver microsomes, erythrocyte lysates and reducing agents)	+*	Petrilli & De Flora (1978b)
	none tested		$Na_2Cr_2O_7$ (*mutagenicity decreased by preincubation with human gastric juice)	+*	De Flora et al. (1979) (abstract)
	none tested		chromate and dichromate (*mutagenicity decreased by addition of rat liver microsomes)	+*	Löfroth (1978)
	chromic salts	−	chromate and dichromate	+	Löfroth & Ames (1978)
	none tested		$PbCrO_4$; CrO_3 (*mutagenicity unaffected by addition of rat liver microsomes)	+*	Nestmann et al. (1979)
Forward mutation: E. coli K-12/343/113(λ) gal+	none tested		$PbCrO_4$	−	Nestmann et al. (1979)
Differential killing: ('DNA-repair') B. subtilis rec+/rec−	$CrCl_3$	−	$K_2Cr_2O_7$; K_2CrO_4 (*mutagenicity suppressed by addition of reducing agents)	+*	Nishioka (1975)

Table 9 (contd)

Bacterial assay system	Trivalent chromium[a] Test compound(s)	Result	Hexavalent chromium Test compound(s)	Result	Reference
	$CrCl_3$	—			Nakamuro et al. (1978)
	$Cr(OOCCH_3)_3$	+	$K_2Cr_2O_7$; K_2CrO_4; CrO_3	+	
	$Cr_2(SO_4)_3$	—	CrO_3; K_2CrO_4; $K_2Cr_2O_7$	+	Kada et al. (1980)
E. coli polA$^+$/polA$^-$	none tested		$PbCrO_4$	—	Nestmann et al. (1979)

[a]Because most anhydrous Cr[III] compounds are insoluble, those listed in this table were used in various hydrated forms.

Table 10. Summary of cytogenetic effects of chromium compounds on cultured mammalian cells

Cell type	Trivalent chromium			Hexavalent chromium			Reference
	Test compound	Dose range (x10^-6 M)	Result[a]	Test compound	Dose range (x10^-6 M)	Result[a]	
Primary Syrian hamster embryo cells	$CrCl_3$ $Cr_2(SO_4)_3$	6.8-68 3.5-35	— —	$K_2Cr_2O_7$ (* effect abolished by addition of a reducing agent)	0.3-1.7	+*	Tsuda & Kato (1976, 1977)
Human peripheral blood lympho-cytes	$CrCl_3$	1500-2255	+	CrO_3 CrO_3	0.7-3.4 20-60	+ +	Kaneko (1976)
Primary mouse fetal cells	$CrCl_3$	8 (as Cr)	+	$K_2Cr_2O_7$	0.3-2 (as Cr)	+	Raffetto et al. (1977)
Human embryonic fibroblasts	none tested			$K_2Cr_2O_7$	0.5	+	Bigaliev et al. (1977, 1978)
Human peripheral blood lympho-cytes	$Cr(OOCCH_3)_3$ $CrCl_3$	16-32 32	+ —	$K_2Cr_2O_7$ K_2CrO_4	0.5-4 4-8	+ +	Nakamuro et al. (1978)
Chinese hamster V79/4 cell line	none tested			$K_2Cr_2O_7$	1.7-2.7	+	Newbold et al. (1979)
Fm3A (mouse mammary car-cinoma)	$Cr_2(SO_4)_3$	32-1000	—	K_2CrO_4 $K_2Cr_2O_7$ CrO_3	3.2-10 0.6-3.2 1-10	+ + +	Umeda & Nishimura (1979)
Chinese hamster cell line CHO	$CrCl_3$ $CrK(SO_4)_2$ $Cr(OOCCH_3)_3$	960 (as Cr) 2885 96-385	+ + +	$K_2Cr_2O_7$ $Na_2Cr_2O_7$ K_2CrO_4 Na_2CrO_4 CrO_3 $CaCrO_4$	2-20 (as Cr) 2-20 (as Cr) 5 (as Cr) 5-10 (as Cr) 2-5 (as Cr) 10 (as Cr)	+ + + + + +	Levis & Majone (1979)

[a] In all these studies, '+' indicates the induction of significant increases in chromatid breaks and fragments, and in some cases rearrangements.

Several Cr[VI] compounds (at 10^{-6} M) (listed in Table 10 under Levis & Majone, 1979) doubled the frequency of sister-chromatid exchanges in Chinese hamster CHO cells, whereas Cr[III] compounds were completely inactive even when used at concentrations 500 times higher (Levis & Majone, 1979; Majone & Levis, 1979). Cr[VI] compounds (potassium chromate, potassium dichromate, 10^{-6} M, 48-hr exposure) quadrupled the frequency of sister-chromatid exchanges in cultured human fibroblasts; 10^{-6} M potassium chromate trebled the frequency in Chinese hamster CHO cells, whereas no increase was induced by 10^{-5} M chromic [III] chloride (MacRae *et al.*, 1979).

At equitoxic doses, hexavalent chromium (potassium dichromate), but not trivalent chromium (chromic chloride), induced unscheduled DNA synthesis in an established mouse cell line (Raffetto *et al.*, 1977). Potassium chromate [VI] but not chromic [III] glycine induced DNA damage (as determined by alkaline sucrose sedimentation) and unscheduled DNA synthesis in cultured human fibroblasts (Whiting *et al.*, 1979).

Hexavalent chromium induced morphological transformation in Syrian baby hamster kidney (BHK 21) cells (calcium chromate: Fradkin *et al.*, 1975), Syrian hamster primary embryonic cells (potassium dichromate: Tsuda & Kato, 1977), mouse tertiary fetal cells (potassium dichromate: Raffetto *et al.*, 1977; trivalent chromium as chromic chloride was also positive in this test) and Syrian hamster secondary embryo cells (sodium chromate: DiPaolo & Casto, 1979). Hexavalent chromium (potassium, calcium, lead and zinc chromates) also enhanced the viral transformation of Syrian hamster secondary embryo cells by simian adenovirus SA7 (Casto *et al.*, 1979) [The ability of cells, morphologically transformed by hexavalent chromium, to produce tumours when transplanted to appropriate animals was not tested in any of these studies].

Potassium chromate [VI] induced a significant and dose-related increase in micronucleated polychromatic erythrocytes (micronuclei) in the bone marrow of NMRI mice following 2 i.p. injections of doses ranging from 12-48 mg/kg bw (Wild, 1978).

Potassium dichromate [VI], administered chronically by i.p. injection to rats at a dose of 1 mg/kg bw, caused a significant increase in chromosomal aberrations in the bone marrow (approximately 13% of cells with aberrations compared with less than 2% in controls). A single i.p. dose of 15 mg/kg bw sodium dichromate [VI] induced aberrations in 6% of bone-marrow cells (Bigaliev *et al.*, 1978).

(b) Humans

Toxic effects

The lethal dose of various forms of hexavalent chromium compounds by ingestion has been estimated to be in the range 1.5-16 g (Langård, 1980). In such fatal poisoning cases, haemorrhagic changes have been found in various organs, and particularly in the gastro-intestinal tract; bleeding is thus one of the reasons for shock and death. Pathological lesions were also observed in the kidneys, particularly in the tubules. Sharma *et al.* (1978) reported a case of acute poisoning with intravascular haemolysis and acute renal failure after ingestion of 'a few grams' of potassium dichromate [VI].

Chronic ulcers (Maloof, 1955), acute irritative dermatitis and allergic eczematous dermatitis have occurred in workers in contact with chromium compounds. The hexavalent chromium compounds are particularly active, the role of trivalent compounds being questionable (Nater, 1962). Chromate dermatitis may be aggravated by ingestion of chromate (Kaaber & Veien, 1978).

Contact hypersensitivity due to chromium compounds has been reviewed by Polak *et al.* (1973). It is caused by a direct effect of a hapten on the skin, where chromium is conjugated with autologous proteins. Cr[VI] is reduced to Cr[III] in the skin, chiefly by sulphydryl groups of aminoacids; only Cr[III] is then able to conjugate with proteins. Cr[III] is therefore probably bound to proteins to build the full antigen.

Exposure to airborne Cr[VI] compounds may give rise to a corrosive reaction in the nasal septum leading to perforation (Cavazzani & Viola, 1970; Kleinfeld & Rosso, 1965). Bronchitis has been reported to be more frequent among electric welders using electrodes containing chromium than in controls (Jindrichova, 1978). Bovet *et al.* (1977) detected an obstructive respiratory syndrome among workers in the chromium electroplating industry. Bronchial asthma may occur as a result of inhalation of chromate dust or chromium [VI] trioxide fumes (Meyers, 1950).

Franchini *et al.* (1978) reported on the excretion of β-glucuronidase, protein and lysozyme in the urine of a total of 99 workers exposed to chromium compounds. No abnormal levels were found among 39 stainless-steel welders; 8/22 workers using special electrodes when welding on armoured steel had increased urinary levels of β-glucuronidase, and 3 of these workers had proteinuria. Among 24 workers engaged in chromium plating, 9 had increased β-glucuronidase and 4 had elevated levels of protein in urine.

Effects on reproduction and prenatal toxicity

It was mentioned in an abstract that no significant correlation was found between the chromium content of water samples collected from houses in 48 areas of South Wales and the frequency of malformations of the central nervous system (Morton & Elwood, 1974).

A mean value of 111 µg/l Cr was found in maternal blood, 124 µg/l in cord blood and 63 mg/kg in placental tissues. Although the blood Cr content of people from various areas differed by a factor of two, the ratio of the Cr content in maternal:cord blood (0.85-0.98) was relatively constant (Creason *et al.*, 1976).

Absorption, distribution and excretion

Chromates [VI] are absorbed from the gastrointestinal tract at a rate of about 2%. When ^{51}Cr[VI] was administered intraduodenally, approximately half of the administered radioactivity appeared to be absorbed, on the basis of faecel excretion, while 10% appeared in the urine during the first 24 hours. These values are based on urinary excretion levels, however, and may be an underestimation, since the gastrointestinal tract also takes part in chromium excretion (Donaldson & Barreras, 1966).

In workers exposed to chromium during chromium-plating and subsequent polishing of the plated surface or to chromium in welding fumes, the chromium is rapidly absorbed *via* the respiratory tract and excreted in the urine (Franchini *et al.*, 1975; Mutti *et al.*, 1979b).

High concentrations of chromium have been detected in fetuses immediately after birth, indicating placental transfer during pregnancy (Schroeder *et al.*, 1962).

Mutagenicity and other short-term tests

A cytogenetic examination of workers exposed to Cr[VI] compounds by inhalation of aerosols revealed that exposure caused an increase in chromosomal aberrations in peripheral blood lymphocytes (3.6-9.4% cells with aberrations compared with 1.9% in unexposed controls) (Bigaliev *et al.*, 1977). Bigaliev *et al.* (1978) also observed an increase in chromosomal aberrations in peripheral blood leucocytes of workers handling different chromium compounds.

Maltoni (1976b) carried out sputum cytological examinations among 116 workers in the chromate production industry exposed to dichromates and chromium pigments. The cytological samples were classified using the Papanicolaou system: none were in the tumorous stages (classes IV and V), but intermediate stage lesions (classes III and III-IV, i.e., dystypical adenomatous proliferation, squamous-cell dysplasia and basal-cell dysplasia) were found in 30 of the workers.

3.3 Case reports and epidemiological studies

(a) Case reports

Korallus *et al.* (1974a,b) studied workers in two plants that manufactured chromic [III] oxide and chromium [III] sulphates. Although the workers were predominantly exposed to trivalent chromium compounds, the chromium [III] sulphate manufacturers also worked at a chromic acid (chromium [VI] trioxide) plant involving exposure to hexavalent dichromates. Of 32 deaths among the workers, 10 were from cancer, including 3 from bronchial tumours (1 sarcoma, 2 carcinomas). The authors concluded that this study did not indicate a carcinogenic effect of Cr[III].

Ohsaki *et al.* (1974, 1978) reported 14 cases of lung cancer (10 carcinomas, 4 unspecified) among 133 workers from a Japanese chromate production factory that had operated between 1936 and 1973. Workers, who were followed up through 1976, had been exposed to chromium [VI] trioxide, water-insoluble trivalent chromium compounds and water-soluble hexavalent chromium compounds, including dichromates of sodium and potassium.

Hanslian *et al.* (1967) carried out an otorhinolaryngological examination survey of 77 workers from 8 chromium-plating factories. The workers were exposed to a hexavalent chromium trioxide aerosol at levels ranging from 23-681 μg/m^3. Sixteen papillomas of the upper respiratory tract were found in 14 of the 77 workers. The authors compared this prevalence of papillomas of the oral cavity with that of other workers surveyed (10/208) and with that of clinical patients (1/40).

Five cases of lung carcinomas, two cases of carcinoma of the upper jaw and one case each of cancer of the liver and pancreas were reported in chromate production workers or chromium platers (Sano, 1978; Takemoto *et al.*, 1977).

(b) Epidemiological studies

(The epidemiological studies of cancer in workers in various industries in which exposure to different forms of chromium compounds occurs are summarized in Tables 11-15).

(1) Chromate-producing industries: Clinical observations from Germany in the 1930s raised the suspicion that workers in chromate production plants were prone to lung cancer (reviewed by Baetjer, 1950a). Machle & Gregorius (1948) demonstrated a high relative frequency of death from respiratory cancer among workers in the chromate-producing industry. Among 193 deaths from all causes at 7 chromate-producing plants in the US, 21.8% resulted from respiratory cancer, as compared with an expected frequency of 1.4% in a control group from other industries. In a study of medical records from two hospitals

near a chromate-producing plant, Baetjer (1950b) found that 3.8% of the 290 lung cancer patients were chromate workers; this figure was significantly higher than among a random sample of other hospital admissions. Mancuso & Hueper (1951) reported that among 33 deaths from all causes in men who had worked for at least one year at a chromate-producing plant in Ohio, 18.2% were attributed to respiratory cancer, as contrasted with an expected frequency of 1.2% for the male population in the county where the plant was located.

The US Public Health Service (Gafafer, 1953) conducted a health examination survey of workers in 7 US chromium manufacturing plants and collected data on death claims submitted to the sick-benefit plans of the plants. The following groups of chromate workers were excluded from the cancer mortality study: (1) workers who were not members of sick-benefit plans; (2) workers who had terminated employment with the chromate industry; (3) workers who had died more than a year after the onset of disability from cancer; and (4) workers who were known to have had lung cancer but for whom lung cancer was not listed on their death certificates. Thus, the mortality study cohort consisted of active male workers employed during 1940-1950 who were members of the sick-benefit associations. Comparison was made to age-specific, race-specific US male mortality rates during 1940-1948. The denominator for the population at risk was composed of a total of 5522 chromate person-years of membership in the sick-benefit associations. For the white employees, 10 deaths from lung cancer were observed as compared with 0.7 expected [Standardized Mortality Ratio (SMR)=1429]. For the black employees, 16 deaths from lung cancer were observed as compared with 0.2 expected (SMR=8000). There was no excess risk for cancer at other sites, with a total of 6 observed *versus* 6.3 expected in the combined group. In the second phase of this study, a health survey team conducted a cross-sectional examination survey of 897 workers, 10 of whom were judged to have bronchogenic carcinoma. Comparison was made with data based upon a Boston X-ray survey of 259,072 males in whom 54 cases of lung cancer were identified. The chromate production workers had a lung cancer prevalence rate of 1115 per 100,000, while the X-ray survey population had a prevalence rate of 20.8 per 100,000. The excess of lung cancer among chromate production workers started to appear in the age group 40-49, in which there was a prevalence rate of 1429 per 100,000, as compared with the Boston prevalence rate of 4.4 per 100,000 in that age group. Excesses also occurred in older age groups [The lung cancer mortality rates were considered by the Working Group to be underestimated because of the exclusion of the four groups of workers described above, the largest group of which was terminated and retired workers who would not have belonged to the sick-benefit plan. The actual numbers of workers in the population at risk were not stated].

Bidstrup & Case (1956) followed 723 workers from three UK chromate-producing factories and reported a significantly higher lung cancer (carcinoma) mortality: 12 deaths as compared with the 3.3 expected on the basis of national death rates. The investigators discussed the possibility that the increased risk of lung cancer among the workers was related to diagnostic bias, place of residence, social class or smoking, but they made no adjustment for these variables. For cancer at other sites, the observed and expected numbers of deaths were similar.

Taylor (1966) studied 1212 male workers who had been employed in 3 US chromate production plants for 3 months or more during 1937 to 1940. The study cohort, constructed from the earnings reports in Old Age and Survivors Disability Insurance records, was restricted to males born during or after 1890. Vital status was ascertained through 1960 by searching the death claim files of the records; death certificates were subsequently obtained for workers for whom death claims had been filed. Comparison was made to age-specific mortality of US males for the calendar years 1950, 1953 and 1958. The chromate production workers experienced a large excess of cancer of the respiratory system (ICD codes 160-165) during the observation period 1937-1960 (71 observed deaths *versus* 8.3 expected; SMR=851) and an excess of nonmalignant respiratory disease (19 observed deaths *versus* 7.8 expected; SMR=242).

Enterline (1974) reanalysed more complete data from the study of Taylor (1966) for the time period 1941-1960. On the basis of US mortality rates, 7.3 deaths from respiratory system cancer (ICD codes 160-164) would have been expected as compared with 69 deaths observed (SMR=943). Two of the 69 deaths were from maxillary sinus cancer. Furthermore, a small excess of deaths from cancer of the digestive system (16 observed *versus* 10.4 expected; SMR=153) was reported, although this difference was not significant.

Mancuso (1975) reported a further study of a chromate-producing plant investigated earlier (Mancuso & Hueper, 1951). Using hygiene data collected in 1949, weighted average exposures to soluble, insoluble and total chromium, combined with length of exposure, were computed, and death rates for the 1931-1937 cohort of workers were applied to these dose/time subdivisions. The analysis was confined to the 41 deaths from lung cancer that occurred during this period (1931-1974), and rates were computed using a direct standardization, with the entire plant population as the standard. In the 1930-1937 cohort, a clustering of cases of lung cancer was observed in those with 27-36 years since first exposure. Increasing mortality from lung cancer was noted with years of observation, age at time of death and exposure to insoluble chromium, soluble chromium and total chromium. For a given exposure to insoluble chromium, an increase in exposure to total chromium resulted in an increased death rate from lung cancer for 4 of the 5 total chromium exposure categories. For each total chromium exposure, increasing exposure to insoluble chromium led to a decreased death rate from lung cancer in 3 of the 5 categories. The author concluded that 'carcinogenic potential extends to all forms of chromium' [The Working Group noted that this study showed a dose-response effect for lung cancer deaths with increasing chromium exposure indices. Both soluble and insoluble chromium appear to be implicated in carcinogenesis, but it was considered that the author's conclusion that all chromium compounds must be regarded as suspect is not justified on the basis of the data presented].

Hill & Ferguson (1979), using 'probability window analysis', suggested that risk for lung cancer in chromate production workers has been reduced by improvements in the process and by reduced exposure to chromium [The Working Group noted that the method of analysis does not use rates of lung cancer for comparison and does not make allowance for the fact that insufficient time had elapsed for the onset of lung cancer to be seen in the newer workers employed after process improvement. Therefore, no conclusions on the safety of current exposures can be made].

Hayes et al. (1979) studied the same plant reported on by Baetjer (1950b) and by Hill & Ferguson (1979) in order to determine whether workers newly employed in facilities constructed to reduce hazardous exposures experienced a reduction in respiratory cancer relative to workers concurrently employed at an older facility. The study cohort consisted of 2101 workers newly employed for at least 90 days between 1945 and 1974. By July 1977, the vital status had been ascertained for 88% of the cohort by searching death claim files of the Social Security Administration and Veterans Administration and by tracing persons using the post, telephone, house visits, voter lists and motor vehicle registration lists. Individuals lost to follow-up were assumed to be alive until the end of the study period. SMRs for the 1803 hourly employees were calculated from expected values derived from the age-, race- and time-specific mortality rates of Baltimore City males. Statistical significance was tested using the Poisson probability distribution. The overall SMR for cancer of the trachea, bronchus and lung (ICD code 162) was 202, based on 59 observed deaths *versus* 29.16 expected [significant difference]. Workers hired between 1945 and 1949 who were employed for less than 3 years had an SMR for lung cancer of 180, based on 20 observed deaths [significant difference]. Those workers with 3 or more years of employment who were hired between 1945-1949 had an SMR of 300, based on 13 observed deaths [significant difference]. The SMR for lung cancer among workers hired between 1950 and 1959 with a short (less than 3 years) duration of employment at a new facility, a mill and roast and dichromate plant put into operation in 1950-1951, was 70 (based on 2 observed deaths), while short-term workers hired between 1950 and 1959 at the older facility had an SMR of 180 (based on 12 observed deaths) [not significant]. The long-term (3 or more years) workers in the new facility who were hired between 1950 and 1959 had a lung cancer SMR of 400, based on 3 observed deaths (95% confidence limits; 0.8-11.7) [not significant], while their counterparts in the older facility had an SMR of 340, based on 9 observed deaths (95% confidence limits; 1.6-6.5) [significant]. Thus, the risk for lung cancer was not eliminated for workers at the facility constructed in 1950-1951. A dose-response relationship as estimated by duration of employment is demonstrated by the increased SMR for lung cancer among long-term workers at both facilities. Additional case-control analyses were conducted to determine whether specific work areas were associated with lung cancer. Controls who had died from nonmalignant causes were matched individually by race, hire date, age at initial employment and duration of employment to the 66 employees who had died from lung cancer. A significant ($P < 0.05$) elevation of lung cancer risk was found in employees who had worked in the 'special products' and dichromate areas where soluble hexavalent chromium compounds were produced and packaged. While no deaths from lung cancer occurred in the group of workers newly hired between 1960 and 1974 at both the old and new facilities, the small number of person-years and short observation period make assessment of the cancer risk impossible at this time for these workers.

(2)   Chromate pigment industries: Several researchers have attempted to determine whether an excess risk of lung cancer occurs in workers exposed to the manufacturing and use of chromate pigments. Langård & Norseth (1975) studied a small Norwegian company producing chromate pigments since 1948. The work force was exposed to lead chromate [VI], zinc chromate [VI], sodium dichromate [VI], zinc oxide and other components of the pigment manufacturing processes. Twenty-four male workers were selected for study because they had more than 3 years of employment with the company up to 1972. Using the Cancer Registry of Norway, 3 workers were identified as having had bronchial carcinoma between 1951 and 1972 and 1 a gastrointestinal cancer. On the basis of 0.079 expected lung cancers from Cancer Registry data, the relative risk of lung cancer in these workers was 38 ($P<0.1$). While past levels of exposure to hexavalent chromium are unknown, present exposures to chromium ranged from 0.01-1.35 mg/m^3. The authors estimate that the lung cancer cases were probably exposed to concentrations of 0.5-1.5 mg/m^3 Cr during their 6-8 years of employment.

Davies (1978, 1979) studied mortality at 3 factories in the UK where chromate pigments were manufactured. A significant excess of lung cancer deaths was found among male workers with 'high' and 'medium' exposures [as defined by the author] in 2 of the factories, when compared with the number of lung cancer deaths expected on the basis of calendar time period and sex- and age-specific rates in the UK. In these same 2 factories, no excess of lung cancer deaths was observed in workers considered to have had 'low' exposures. The men were followed through mid-1977. Exposure to the substances used in the production of lead chromate [VI] occurred in all of the factories; workers in 2 of them (A and B) were additionally exposed to the zinc chromate [VI] manufacturing process. Exposure levels were not specified. Twenty lung cancer deaths occurred among the 252 workers at factory A who were initially employed sometime between 1932 and 1954 and who had been employed for more than 1 year. Of 175 workers in the factory who were judged to have had 'high' and 'medium' exposures to chromates, 18 died from lung cancer, as compared with 8.17 expected lung cancer deaths ($P<0.01$), but there was no excess in those with 'low' exposure. In factory B, 7 lung cancer deaths occurred among 116 workers with all durations of employment and with 'high' and 'medium' exposure to chromate who were first employed sometime between 1948-1967, as compared with 1.43 expected deaths from lung cancer ($P<0.001$). No excess of lung cancer was observed among 114 workers at factory C who were exposed only to the substances used in the production of lead chromate and first employed sometime between 1946-1967. The data from factory A indicate that the excess of lung cancer deaths occurred among individuals first employed less than 25 years before and that the excess disappeared in those with more than 25 years since first employment [The Working Group considered that the latter finding is difficult to assess without further data].

(3) Chromium-plating industries: Investigations of carcinogenic risk in the chromium-plating industry have been conducted in the UK, Japan and Czechoslovakia.

Waterhouse (1975) reported in an abstract that there was a significant (P<0.05) excess of lung cancer deaths in male employees hired since 1946 in a UK chromium-plating factory (49 deaths observed, 34.88 deaths expected). No specific compounds or exposure levels were cited [The Working Group noted the incomplete reporting of the study].

Royle (1975a,b) conducted a historical retrospective and prospective mortality study of past and current workers with 3 months or more of consecutive employment in 54 chromium-plating plants in Yorkshire, UK. The study covered 1238 chromium-plating workers, 142 of whom had died by 31 May 1974; 1056 were male and 182 were female. A control population of 1284 manual workers, consisting of 1099 males and 185 females, was drawn from non-chromium-plating departments of the larger firms and from the past and current work force of two industrial companies located in the same geographic region of the UK. They were matched individually to the platers by sex, age, date when last known to be alive and, for current workers, by smoking habits [The study populations represented 91% of the total exposed population and 93% of the controls]. Vital status was ascertained through May 1974 by means of interviews and searches of the National Health Service Central Register and offices of Registrars of Births and Deaths. Compared with the controls, the chromium platers experienced a significant excess of deaths from total malignant diseases (51 *versus* 24 in male and female controls; P<0.01) [The excess was statistically significant only for individuals who had been platers for more than 1 year]. In male chromium platers, 24 lung cancer deaths (ICD codes 162, 163) were observed *versus* 13 in controls; this difference of almost two-fold was not statistically significant. The mean latent period for intrathoracic cancer in platers was 13.6 years and that for all forms of cancer was 16.4 years. Cancers of the gastrointestinal tract and of other sites in males also occurred in excess, but the differences were not significant (8 in cases *versus* 4 in controls, and 12 in cases *versus* 5 in controls, respectively). Data on smoking histories and work histories were collected by a questionnaire survey of 997 living platers and 1117 living controls included in the mortality study. The smoking habits, with respect to prevalence of smoking, type of tobacco consumed (cigarette, pipe, cigar), inhalation patterns and amount smoked, were considered to be very similar in platers and controls. Differences in work history patterns were observed, however: a significantly higher proportion of controls had worked in asbestos processing, while more platers had worked in coal mines, foundries, potteries, manufacturing and cotton, flax or hemp mills. The author attempted to exclude from the study population all workers who had had extensive exposure to nickel or cadmium plating.

Okubo & Tsuchiya (1977) studied the mortality of 952 Tokyo chromium platers. The cohort was constructed from 1970-1976 records of the Tokyo Health Insurance Society of the Plating Industry and consisted of chromium platers (889 males and 63 females) who were born prior to 31 May 1937, had more than 6 months of work experience in chromium plating, and had a work history record. Vital status was ascertained by questionnaires sent to the management of the plating firms and, for retired workers, by contacting family registers. A control group (2514 males and 1722 females) was selected from workers not involved in chromium plating; however, the expected values were derived from the age-, sex- and year-specific death rates of the Tokyo general population, as applied to the distribution of person-years of observation of the chromium platers and to the industrial control group. Among the chromium platers, 21 deaths from all causes were observed as compared with 38.5 that would have been expected. No deaths were reported to have occurred from lung cancer among the chromium platers, although 1.2 would have been expected in males and more in females. Among male controls, small excesses of deaths were seen from liver cancer (5 observed deaths *versus* 1.7 expected) and from pancreatic cancer (3 observed deaths *versus* 1 expected) [The Working Group considered that the negative findings of this study may have been due to incomplete ascertainment of the vital status of the population; secondly, it seemed likely that the controls employed in the smaller firms may have had exposures similar to those of the platers].

(4)   Ferrochromium industries: Pokrovskaya & Shabynina (1973) studied a cohort of male and female factory workers engaged in the production of chromium ferroalloys between 1955 and 1969 in the USSR. Workers were exposed to hexavalent chromium, trivalent chromium and benzo[a]pyrene. Death certificates were obtained from the municipal vital statistics office, and comparison was made with city mortality rates by sex and by ten-year age group. The availability of complete occupational histories made it possible to exclude from the control cohort subjects who had been exposed to chromium in other plants. Male chromium workers aged 50-59 experienced significant (P=0.001) increases in death rates from all malignancies, from lung cancer and from oesophageal cancer as compared with the municipal population. The relative risk for lung cancer in males was reported to range from a low of 4.4 in the 30-39-year age group to a high of 6.6 in the 50-59-year age group. A large proportion of the excess in lung cancer mortality occurred in workers exposed to high concentrations of dust (cinder pit workers, metal crushers, smelter workers), including workers who were not exposed to benzo[a]pyrene in areas of furnace charge and finished product preparation [The Working Group noted that the number of workers and the number of cancers by specific site were not reported].

Axelsson *et al.* (1980) studied the employees of a ferrochromium plant in Sweden producing ferrochromium alloys by ore furnace reduction of chromite ore, quartz, lime and coke. The study population was defined as all males employed for at least 1 year during the period 1 January 1930 to 31 December 1975. Employee records were available for all of the employees who had worked since 1913. Individuals were classified according to length and site of employment in the plant. Death certificates were obtained from the National Central Bureau of Statistics and cancer incidence from a manual search of Cancer Registry files. Expected numbers for both cancer deaths and cancer cases were calculated using a life-table method, with an assumed 15-year latent period from onset of employment. An analysis was made of the 380 deaths among 1876 persons by cause: there were 69 observed tumour deaths, compared with 76.7 expected; for trachea, bronchus and lung cancer (ICD 162, 163), the observed/expected figures were 5 *versus* 7.2; and for gastrointestinal tract cancer (ICD 151-153), they were 18 *versus* 20. No excess of cancer deaths was noted among arc furnace workers, who are at greatest risk of exposure to Cr[III] and Cr[VI]. Similarly, no increase in observed to expected cases was seen for tumour incidence in transport, metal grinding, sampling and office storage area workers, except for maintenance workers, who experienced 4 cases of cancer of the lung, trachea or bronchus whereas 1 was expected (P=0.038). Further analysis revealed that two of these tumours were mesotheliomas; one arc furnaceman also developed a mesothelioma. Asbestos was used in the insulation of the furnace area. The authors concluded that there was no increased risk of cancer mortality or incidence in workers exposed to chromium of both oxidation states in an industry in which exposure to Cr[III] was higher than that to Cr[VI] : levels of Cr[III] ranged from 0-2.5 mg/m³ and those of Cr[VI] from 0-0.25 mg/m³.

Langård *et al.* (1980) studied a ferrochromium and ferrosilicon production plant in Norway. The study included all present and retired workers employed at the factory for more than 1 year between 1928 and 1977. Cancer incidence was determined from the Cancer Registry for 976 persons who started work before 1 January 1960. Overall mortality was lower than expected (182 observed, 228.2 expected), but there were 7 cases of lung cancer in the ferrochromium subpopulation compared with 3.1 expected (P=0.08) from the national rates; the expected cases were reduced to 1.8 if local rates were applied (P=0.06) and to 0.31 if an internal reference population was used (P=0.03). An excess of prostate cancer was also seen in the entire worker population (20 observed, 13 expected; P=0.06). Hygiene studies in the plant in 1975 indicated the presence of Cr[III] and Cr[VI] in the environment: the atmosphere contained 0.01-0.29 mg/m³ chromium, of which 11-33% was water-soluble Cr[VI]. The authors concluded that although the incidence of lung cancer was increased, the results do not permit examination of the hypothesis that Cr [III] compounds are carcinogenic, in view of concomitant exposure to Cr[VI].

(5) Other industries with exposure to chromium compounds: Bittersohl (1971) studied cancer experience among workers employed in a chemical manufacturing complex which included a chromate factory in which individuals were exposed to chromium [VI] trioxide, iron oxide and nitric acid. When compared with an undefined group of workers, the incidence of neoplasms in chromate workers diagnosed during the years 1958-1970 was reported to be 6-8 times greater, using only crude rates of comparison. For all workers, including those exposed to chromate, the crude incidence rates for lung cancer and stomach cancer were approximately 250 per 10,000 and 300 per 10,000, respectively [The Working Group considered that the data are difficult to interpret, because of lack of information on population size, numbers of deaths, age distribution and methods of calculating rates].

Table 11. Epidemiological studies of cancer in workers in chromate-producing industries

Study population	Comparison population	Respiratory cancers			Other cancers			Notes	Reference
		Site	Number	Estimated relative risk	Site	Number	Estimated relative risk		
Six chromate plants[a]: - active employees; - 4-17 years before 1948; 156 deaths	Cancer mortality in oil-refining company, 1933-1938	Bronchus and lung	32	25	Digestive	13	2	0.01-21.0 mg/m³ (total Cr)	Machle & Gregorius (1948)
Case-control; lung cancer; 290 cases near US chromium plant	Random sample of hospital admissions	Lung	11[b]	*				Levels determined in 1947: 25-6865 µg/m³	Baetjer (1950b)
Cohort study; US chromate-producing plant; workers employed 1 or more years 1931-1949; 33 deaths	Proportionate mortality for county		6	15[c]					Mancuso & Hueper (1951)
Seven US chromium plants; active employees 1940-1950; 5522 person-years	US males white black	Lung	10 16	14.3* 80.0	Other sites	6	1 NS		Gafafer (1953)
Health survey 897 workers	Boston X-ray survey		10	53 (prevalence ratio)					
Three UK factories; 723 men employed 1949-1955	Cancer mortality England and Wales, 1951-1953	Lung	12	3.6*	All other sites	no excess			Bidstrup & Case (1956)
Three US chromate-producing plants; 1212 males employed 3 or more months between 1937-1940; status to 1960	Cancer mortality US males, 1950, 1953, 1958		71	8.5*	All other sites	32	1.3		Taylor (1966)

Study population	Comparison population	Respiratory cancers			Other cancers			Notes	Reference
		Site	Number	Estimated relative risk	Site	Number	Estimated relative risk		
Same populations as Taylor (1966); 1941-1960	Cancer mortality US males, 1950, 1953, 1958		69 (2 maxillary sinus)	9.4*	Digestive system	16	1.5 NS		Enterline (1974)
Same plant as Mancuso & Hueper (1951); employed 1 or more years 1931-1937; all jobs related to exposure to total and soluble/insoluble chromium; lifetime exposure in months calculated	No independent comparison group	Lung	41	Crude Hoyeau rate: 369.7/100,000				[Tables show increased lung cancer risk with increasing total Cr when insoluble level constant and suggest increasing lung cancer with increasing soluble Cr when total constant; exposure into solubility categories may be questioned]	Mancuso (1975)
Same US plant as Baetjer (1959b); 2101 workers employed 3 or more months 1945-1974; status 1977 (88% complete). Populations working in new and/or old production sites	Baltimore City mortality	Lung (162) Cohort 1940-1949 Cohort 1950-1959 <3 years' work: new old >3 years' work: new old	59 13 2 12 3 9	2* 3* 0.7 1.8 NS 4 NS 3.4*				New sites with better controls: 2-17 $\mu g/m^3$ Cr in 1973-1975. Significant excess of lung cancer for workers in 'special products' and dichromates (soluble Cr[VI]); case-control	Hayes et al. (1979)

[a]One plant, with 37 deaths and 10 respiratory cancers but with no adequate employment records available, has been excluded.

[b]Only 11 cases had been exposed to chromium compounds versus none in controls.

[c]Significant if x^2 is applied, but the small number of cancers due to chromate makes use of this procedure questionable.

* - significant

NS - not significant

Others not known or not tested

Table 12. Epidemiological studies of cancer in workers in chromate-pigment industries

Study population	Comparison population	Respiratory cancers			Other cancers			Notes	Reference
		Site	Number	Estimated relative risk	Site	Number	Estimated relative risk		
Norwegian pigment production since 1948; 24 males with over 3 years' employment to 1972	Cancer Registry of Norway	Lung	3	38*	Gastro-intestinal	1		Exposures to Cr in mg/m³: current, 0.01-1.35; estimated lifetime, 0.5-1.5. Materials: $PbCrO_4$, $ZnCrO_4$, $Na_2Cr_2O_7$	Langård & Norseth (1975)
UK chromate pigment factories: A, lead & zinc chromate; B, lead & zinc chromate; C, lead chromate; followed to 1977	UK mortality rates	Lung High & medium exposure						Lung cancer occurred with latency < 25 years; excess disappeared after 25 years	Davies (1978, 1979)
		A (1932-54), 175 wkrs	18	2.2*					
		B (1948-67), 116 wkrs	7	5.0*					
		A & B, low exposure	2	1					
		C (1946-67), all exposures	2	0.7					

* - significant
NS - not significant
Others not known or not tested

Table 13. Epidemiological studies of cancer in workers in chromium-plating industries

Study population	Comparison population	Respiratory cancers Site	Number	Estimated relative risk	Other cancers Site	Number	Estimated relative risk	Notes	Reference
UK chromium-plating workers since 1946	Not stated	Lung	49	1.4*				Incomplete information	Waterhouse (1975)
54 UK chromium-plating plants; 1056 male platers; 1099 male controls	Nonexposed workers in plants and in 2 non-plating industries		24	1.8 NS	Total cancer Gastro-intestinal Other sites	44 8 12	2.0* 2.0 NS 2.4 NS	Current exposure to 0-> 0.1 mg/m³ chromium trioxide. Exposure to several metals including Ni	Royle (1975a,b)
Japanese chromium-plating industry; 952 workers with > 6 months' exposure	4236 nonexposed workers from same industry		0	< 1	Total cancer	5	< 1	The very low relative risks suggest incomplete follow-up.	Okubo & Tsuchiya (1977)

* - significant
NS - not significant
Others not known or not tested

Table 14. Epidemiological studies of cancer in workers in ferrochromium industries

Study population	Comparison population	Respiratory cancers			Other cancers			Notes	Reference
		Site	Number	Estimated relative risk	Site	Number	Estimated relative risk		
Soviet workers in 1955-1969 in the ferrochromium alloy industry	City mortality	Lung	not given	(males) 4.4-6.6* by age	Total cancer Oesophageal	not given not given	(males) 0.5-3.3* 2.0*-11.3*	Exposed to Cr[III], Cr[VI] and benzo[a]pyrene; highest risk with dust exposure; no numbers provided	Pokrovskaya & Shabynina (1973)
Swedish ferrochromium plant; ferroalloys; 1876 workers for 1 year or more 1930-1975; traced by parish lists and cancer registry; 380 deaths	Classification of work areas by exposure to Cr [III] and Cr [VI]; comparison with county or national statistics	Mortality study of all workers Maintenance workers	5 4 (2 mesotheliomas)	<1 4.0*	Prostate (all workers)	23	1.2 NS	Asbestos exposure	Axelsson et al. (1980)
Norwegian; ferrochromium and ferrosilicon; 976 workers employed 1928-1960	General population; internal comparison with nonexposed	Lung (ferrochromium workers)	7	A[a]2.3 NS B[b]8.5*	Stomach (ferrochromium workers) Prostate (all workers)	5 20	1.5 NS 1.5 NS		Langård et al. (1980)

* - significant

NS - not significant

Others not known or not tested

[a] On the basis of national rates

[b] On the basis of an internal reference population

Table 15. Epidemiological studies of workers in other industries with exposure to chromium compounds

Study population	Comparison population	Respiratory cancers			Other cancers			Notes	Reference
		Site	Number	Estimated relative risk	Site	Number	Estimated relative risk		
Chemical manufacture; 30,000 employees; cases 1958-1970	Non exposed workers; used crude incidence		Not given		All malignant neoplasms for chromate factory[a]	852/ 10,000	10.1	Exposure to chromium trioxide, iron oxide, nitric acid	Bittersohl (1971)

[a]Numbers calculated by National Institute for Occupational Safety & Health (1975) from a histogram. This study was done in a big chemical manufacture industry, and the numbers of total malignant neoplasms associated with exposure to different compounds are given.

4. Summary of Data Reported and Evaluation

4.1 Experimental data

Calcium chromate [VI] is carcinogenic in rats when given by several routes, producing tumours at the sites of administration. Lead chromate [VI], sintered calcium chromate [VI], zinc chromate [VI], strontium chromate [VI], sintered chromium [VI] trioxide, lead chromate [VI] oxide and cobalt-chromium alloy produce sarcomas at the sites of their subcutaneous, intramuscular and/or intrapleural administration in rats; lead chromate [VI] also produced renal carcinomas following its intramuscular administration in rats.

Experiments in mice, rats, hamsters, guinea-pigs and rabbits to investigate the carcinogenicity of chromic [III] acetate, chromic [III] oxide, mixed chromate [VI] dust, potassium dichromate [VI], chromium [VI] trioxide, chromium metal, potassium chromate [VI], sodium chromate [VI], roasted chromite [III] ore, sodium dichromate [VI], barium chromate [VI], chromium [III] sulphate, chromium [III] carbonyl, chromite [III] ore, zinc potassium chromate [VI] and zinc yellow [VI] were inadequate to evaluate the carcinogenicity of these chromium compounds.

Chromium [VI] compounds cause mutations and allied effects in a very wide range of prokaryotic and eukaryotic systems, both *in vitro* and *in vivo*. In similar tests, there is good evidence that chromium [III] compounds are not mutagenic: the few positive results in assays for chromosomal aberrations were obtained only with extremely high doses and could be explained by nonspecific toxic effects.

Chromium [III] compounds apparently cross the placenta to only a small extent when administered parenterally to laboratory animals. Some teratogenic effects have been reported with extremely high doses. It is uncertain whether the effects reported represent a direct effect on the embryo or are the result of maternal toxicity. Embryotoxic and teratogenic effects occurred in hamsters following exposure to chromium [VI] trioxide.

4.2 Human data

An increased frequency of chromosomal aberrations has been observed in workers exposed to chromium [VI] compounds.

Several studies of the chromate production industry over the past 10 years have demonstrated a large excess risk of lung cancer. One study has suggested that even the more recently employed workers (who receive lower doses of chromium than workers employed previously) may have an excess risk with long duration of employment. The same study indicated that the highest risk occurs among workers in areas where dichromate [VI], chromium [VI] trioxide and other products are processed.

Studies in other industries in which workers are exposed to chromium products, such as manufacture of ferrochromium alloys, chromium plating and chromate pigment, are few, are inadequately reported and include only small populations of workers. However, the only two studies of the chromate [VI] pigment industry suggest a risk of lung cancer similar to that seen in the production industry. Metal alloy workers also have a risk of respiratory cancers, but some of the observed cancers were mesotheliomas in workers exposed to asbestos in the same work environment. The data from the study of chemical industries in which chromium [III] compounds are used has given conflicting results, while the studies of chromium-plating workers are inconclusive with regard to respiratory cancer risk. The relative contributions of chromium [III] and chromium [VI] compounds to the risk of respiratory cancers in the above manufacturing processes and in the use of chromium products cannot be assessed on the basis of available data.

The original studies of the chromate production industry did not show an excess risk of cancer at sites other than the respiratory tract. Studies of other chromium-using industries have suggested excesses of cancers at all sites (chromium platers) and of both total cancers and oesophageal cancers (metal alloy workers). Prostate cancer and maxillary sinus cancers have been reported in workers in these industries as well; however, the risk of cancers at sites other than the lung cannot be assessed on the basis of current data.

Although the available epidemiological evidence does not permit a clear distinction between the relative carcinogenicity of chromium compounds of different oxidation states or solubilities, it appears that exposure to a mixture of chromium [VI] compounds of different solubilities (as found in the chromate production industry) carries the greatest risk to humans.

4.3 Evaluation

There is *sufficient evidence* for the carcinogenicity of calcium chromate and some relatively insoluble chromium [VI] compounds (sintered calcium chromate, lead chromate, strontium chromate, sintered chromium trioxide and zinc chromate) in rats. There is *limited evidence* for the carcinogenicity of lead chromate [VI] oxide and cobalt-chromium alloy in rats. The data were inadequate for the evaluation of the carcinogenicity of other chromium [VI] compounds and of chromium [III] compounds (see section 4.1). There is *sufficient evidence* of respiratory carcinogenicity in men occupationally exposed during chromate production. Data on lung cancer risk in other chromium-associated occupations and for cancer at other sites are insufficient. The epidemiological data do not allow an evaluation of the relative contributions to carcinogenic risk of metallic chromium, chromium [III] and chromium [VI] or of soluble *versus* insoluble chromium compounds.

5. References

Ackermann, F. (1977) Method of instrumental neutron activation analysis and its application for the determination of trace metals in sediments (Ger.). *Dtsch. Gewaesserkd. Mitt., 21,* 53-60 [*Chem. Abstr., 88,* 15489g]

Al-Badri, J.S., Sabir, S.M., Shehab, K.M., Jalil, M. & Al-Rawi, H. (1977) Determination of inorganic elements in Iraqi tobacco leaves and cigarets by neutron activation analysis. *Iraqi J. Sci., 18,* 34-44

Allied Chemical (1960) *Chromium Chemicals. Technical and Engineering Service Bulletin No. 52,* Morristown, NJ, p. 58

Allied Chemical (1973a) *Product Bulletin, Potassium Bichromate,* Morristown, NJ

Allied Chemical (1973b) *Product Bulletin, Sodium Bichromate,* Morristown, NJ

Anon. (1978) Chromic acid. *Chem. Mktg Rep., 213,* 6 March, p. 9

Anon. (1979) Sodium bichromate. *Chem. Mktg Rep., 216,* 9 July, p. 9

Arpadzhyan, S. & Kachov, I. (1978) Atomic absorption determination of cadmium, chromium and zinc in blood serum (Ger.). *Zentralbl. Pharm., 117,* 237-240 [*Chem. Abstr., 89,* 55862a]

Astapova, T.I., Kutepova, A.I., Ovsyannikova, L.V. & Ruban, S.G. (1978) Gas-chromatographic determination of chromium in carbon monoxide conversion catalysts (Russ.). *Zh. anal. Khim., 33,* 2065-2066 [*Chem. Abstr., 90* 80288w]

Axelsson, G., Rylander, R. & Schmidt, A. (1980) Mortality and incidence of tumours among ferrochromium workers. *Br. J. ind. Med., 37,* 121-127

Bacon, F.E. (1964) *Chromium and chromium alloys.* In: Kirk, R.E. & Othmer, D.F., eds, *Encyclopedia of Chemical Technology,* 2nd ed., Vol. 5, New York, NY, John Wiley & Sons, pp. 453-464

Baetjer, A.M. (1950a) Pulmonary carcinoma in chromate workers. I. A review of the literature and report of cases. *Arch. ind. Hyg. occup. Med., 2,* 487-504

Baetjer, A.M. (1950b) Pulmonary carcinoma in chromate workers. II. Incidence on basis of hospital records. *Arch ind. Hyg. occup. Med., 2,* 505-516

Baetjer, A,M. (1956) *Relation of chromium to health.* In: Udy, M.J., ed., *Chromium,* Vol. 1, New York, NY, Reinhold, pp. 76-104

Baetjer, A.M., Damron, C. & Budacz, V. (1959a) The distribution and retention of chromium in men and animals. *Arch. ind. Health, 20*, 136-150

Baetjer, A.M., Lowney, J.F., Steffee, H. & Budacz, V. (1959b) Effect of chromium on incidence of lung tumors in mice and rats. *Arch. ind. Health, 20*, 124-135

Barium & Chemicals, Inc. (1978a) *Data Sheet, Barium Chromate*, Steubenville, OH

Barium & Chemicals, Inc. (1978b) *Data Sheet, Calcium Chromate*, Steubenville, OH

Barium & Chemicals, Inc. (1978c) *Data Sheet, Strontium Chromate*, Steubenville, OH

Bianchi, V., Levis, A.G. & Saggioro, D. (1979) Differential cytotoxic activity of potassium dichromate on nucleoside uptake in BHK fibroblasts. *Chem.-biol. Interactions, 24*, 137-151

Bidstrup, P.L. & Case, R.A.M. (1956) Carcinoma of the lung in workmen in the bichromates-producing industry in Great Britain. *Br. J. ind. Med., 13*, 260-264

Bigaliev, A.B., Elemesova, M.S. & Turebaev, M.N. (1977) Evaluation of the mutagenous activity of chromium compounds. *Gig. Tr. Prof. Zabol., 6*, 37-40

Bigaliev, A.B., Elemesova, M.S., Turebaev, M.N. & Bigalieva, R.K. (1978) Cytogenetic study of the mutagenic activity of industrial substances (Russ.). *Zdravookhr. Kaz., 8*, 48-50 [*Chem. Abstr., 89*, 191930j]

Bittersohl, G. (1971) Epidemiology of carcinomatosis in the chemical industry (Ger.). *Arch. Geschwulstforsch., 38*, 198-209

Blokin, V.S. & Trop, F.S. (1977) *Dynamics of the morphological changes in animals subjected to inhalational dust treatment using chromium oxide and trisubstituted chromium phosphate.* In: Dubinin, N.P., ed., *Genetic Effect of the Pollution of the Environment*, Moscow, Nauka, pp. 173-176

Bonatti, S., Meini, M. & Abbondandolo, A. (1976) Genetic effects of potassium dichromate in *Schizosaccharomyces pombe. Mutat. Res., 38*, 147-150

Bourne, H.G., Jr & Yee, H.T. (1950) Occupational cancer in a chromate plant - an environmental appraisal. *Ind. Med. Surg., 19*, 563-567

Bovet, P., Lob, M. & Grandjean, M. (1977) Spirometric alterations in workers in the chromium electroplating industry. *Int. Arch. occup. environ. Health, 40*, 25-32

Buckell, M. & Harvey, D.G. (1951) An environmental study of the chromate industry. *Br. J. ind. Med., 8*, 298-301

Casto, B.C., Meyers, J. & DiPaolo, J.A. (1979) Enhancement of viral transformation for evaluation of the carcinogenic or mutagenic potential of inorganic metal salts. *Cancer Res., 39*, 193-198

Cavazzani, M. & Viola, A. (1970) Clinical and cytological study of the rhinopathology of chromium (Ital.). *Med. Lav., 61*, 168-173

Chalupski, V.H. (1956) *The manufacture and properties of chromium pigments.* In: Udy, M.J., ed., *Chromium.* Vol. 1, New York, NY, Reinhold, pp. 364-376

Copson, R.L. (1956) *Production of chromium chemicals.* In: Udy, M.J., ed., *Chromium,* Vol. 1, New York, NY, Reinhold, pp. 262-282

Creason, J.P., Svendsgaard, D., Bumgarner, J., Pinkerton, C. & Hinners, T. (1976) Maternal-fetal tissue levels of 16 trace elements in 8 selected continental United States communities. *Trace Subst. environ. Health, 10*, 53-62

Cross, H. (1956) *Chromium in cobalt-base alloys.* In: Udy, M.H., ed., *Chromium,* Vol. 2, *Metallurgy of Chromium and Its Alloys,* New York, NY, Reinhold, pp. 304-309

Darrin, M. (1956) *Chromium chemicals - their industrial use.* In: Udy, M.J., ed., *Chromium,* Vol. 1, New York, NY, Reinhold, pp. 251-261

Davies, J.M. (1978) Lung-cancer mortality of workers making chrome pigments (letter to the Editor). *Lancet, i*, 384

Davies, J.M. (1979) Lung cancer mortality in workers in chromate pigment manufacture: an epidemiological survey. *J. Oil Color. chem. Assoc., 62*, 157-163

Davis, G.K. (1956) *Chromium in soils, plants, and animals.* In: Udy, M.J., ed., *Chromium,* Vol. 1, New York, NY, Reinhold, pp. 105-109

Davis, J.M.G. (1972) The fibrogenic effects of mineral dusts injected into the pleural cavity of mice. *Br. J. exp. Pathol., 53*, 190-201

De Flora, S., Boido, V. & Picciotto, A. (1979) *Metabolism of mutagens in the gastric environment* (abstract). In: *Abstracts of the 9th Annual Meeting of the European Environmental Mutagen Society, Tučepi-Makarska, Yugoslavia, 1979,* p. 50

DiPaolo, J.A. & Casto, B.C. (1979) Quantitative studies of *in vitro* morphological transformation of Syrian hamster cells by inorganic metal salts. *Cancer Res., 39*, 1008-1013

Dixit, M.N., Bhale, G.L. & Thomas, A. (1976) Emission spectrographic determination of trace elements in plant materials. *Indian J. pure appl. Phys., 14*, 485-487

Donaldson, R.M., Jr & Barreras, R.F. (1966) Intestinal absorption of trace quantities of chromium. *J. lab. clin. Med., 68*, 484-493

Dunstan, L.P. & Garner, E.L. (1977) Chemical preparation of biological materials for accurate chromium determination by isotope dilution mass spectrometry. *Trace Subst. environ. Health, 11*, 334-337

Dvizhkov, P.P. & Fedorova, V.I. (1967) On blastomogenic properties of chromic oxide. *Vop. Onkol., 13*, 57-62

EEC (1975) Council directive of 16 June 1975, concerning the quality required of surface water intended for the abstraction of drinking-water in the Member States. *Off. J. Eur. Comm., L 194*, 26-31

Enterline, P.E. (1974) Repsiratory cancer among chromate workers. *J. occup. Med., 16*, 523-526

Falk, H.L. (1970) *Chemical definitions of inhalation hazards.* In: Hanna, M.G., Jr, Nettesheim, P. & Gilbert, J.R., eds, *Inhalation Carcinogenesis (US Atomic Energy Commission Symposium Series No. 18)*, Oak Ridge, TN, US Atomic Energy Commission, Division of Technical Information Extension, pp. 13-26

Fishbein, L. (1976) Environmental metallic carcinogens: an overview of exposure levels. *J. Toxicol. environ. Health, 2*, 77-109

Fradkin, A., Janott, A., Lane, B.P. & Kuschner, M. (1975) *In vitro* transformation of BHK 21 cells grown in the presence of calcium chromate. *Cancer Res., 35*, 1058-1063

Franchini, I., Mutti, A., Gardini, F. & Borghetti, A. (1975) *Excretion and renal elimination of chromium compared to degree and length of occupational exposure* (Fr.). In: Roche, L. & Traeger, J., eds, *Rein et Toxique*, Paris, Masson

Franchini, I., Mutti, A., Cavatorta, A., Corradi, A., Cosi, A., Olivetti, G. & Borghetti, A. (1978) Nephrotoxicity of chromium. Remarks on an experimental and epidemiological investigation. *Contr. Nephrol., 10*, 98-110

Furst, A., Schlauder, M. & Sasmore, D.P. (1976) Tumorigenic activity of lead chromate. *Cancer Res., 36*, 1779-1783

Gafafer, W.M., ed. (1953) *Health of Workers in Chromate Producing Industry: A Study (US Public Health Service, Division of Occupational Health Publication No. 192)*, Washington DC, US Public Health Service

Gahler, A.R. (1962) *Chromium*; In: Furman, N.H., ed., *Standard Methods of Chemical Analysis*, Vol. 1, 6th ed., New York, Van Nostrand-Reinhold, pp. 350-376

Gale, T.F. (1974) Effects of chromium on the hamster embryo (abstract). *Teratology, 9*, A-17

Gale, T.F. (1978) Embryotoxic effects of chromium trioxide in hamsters. *Environ. Res., 16*, 101-109

Gomes, E.R. (1972) Incidence of chromium-induced lesions among electroplating workers in Brazil. *Ind. Med., 41*, 21-25

Green, M.H.L., Muriel, W.J. & Bridges, B.A. (1976) Use of a simplified fluctuation test to detect low levels of mutagens. *Mutat. Res., 38*, 33-42

Gresh, J.T. (1944) Chromic acid poisoning resulting from inhalation of mist developed from five per cent chromic acid solution. II. Engineering aspects of chromic acid poisoning from anodizing operations. *J. ind. Hyg. Toxicol., 26*, 127-130

Guillemin, M.P. & Berode, M. (1978) A study of the difference in chromium exposure in workers in two types of electroplating process. *Ann. occup. Hyg., 21*, 105-112

Hanslian, L., Navratil, J., Jurak, J. & Kotrle, M. (1967) The impairment of higher respiratory pathways by chromic acid aerosol (Czech.). *Prav. lek., 19*, 294-298

Hartford, W.H. (1963) *Chromium*. In: Kolthoff, I.M. & Elving, P.J., eds, *Treatise on Analytical Chemistry*, Part II, Vol. 8, New York, London, John Wiley & Sons, pp. 273-377

Hartford, W.H. (1979) *Chromium compounds*. In: Kirk, R.E., Othmer, D.F., Grayson, M. & Eckroth, D., eds, *Encyclopedia of Chemical Technology*, 3rd ed., Vol. 6, New York, NY, John Wiley & Sons, pp. 82-86, 97-98, 101, 105-110, 113, 115

Hartford, W.H. & Copson, R.L. (1964) *Chromium compounds*. In: Kirk, R.E. & Othmer, D.F., eds, *Encyclopedia of Chemical Technology*, 2nd ed., Vol. 5, New York, NY, John Wiley & Sons, pp. 485-486, 494, 499, 510

Hawley, G.G., ed. (1977) *The Condensed Chemical Dictionary*, 9th ed., New York, NY, Van Nostrand-Reinhold, pp. 206-207, 788, 938, 942

Hayes, R.B., Lilienfeld, A.M. & Snell, L.M. (1979) Mortality in chromium chemical production workers: a prospective study. *Int. J. Epidemiol., 8*, 365-374

Haynes, E. (1907) Metal alloy. *US Patent 873, 745*, 23 April

Heath, J.C., Freeman, M.A.R. & Swanson, S.A.V. (1971) Carcinogenic properties of wear particles from prostheses made in cobalt-chromium alloy. *Lancet, i,* 564-566

Heigl, A. (1978) Polarographic determination of copper, lead, tin, cadmium, nickel, zinc, iron, cobalt and chromium in waste water (Ger.). *Chimia, 32*, 339-344 [*Chem. Abstr., 90*, 76081f]

Hercules Inc. (1978) *Imperial Colorants, Comments*, Wilmington, DE

Herrmann, H. & Speck, L.B. (1954) Interaction of chromate with nucleic acids in tissues. *Science, 119*, 221

Hill, W.J. & Ferguson, W.S. (1979) Statistical analysis of epidemiological data from a chromium chemical manufacturing plant. *J. occup. Med., 21*, 103-106

Howarth, C.L. (1956) *Chromium chemicals in the textile industry*. In: Udy, M.J., ed., *Chromium*, Vol. 1, New York, NY, Reinhold, pp. 283-290

Hueper, W.C. (1955) Experimental studies in metal cancerigenesis. VII. Tissue reactions to parenterally introduced powdered metallic chromium and chromite ore. *J. natl Cancer Inst., 16*, 447-462

Hueper, W.C. (1958) Experimental studies in metal cancerigenesis. X. Cancerigenic effects of chromite ore roast deposited in muscle tissue and pleural cavity of rats. *Arch. ind. Health, 18*, 284-291

Hueper, W.C. (1961) Environmental carcinogenisis and cancers. *Cancer Res., 21*, 842-857

Hueper, W.C. & Payne, W.W. (1959) Experimental cancers in rats produced by chromium compounds and their significance to industry and public health. *Am. ind. Hyg. Assoc. J., 20*, 274-280

Hueper, W.C. & Payne, W.W. (1962) Experimental studies in metal carcinogenesis. Chromium, nickel, iron, arsenic. *Arch. environ. Health, 5*, 445-462

Huff, J.W., Sastry, K.S., Gordon, M.P. & Wacker, W.E.C. (1964) The action of metal ions on tobacco mosaic virus ribonucleic acid. *Biochemistry, 3*, 501-506

IARC (1973) *IARC Monographs on the Evaluation of Carcinogenic Risk of Chemicals to Man*, Vol. 2, *Some Inorganic and Organometallic Compounds*, Lyon, pp. 100-125

Iijima, S., Matsumoto, N., Lu, C.C. & Katsunuma, H. (1975) Placental transfer of $CrCl_3$ and its effects on foetal growth and development in mice (abstract). *Teratology, 12*, 198

Il'inykh, S.V. (1977) *Method for the determination of chromium in canned food packed into cans made of chrome-plated tin* (Russ.). In: *Hygienic Aspect of Defence of Health of Workers*, Moscow, Erismana Institute of Hygiene, pp. 193-194 [*Chem. Abstr., 89*, 88934d]

Ivankovic, S. & Preussmann, R. (1975) Absence of toxic and carcinogenic effects after administration of high doses of chromic oxide pigment in subacute and long-term feeding experiments in rats. *Food Cosmet. Toxicol., 13*, 347-351

Jett, R., Jr, Pierce, J.O., II & Stemmer, K.L. (1968) Toxicity of alloys of ferrochromium. III. Transport of chromium (III) by rat serum protein studied by immunoelectrophoretic analysis and autoradiography. *Arch. environ. Health, 17*, 29-34

Jindrichova, J. (1978) Harmful effects caused by chromium in electric welders (Ger.). *Zeitschr. ges. Hyg., 24*, 86-88

Johnson, R.F. (1974) *Chromium*. In: *Canadian Minerals Yearbook Preprints*, Ottawa, Department of Energy, Mines and Resources, pp. 1-8

Jones, T.S. (1978) *Ferroalloys*. In: *Minerals Yearbook, 1976*, Vol. 1, *Metals, Minerals and Fuels*, Washington DC, Bureau of Mines, US Government Printing Office, pp. 533-550

de Jong, G.J. & Brinkman, U.A.T. (1978) Determination of chromium (III) and chromium (VI) in sea water by atomic absorption spectrometry. *Anal. chim. Acta, 98*, 243-250

Kaaber, K. & Veien, N.K. (1978) Chromate ingestion in chronic chromate dermatitis. *Contact Dermatitis, 4*, 119-120

Kada, T., Hirano, K. & Shirasu, Y. (1980) Screening of environmental chemical mutagens by the *rec*-assay system with *Bacillus subtilis*. *Chem. Mutagens, 6* (in press)

Kaneko, T. (1976) Chromosome damage in cultured human leukocytes induced by chromium chloride and chromium trioxide (Jpn.). *Jpn. J. ind. Health, 18*, 136-137

Kayne, F.J., Komar, G., Laboda, H. & Vanderlinde, R.E. (1978) Atomic absorption spectrophotometry of chromium in serum and urine with a modified Perkin-Elmer 603 atomic absorption spectrophotometer. *Clin. Chem., 24*, 2151-2154 [*Chem. Abstr., 90*, 50905c]

Kleinfeld, M. & Rosso, A. (1965) Ulcerations of the nasal septum due to inhalation of chromic acid mist. *Ind. Med. Surg., 34*, 242-243

Kolihova, D., Sychra, V. & Dudova, N. (1978) Atomic absorption spectrometric analysis of ilmenite and inorganic pigments based on titanium dioxide. III. Determination of copper, manganese, chromium and iron by atomic absorption spectrometry with electrothermic atomization (Czech.). *Chem. Listy, 72*, 1081-1087 [*Chem. Abstr., 90*, 40259f]

Korallus, U., Ehrlicher, H. & Wüstefeld, E. (1974a) Trivalent chromium compounds. Results of a study in occupational medicine. I. General; technology; preliminary study (Ger.). *Arbeitsmed. Sozialmed. Präventivmed., 9*, 51-54

Korallus, U., Ehrlicher, H. & Wüstefeld, E. (1974b) Trivalent chromium compounds: results of a study in occupational medicine. II. Disease status analysis (Ger.). *Arbeitsmed. Sozialmed. Präventivmed., 9*, 76-79

Kovalchuk, N.D. (1966) The behaviour of Cr^{51} in the animal organism following its intravenous injection (Russ.). *Med. Radiol. (USSR), 11*, 30-35

Kretzschmar, J.G., Delespaul, I., De Rijck, T. & Verduyn, G. (1977) The Belgian network for the determination of heavy metals. *Atmos. Environ., 11*, 263-271

Kroner, C.R. (1973) *The occurrence of trace metals in surface waters*. In: Sabadell, J.E., ed., *Proceedings of a Symposium on Traces of Heavy Metals in Water Removal Processes and Monitoring*, Springfield, VA, National Technical Information Service, pp. 311-322

Kubinski, H., Zeldin, P.E. & Morin, N.R. (1977) Survey of tumor-producing agents for their ability to induce macromolecular complexes (abstract). *Proc. Am. Assoc. Cancer Res., 18*, 16

Kushner, M. & Laskin, S. (1971) Experimental models in environmental carcinogenesis. *Am. J. Pathol., 64*, 183-196

Laboratorio Provinciale di Igiene e Profilatti (1975) *La Tutela della Salute nella Fabbriche*, Vol. 2, Pisa

Lalor, E. (1973) *Zinc and strontium chromates*. In: Patton, T.C., ed., *Pigment Handbook*, Vol. 1, New York, John Wiley & Sons, pp. 847-859

Lane, B.P. & Mass, M.J. (1977) Carcinogenicity and cocarcinogenicity of chromium carbonyl in heterotopic tracheal grafts. *Cancer Res., 37*, 1476-1479

Langård, S. (1980) *Chromium*. In: Waldron, H.A., ed., *Metals in the Environment*, London, Academic Press (in press)

Langård, S. & Norseth, T. (1975) A cohort study of bronchial carcinomas in workers producing chromate pigments. *Br. J. ind. Med., 32*, 62-65

Langård, S. & Norseth, T. (1979) *Chromium*. In: Friberg, L., Nordberg, G.F. & Vouk, V.B., eds, *Handbook on the Toxicology of Metals*, Amsterdam, Elsevier, pp. 383-397

Langård, S., Gundersen, N., Tsalev, D.L. & Gylseth, B. (1978) Whole blood chromium level and chromium excretion in the rat after zinc chromate inhalation. *Acta pharmacol. Toxicol., 42*, 142-149

Langård, S., Andersen, A. & Gylseth, B. (1980) Incidence of cancer among ferrochromium and ferrosilicon workers. *Br. J. ind. Med., 37*, 114-120

Laskin, S. (1972) *Research in Environmental Sciences*, Washington DC, Institute of Environmental Medicine, pp. 92-97

Laskin, S., Kuschner, M. & Drew, R.T. (1970) *Studies in pulmonary carcinogenesis*. In: Hanna, M.G., Jr, Nettesheim, P. & Gilbert, J.R., eds, *Inhalation Carcinogenesis (US Atomic Energy Commission Symposium Series No. 18)* Oak Ridge, TN, US Atomic Energy Commission, Division of Technical Information Extension, pp. 321-351

Levis, A.G. & Majone, F. (1979) Cytotoxic and clastogenic effects of soluble chromium compounds on mammalian cell cultures. *Br. J. Cancer, 40*, 523-533

Levis, A.G., Buttignol, M., Bianchi, V. & Sponza, G. (1978a) Effects of potassium dichromate on nucleic acid and protein syntheses and on precursor uptake in BHK fibroblasts. *Cancer Res., 38*, 110-116

Levis, A.G., Bianchi, V., Tamino, G. & Pegoraro, B. (1978b) Cytotoxic effects of hexavalent and trivalent chromium on mammalian cells *in vitro*. *Br. J. Cancer, 37*, 386-
396

Levy, L.S. & Venitt, S. (1975) Carcinogenic and mutagenic activity of chromium containing materials. *Br. J. Cancer, 32*, 254-255

Li, M.-C., Sheng, K.-L., Ching, C.-F., Chen, C.-H., Chin, P.-K., Jung, T.-W. & Wang, H.-P.
(1979) Determination of trace elements in environmental samples by proton-induced
X-ray emission analysis (Chin.). *K'o Hsueh Tung Pao, 24*, 19-21 [*Chem. Abstr., 90*,
145297v]

Lilien, D.L., Spivak, J.L. & Goldman, I.D. (1970) Chromate transport in human leukocytes.
J. clin. Invest., 49, 1551-1557

Löfroth, G. (1978) The mutagenicity of hexavalent chromium is decreased by microsomal
metabolism. *Naturwissenschaften, 65*, 207-208

Löfroth, G. & Ames, B.N. (1978) Mutagenicity of inorganic compounds in *Salmonella typhimurium*: arsenic, chromium and selenium. *Mutat. Res., 53*, 65-66

Luciani, S., Dal Toso, R., Rebellato, A.M. & Levis, A.G. (1979) Effects of chromium compounds on plasma membrane Mg^{2+}-ATPase activity of BHK cells. *Chem.-biol. Interactions, 27*, 59-67

Lumbio, J.S. (1953) Lesions in the upper respiratory tract of chromium platers (Swed.).
Nord. Hyg. Tidskr., 5-6, 86-91

Machle, W. & Gregorius, F. (1948) Cancer of the respiratory system in the United States
chromate producing industry. *Publ. Health Rep. (Wash.), 63*, 1114-1127

MacRae, W.D., Whiting, R.F. & Stich, H.F. (1979) Sister chromatid exchanges induced in
cultured mammalian cells by chromate. *Chem.-biol. Interactions, 26*, 281-286

Majone, F. (1977) Effects of potassium dichromate on mitosis of cultured mammalian cells.
Caryologia, 30, 469-481

Majone, F. & Levis, A.G. (1979) Chromosomal aberrations and sister chromatid exchanges
in Chinese hamster cells treated *in vitro* with hexavalent chromium compounds.
Mutat. Res., 67, 231-238

Makarov-Zemlyanskii, Y.Y., Men'shikov, B.I. & Strakhov, I.P. (1978) Persulphate method for determining chromium (III) in solutions with a 'silver free' catalyst (Russ.). *Kozh.-Obuvn. Prom-st., 20*, 43-45 [*Chem. Abstr., 89*, 76343x]

Maloof, C.C. (1955) Use of edathamil calcium in treatment of chrome ulcers of the skin. *Arch. ind. Health, 11*, 123-125

Maltoni, C. (1974) Occupational carcinogenesis. *Excerpta Med. Int. Congr. Ser., 322*, 19-26

Maltoni, C. (1976a) Predictive value of carcinogenesis bioassays. *Ann. N.Y. Acad. Sci., 271*, 431-443

Maltoni, C. (1976b) Precursor lesions in exposed populations as indicators of occupational cancer risk. *Ann. N.Y. Acad. Sci., 271*, 444-447

Mancuso, T.F. (1975) *Consideration of chromium as an industrial carcinogen.* In: Hutchinson, T.C., ed., *Proceedings of the International Conference on Heavy Metals in the Environment, Toronto, 1975*, Toronto, Institute for Environmental Studies, pp. 343-356

Mancuso, T.F. & Hueper, W.C. (1951) Occupational cancer and other health hazards in a chromate plant: a medical appraisal. I. Lung cancers in chromate workers. *Ind. Med. Surg., 20*, 358-363

Matsumoto, N., Iijima, S. & Katsunuma, H. (1976) Placental transfer of chromic chloride and its teratogenic potential in embryonic mice. *J. toxicol. Sci., 2*, 1-13

Matthews, N.A. (1976) *Ferroalloys.* In: *Mineral Facts and Problems,* Washington DC, US Bureau of Mines, US Government Printing Office, p. 365

McGean Chemical Co., Inc. (1978) *Data Sheet. Speciality Chromium Chemicals*, Cleveland, OH

Mellor, J.W. (1931) *A Comprehensive Treatise on Inorganic and Theoretical Chemistry*, Vol. 11, Chapt. 60, *Chromium*, London, Longmans, Green & Co.

Mertz, W. (1969) Chromium occurrence and function in biological systems. *Physiol. Rev., 49*, 163-239

Mertz, W. (1975) Effects and metabolism of glucose tolerance factor. *Nutr. Rev., 33*, 129-135

Mertz, W., Roginski, E.E., Feldman, F.J. & Thurman, D.E. (1969) Dependence of chromium transfer into the rat embryo on the chemical form. *J. Nutr., 99*, 363-367

Meyers, J.B. (1950) Acute pulmonary complications following inhalation of chromic acid mist. *Arch. ind. Hyg. occup. Med., 2*, 742-747

Min, B.C. (1976) A study on the concentration of heavy metals in the tributaries of Han river (Kor.). *Kongjung Poken Chapchi, 13*, 337-347 [*Chem. Abstr., 90*, 92066k]

Ministry of Health & Welfare (1978) *Drinking Water Standards*, Tokyo

Morning, J.L. (1975) *Chromium. Preprint from Bulletin 667, Bureau of Mines,* Washington DC, US Department of the Interior, pp. 1-12

Morning J.L. (1976) *Chromium.* In: *Mineral Facts and Problems,* Washington DC, US Bureau of Mines, US Government Printing Office, pp. 1-12

Morning, J.L. (1977) *Chromium.* In: *Mineral Commodity Profiles,* MCP-1, May 1977, Washington DC, Bureau of Mines, US Government Printing Office, p. 3

Morning, J.L. (1978) *Chromium.* In: *Minerals Yearbook - 1976,* Vol. 1, *Metals, Minerals and Fuels,* Washington DC, Bureau of Mines, US Government Printing Office, pp. 297-308

Morton, M.S. & Elwood, P.C. (1974) CNS malformations and trace elements in water (abstract). *Teratology, 10*, 318

Mosinger, M. & Fiorentini, H. (1954) On the pathology of chromates. First experimental researches. *Arch. Mal. prof. Méd. Trav. Sécur. Soc., 15*, 187-199

Mueller, G. (1977) Pollution research on dated sediment cores from Lake Constance. II. Historical evolution of heavy metals - relationship to the evolution of polycyclic aromatic hydrocarbons (Ger.). *Z. Naturforsch., 32c*, 913-919 [*Chem. Abstr., 88*, 78774s]

Mukubo, K. (1978) Studies on experimental lung tumor by the chemical carcinogens and inorganic substances. III. Histopathological studies on lung tumors in rats induced by pertracheal vinyl tube infusion of 20-methylcholanthrene combined with chromium and nickel powders. *J. Nara med. Assoc., 29*, 321-340

Mutti, A., Cavatorta, A., Borghi, L., Canali, M., Giaroli, C. & Franchini, I. (1979a) Distribution and urinary excretion of chromium. Studies on rats after administration of single and repeated doses of potassium dichromate. *Med. Lav., 3,* 171-179

Mutti, A., Cavatorta, A., Pedroni, C., Borghi, A., Giaroli, C. & Franchini, I. (1979b) The role of chromium accumulation in the relationship between airborne and urinary chromium in welders. *Int. Arch. occup. environ. Health, 43,* 123-133

Nakamuro, K., Yoshikawa, K., Sayato, Y. & Kurata, H. (1978) Comparative studies of chromosomal aberration and mutagenicity of trivalent and hexavalent chromium. *Mutat. Res., 58,* 175-181

Nater, J.P. (1962) Possible causes of chromate eczema. *Ned. Tijdschr. Geneeskd., 106,* 1429-1431

National Academy of Sciences (1974) *Chromium,* Washington DC

National Institute for Occupational Safety & Health (1973) *Criteria for a Recommended Standard... Occupational Exposure to Chromic Acid,* Washington DC, US Department of Health, Education, & Welfare

National Institute for Occupational Safety & Health (1975) *Criteria for a Recommended Standard... Occupational Exposure to Chromium (VI),* Washington DC, US Department of Health, Education, & Welfare

Nestmann, E.R., Matula, T.I., Douglas, G.R., Bora, K.C. & Kowbel, D.J. (1979) Detection of the mutagenic activity of lead chromate using a battery of microbial tests. *Mutat. Res., 66,* 357-365

Nettesheim, P., Hanna, M.G., Jr, Doherty, D.G., Newell, R.F. & Hellman, A. (1971) Effect of calcium chromate dust, influenza virus and 100 R whole-body X radiation on lung tumor incidence in mice. *J. natl Cancer Inst., 47,* 1129-1138

Newbold, R.F., Amos, J. & Connell, J.R. (1979) The cytotoxic, mutagenic and clastogenic effects of chromium-containing compounds on mammalian cells in culture. *Mutat. Res., 67,* 55-63

Nishioka, H. (1975) Mutagenic activities of metal compounds in bacteria. *Mutat. Res., 31,* 185-189

Nissing, W. (1975) Trace-element pollution of the Lower Rhine and their significance in drinking-water supply (Ger.). *Ber. Arbeitsgem. Rheinwasserwerke., 32*, 83-94 [*Chem. Abstr., 88*, 176854n]

Ohsaki, Y., Abe, S., Homma, Y., Yozawa, K., Kishi, F. & Murao, M. (1974) High incidence of lung cancer in chromate workers (Jpn.). *J. Jpn. Soc. intern. Med., 63*, 1198-1203

Ohsaki, Y., Abe, S., Kimura, K., Tsuneta, Y., Mikami, H. & Murao, M. (1978) Lung cancer in Japanese chromate workers. *Thorax, 33*, 372-374

Okubo, T. & Tsuchiya, K. (1977) An epidemiological study on lung cancer among chromium plating workers. *Keio J. Med., 26*, 171-177

Onkelinx, C. (1977) Compartment analysis of metabolism of chromium [III] in rats of various ages. *Am. J. Physiol., 232*, E 478-E 484

Osaki, S., Osaki, T., Shibata, S. & Takashima, Y. (1976) Determination of hexavalent and total chromium in sea water by isotope dilution mass spectrometry (Jpn.). *Bunseki Kagaku, 25*, 358-362 [*Chem. Abstr., 86*, 126960g]

Paradellis, T. (1977) Determination of trace elements in whole blood by photon-induced x-ray fluorescence. *Eur. J. nucl. Med., 2*, 277-279

Payne, W.W. (1960a) Production of cancers in mice and rats by chromium compounds. *Arch. ind. Health, 21*, 530-535

Payne, W.W. (1960b) The role of roasted chromite ore in the production of cancer. *Arch. environ. Health, 1*, 20-26

Petrilli, F.L. & De Flora, S. (1977) Toxicity and mutagenicity of hexavalent chromium on *Salmonella typhimurium. Appl. environ. Microbiol., 33*, 805-809

Petrilli, F.L. & De Flora, S. (1978a) Oxidation of inactive trivalent chromium to the mutagenic hexavalent form. *Mutat. Res., 58*, 167-173

Petrilli, F.L. & De Flora, S. (1978b) Metabolic deactivation of hexavalent chromium mutagenicity. *Mutat. Res., 54*, 139-147

Pokrovskaya, L.V. & Shabynina, N.K. (1973) Carcinogenous hazards in the production of chromium ferroalloys (Russ.). *Gig. Tr. Prof. Zabol., 10*, 23-26

Polak, L., Turk, J.L. & Frey, J.R. (1973) Studies on contact hypersensitivity to chromium compounds. *Prog. Allergy, 17*, 145-226

PPG Industries (1978) *Bulletin 40C, Sodium Chromate*, Pittsburg, PA

Raffetto, G., Parodi, S., Parodi, C., De Ferrari, M., Troiano, R. & Brambilla, G. (1977) Direct interaction with cellular targets as the mechanism for chromium carcinogenesis. *Tumori, 63*, 503-512

Rainaldi, G., Colella, C. & Piras, A. (1979) *Mutagenicity of $K_2Cr_2O_7$ in Chinese hamster cells* (abstract). In: *Abstracts of the 9th Annual Meeting of the European Environmental Mutagen Society, Tučepi-Makarska, Yugoslavia, 1979*, p. 126

Rasmussen, L. (1977) Epiphytic bryophytes as indicators of the changes in the background levels of airborne metals from 1951-75. *Environ. Pollut., 14*, 37-45

Robertson, D.E. & Carpenter, R. (1972) *Neutron Activation Techniques for the Measurement of Trace Metals in the Marine Environment*, Springfield, VA, National Technical Information Service

Robertson, F.N. (1975) Hexavalent chromium in the ground water in Paradise Valley, Arizona. *Ground Water, 13*, 516-527

Roe, F.J.C. & Carter, R.L. (1969) Chromium carcinogenesis: calcium chromate as a potent carcinogen for the subcutaneous tissues of the rat. *Br. J. Cancer, 23*, 172-176

Roskill Information Services (1974) *Chromium: World Survey of Production, Consumption and Prices*, 2nd ed., London, pp. 8, 80-93

Royle, H. (1975a) Toxicity of chromic acid in the chromium plating industry (1). *Environ. Res., 10*, 39-53

Royle, H. (1975b) Toxicity of chromic acid in the chromium plating industry (2). *Environ. Res., 10*, 141-163

Ryan, T.R. & Vogt, C.R.H. (1977) Determination of physiological levels of Cr (III) in urine by gas chromatography. *J. Chromatogr., 130*, 346-350

Salmon, L., Atkins, D.H.F., Fischer, E.M.R. & Law, D.V. (1977) Retrospective analysis of air samples in the UK 1957-1974. *J. radioanal. Chem., 37*, 867-880

Sanderson, C.J. (1976) The uptake and retention of chromium by cells. *Transplantation,* *21,* 526-529

Sano, T. (1978) Pathology of chromium lesions (Jpn.). *Rodo no Kagaku, 33,* 4-14

Schiek, R.C. (1973) *Lead chromate pigments. Chrome yellow and chrome orange.* In: Patton, T.C., ed., *Pigment Handbook,* Vol. 1, New York, NY, John Wiley & Sons, pp. 357-363

Schroeder, H.A., Balassa, J.J. & Tipton, I.H. (1962) Abnormal trace metals in man - chromium. *J. chron. Dis., 15,* 941-964

Schroeder, H.A., Balassa, J.J. & Vinton, W.H., Jr (1964) Chromium, lead, cadmium, nickel and titanium in mice: effect on mortality, tumors and tissue levels. *J. Nutr., 83,* 239-250

Schroeder, H.A., Balassa, J.J. & Vinton, W.H., Jr (1965) Chromium, cadmium and lead in rats: effects on life span, tumors and tissue levels. *J. Nutr., 86,* 51-66

Sharma, B.K., Singhal, P.C. & Chugh, K.S. (1978) Intravascular haemolysis and acute renal failure following potassium dichromate poisoning. *Postgrad. med. J., 54,* 414-415

Sibley, S.F. (1976) *Cobalt.* In: *Mineral Facts and Problems,* Washington DC, Bureau of Mines, US Government Printing Office, pp. 269-280

Sirover, M.A. & Loeb, L.A. (1976) Infidelity of DNA synthesis *in vitro*: screening for potential metal mutagens or carcinogens. *Science, 194,* 1434-1436

Smith, D.E., Slade, M.D., Spencer, O.K., Roberts, W.L. & Ruckman, J.H. (1976) Metal concentrations in air particulate in the Four Corners area. *Utah Acad. Proc., 53,* 75-83

Sontag, G., Kerschbaumer, M. & Kainz, G. (1977) Determination of toxic heavy metals in effluent Austrian medicinal and table water (Ger.). *Z. Wasser Abwasser Forsch., 10,* 166-169 [*Chem. Abstr., 88,* 110183m]

Steffee, C.H. & Baetjer, A.M. (1965) Histopathologic effects of chromate chemicals. Report of studies in rabbits, guinea pigs, rats and mice. *Arch. environ. Health, 11,* 66-75

Stern, R.M. (1977) *A Chemical, Physical and Biological Assay of Welding Fume. I. Fume Characteristics,* No. 77.05, Copenhagen, The Danish Welding Institute

Stern, R.M. (1980) *A chemical, physical and mutagenic assay of welding fume.* In: *Proceedings of the 1st International Workshop on* in vitro *Effects of Fibrous Dust, Medical Research Council/Pneumoconiosis Research Unit, Cardiff, UK, 1979,* London, Academic Press (in press)

Stoner, G.D., Shimkin, M.B., Troxell, M.C., Thompson, T.L. & Terry, L.S. (1976) Test for carcinogenicity of metallic compounds by the pulmonary tumor response in strain A mice. *Cancer Res., 36,* 1744-1747

Strik, J.J.T.W.A., De Iongh, H.H., VanRijn, J.W.A. & Wuite, T.P. (1975) *Toxicity of chromium [VI] in fish, with special reference to organ's weights, liver and plasma enzyme activities, blood parameters and histological alterations.* In: Koeman, S.H. & Strik, J.J.T.W.A., eds, *Sublethal Effects of Toxic Chemicals on Aquatic Animals,* Amsterdam, Elsevier, pp. 31-41

Sullivan, C.P., Donachie, M.J., Jr & Morral, F.R. (1970) *Cobalt-base Superalloys 1970,* Brussels, Centre d'Information du Cobalt, pp. 1-4, 38-44

Sunderman, F.W., Jr, Lau, T.J. & Cralley, L.J. (1974) Inhibitory effect of manganese upon muscle tumorigenesis by nickel subsulfide. *Cancer Res., 34,* 92-95

Takemoto, K., Kawai, H. & Yoshimura, H. (1977) *Studies on the relation of chromium and pulmonary disease. II. Chromium contamination of lung cancer* (Jpn.). In: *Proceedings of the 50th Annual Meeting of the Japan Association of Industrial Health,* Tokyo, pp. 368-369

Tamaro, M., Banfi, E., Venturini, S. & Monti-Bragadin, C. (1975) *Hexavalent chromium compounds are mutagenic for bacteria* (Ital.). In: *Proceedings of the 17th National Congress of the Italian Society for Microbiology, Padua, 1975,* pp. 411-415

Tamino, G. (1977) Interactions of chromium with nucleic acids of mammalian cells (Ital.). *Atti Assoz. Genet. Ital., 22,* 69-71

Taylor, F.H. (1966) The relationship of mortality and duration of employment as reflected by a cohort of chromate workers. *Am. J. publ. Health, 56,* 218-229

Teherani, D.K., Stehlik, G., Tehrani, N., Schada, H. & Hinteregger, J. (1977) Determination of heavy metals and selenium in fish from Upper Austrian waters. II. Lead, cadmium, scandium, chromium, cobalt, iron, zinc and selenium (Ger.). *Ber. Oesterr. Studienges. Atomenerg.,* SGAE No. 2797, pp. 1-21 [*Chem. Abstr., 88,* 49150e]

Thayer, T.P. (1956) *Mineralogy and geology of chromium.* In: Udy, M.J., ed., *Chromium,* Vol. 1, New York, NY, Reinhold, p. 25

Thomsen, E. & Stern, R.M. (1979) *A Simple Analytical Technique for the Determination of Hexavalent Chromium in Welding Fumes and Other Complex Matrices*, No. 79.01, Copenhagen, The Danish Welding Institute

Tsuda, H. & Kato, K. (1976) Potassium dichromate-induced chromosome aberrations and its control with sodium sulfite in hamster embryonic cells *in vitro. Gann, 67,* 469-470

Tsuda, H. & Kato, K. (1977) Chromosomal aberrations and morphological transformation in hamster embryonic cells treated with potassium dichromate *in vitro. Mutat. Res., 46,* 87-94

Udy, M.C. (1956) *The physical and chemical properties of compounds of chromium.* In: Udy, M.J., ed., *Chromium*, Vol. 1, New York, NY, Reinhold, pp. 165, 206

Udy, M.J. (1956) *History of chromium.* In: Udy, M.J., ed., *Chromium*, Vol. 1, New York, NY, Reinhold, pp. 2-3

Umeda, M. & Nishimura, M. (1979) Inducibility of chromosomal aberrations by metal compounds in cultured mammalian cells. *Mutat. Res., 67,* 221-229

US Department of Commerce (1978) *US Imports for Consumption and General Imports*, FT 246/Annual 1977, Bureau of the Census, Washington DC, US Government Printing Office, pp. 231-233, 247, 293

US Department of Commerce (1979) *US Exports. Schedule E Commodity Groupings. Schedule E Commodity by Country,* FT 410/December 1978, Washington DC, US Government Printing Office, pp. 2-71, 2-238, 2-290

US Environmental Protection Agency (1977) *Environmental Monitoring Near Industrial Sites, Chromium,* PB-271 881, Springfield, VA, National Technical Information Service

US Environmental Protection Agency (1978) Maximum contaminent levels for inorganic chemicals. *US Code Fed. Regul., Title 40*, Part 141.11, p. 218

US Environmental Protection Agency (1979) Facilities engaged in leather tanning and finishing; effluent limitations guidelines, pretreatment standards, and new source performance standards. *Fed. Regist., 44,* 38746-38776

US Occupational Safety & Health Administration (1978) Air contaminants. *US Code Fed. Regul., Title 29*, part 1910.1000, pp. 99-102

Vallee, M. (1969) The transport system for sulfate in *Chlorella pyrenoidosa* and its regulation. IV. Studies with chromate ion (Fr.). *Biochem. biophys. Acta, 173*, 486-500

Venitt, S. & Levy, L.S. (1974) Mutagenicity of chromates in bacteria and its relevance to chromate carcinogenesis. *Nature, 250*, 493-495

Versieck, J., Hoste, J., Barbier, F., Steyaert, H., De Rudder, J. & Michels, H. (1978) Determination of chromium and cobalt in human serum by neutron activation analysis. *Clin. Chem., 24*, 303-308

Vigliani, E.C. & Zurlo, N. (1955) Observations of the Clinica del Lavoro with several maximum operating position concentrations (MAK) of industrial poisons (Ger.). *Arch. Gewerbepathol. Gewerbehyg., 13*, 528-534

Visek, W.J., Whitney, I.B., Kuhn, U.S.G., III & Comar, C.L. (1953) Metabolism of Cr^{51} by animals as influenced by chemical state. *Proc. Soc. exp. Biol. Med., 10*, 610-615

Wacker, W.E.C. & Vallee, B.L. (1959) Nucleic acids and metals. I. Chromium, manganese, nickel, iron and other metals in ribonucleic acid from diverse biological sources. *J. biol. Chem., 234*, 3257-3262

Waterhouse, J.A.H. (1975) Cancer among chromium platers (abstract). *Br. J. Cancer, 32*, 262

Weast, R.C., ed. (1977) *Handbook of Chemistry and Physics*, 58th ed., Cleveland, OH, Chemical Rubber Company, pp. B-74, B-87 - B-88, B-105, B-126, B-141, B-146, B-158

White, L.R., Jakobsen, K. & Østgaard, K. (1979) Comparative toxicity studies of chromium-rich welding fumes and chromium on an established human cell line. *Environ. Res., 20*, 366-374

Whiting, R.F., Stich, H.F. & Koropatnick, D.J. (1979) DNA damage and DNA repair in cultured human cells exposed to chromate. *Chem.-biol. Interactions, 26*, 267-280

Whitney, R.G. & Risby, T.H. (1975) *Selected Methods in the Determination of First Row Transition Metals in Natural Fresh Water*, University Park, PA, Pennsylvania University Press

WHO (1970) *European Standards for Drinking-Water,* 2nd ed., Geneva, World Health Organization, p. 33

Wild, D. (1978) Cytogenetic effects in the mouse of 17 chemical mutagens and carcinogens evaluated by the micronucleus test. *Mutat. Res., 56,* 319-327

Windholz, M., ed. (1976) *The Merck Index*, 9th ed., Rahway, NJ, Merck & Co., pp. 128, 1308

Winell, M. (1975) An international comparison of hygienic standards for chemicals in the work environment. *Ambio, 4,* 34-36

Yarbro, S. & Flaschka, H.A. (1976) Long-path photometry in clinical analysis. I. The determination of chromium using diphenylcarbazide. *Microchem. J., 21,* 415-423

Lead salts were first considered by an IARC Working Group in 1971 (IARC, 1972); lead tetraalkyls were considered in 1972 (IARC, 1973). Since that time, new data have become available, and these are included in the present monograph and have been taken into consideration in the evaluation.

1. Chemical and Physical Data

1.1 Synonyms, trade names and molecular formulae

Table 1. Synonyms (Chemical Abstracts Services names are given in bold), trade names and atomic or molecular formulae of lead and lead compounds

Chemical name	Chem. Abstr. Reg. Serial No.	Synonyms and trade names	Formula
Lead	7439-92-1	C.I. 77575; C.I. pigment metal 4 KS-4; Lead Flake; Lead S2; SO; SI	Pb
Lead acetate	301-04-2	**Acetic acid, lead (2+) salt**; dibasic lead acetate; lead (II) acetate; lead (2+) acetate; lead diacetate; lead dibasic acetate; plumbous acetate Salt of Saturn; Sugar of Lead	$Pb(OOCCH_3)_2$
Lead acetate trihydrate	6080-56-4	**Acetic acid, lead (2+) salt, trihydrate**; lead diacetate trihydrate	$Pb(OOCCH_3)_2 .3H_2O$
Lead carbonate	598-63-0	**Carbonic acid, lead (2+) salt (1:1)**; dibasic lead carbonate; lead (2+) carbonate White lead	$PbCO_3$
Lead chloride	7758-95-4	**Lead chloride [$PbCl_2$]**; lead (II) chloride; lead (2+) chloride; lead dichloride; plumbous chloride	$PbCl_2$
Lead naphthenate	50825-29-1	A complex mixture of lead salts of organic acids obtained during the manufacture of hydrocarbon distillates, principally cyclopentanoic acids	

(Table 1 (contd)

Chemical name	Chem. Abstr. Reg. Serial No.	Synonyms and trade names	Formula
Lead nitrate	10099-74-8	Lead dinitrate; lead (II) nitrate; lead (2+) nitrate; **nitric acid, lead (2+) salt**	$Pb(NO_3)_2$
Lead oxide	1317-36-8	C.I. 77577; C.I. pigment yellow 46; lead monoxide; **lead oxide [PbO]** ; lead oxide yellow; lead (II) oxide; lead protoxide; plumbous oxide Litharge; Litharge Pure; Litharge Yellow L-28; Massicot; Massico-tite; Yellow Lead Ocher	PbO
Lead phosphate	7446-27-7	C.I. 77622; lead *ortho*phosphate; lead phosphate (3:2); lead (2+) phosphate; **phosphoric acid, lead (2+) salt (2:3)**; trilead phosphate Perlex Paste 500; Perlex Paste 600A	$Pb_3(PO_4)_2$
Lead subacetate	1335-32-6	Basic lead acetate; bis (aceto)dihy-droxytrilead; bis(acetato)tetrahy-droxytrilead; lead acetate, basic; **lead, bis(acetato-*O*)tetrahydroxy-tri-**; monobasic lead acetate; subacetate lead	$Pb(OOCCH_3)_2 \cdot 2Pb(OH)_2$
Lead tetroxide	1314-41-6	C.I. pigment red 105; lead *ortho*-plumbate; **lead oxide [Pb_3O_4]** ; lead oxide, red; lead tetraoxide; orange lead; plumboplumbic oxide; red lead; red lead oxide; trilead tetroxide Mineral Orange; Minium; Minium red; Paris red; Saturn red	Pb_3O_4
Tetraethyllead	78-00-2	**Plumbane, tetraethyl-; TEL;** tetraethylplumbane	$Pb(C_2H_5)_4$
Tetramethyllead	75-74-1	**Plumbane, tetramethyl-;** tetra-methylplumbane; TML	$Pb(CH_3)_4$

1.2 Chemical and physical properties of the pure substances

Physical properties of the lead compounds considered in this monograph are given, when available, in Table 2. Information on solubility, from Weast (1977), unless otherwise specified, is given below.

Lead - insoluble in water; reacts with nitric acid and hot sulphuric acid

Lead acetate - soluble in water (443 g/l) and glycerine; slightly soluble in ethanol

Lead acetate trihydrate - soluble in water (456.1 g/l at 15°C); insoluble in ethanol

Lead carbonate - practically insoluble in water (0.0011 g/l at 20°C); soluble in acids and alkali

Lead chloride - slightly soluble in water (9.9 g/l at 20°C), dilute hydrochloric acid and ammonia; insoluble in ethanol

Lead naphthenate - soluble in ethanol (Hawley, 1977)

Lead nitrate - soluble in water (376.5 g/l at 0°C; 1270 g/l at 100°C), 43% ethanol (87.7 g/l at 22°C)

Lead oxide - practically insoluble in water (0.017 g/l at 20°C); soluble in alkali, ammonium chloride and nitric acid

Lead phosphate - practically insoluble in water (0.00014 g/l at 20°C); soluble in alkali and nitric acid

Lead subacetate - soluble in cold water (62.5 g/l) and in boiling water (250 g/l) (Windholz, 1976)

Lead tetroxide - soluble in hydrochloric and acetic acids; insoluble in water and ethanol

Tetraethyllead - insoluble in water; soluble in benzene, ethanol and diethyl ether

Tetramethyllead - insoluble in water; soluble in benzene, ethanol and diethyl ether

Table 2. Physical properties of lead and lead compounds [a]

Chemical name	Atomic/ molecular weight	Melting-point (^{o}C)	Boiling-point (^{o}C)	Density (g/cm^3)	Crystal system
Lead	207.19	327.5	1740	11.3437[16]	cubic
Lead acetate	325.28	280	-	3.25_4^{20}	crystalline
Lead acetate trihydrate	379.33	75 (-H$_2$O)	200 (dec.)	2.55	monoclinic
Lead carbonate	267.20	315 (dec.)	-	6.6	rhombic
Lead chloride	278.10	501	950	5.85	rhombic
Lead naphthenate	-	approx. 100°C[b]	-	1.15[c]	-
Lead nitrate	331.20	470 (dec.)	-	4.53^{20}	cubic or mono-clinic
Lead oxide	223.19	888	-	9.53	tetrahedral
Lead phosphate	811.51	1014	-	6.9-7.3	hexagonal
Lead subacetate	807.75	-	-	-	powder
Lead tetroxide	685.57	500 (dec.)	-	9.1	red crystalline scales or amor-phous powder
Tetraethyllead	323.44	-136.8	200 (dec.)	1.659[11]	liquid
Tetramethyllead	267.33	-27.5	110	1.995	liquid

[a] Data from Weast (1977), unless otherwise specified

[b] Hawley (1977)

[c] Whitaker (1965)

1.3 Technical products and impurities

The specifications of the American Society for Testing and Materials (1977) for common desilverized *lead* are as follows: lead (by difference), 99.85% min; bismuth, 1500 mg/kg max; copper, 25 mg/kg max; arsenic, antimony and tin combined, 50 mg/kg max; iron, 20 mg/kg max; silver, 20 mg/kg max ; and zinc, 20 mg/kg max.

Lead available in Japan has a minimum 99.99% purity and contains the following impurities: bismuth, 50 mg/kg max; antimony and tin combined, 50 mg/kg max; arsenic, 20 mg/kg max; copper, 20 mg/kg max; iron, 20 mg/kg max; silver, 20 mg/kg max; and zinc, 20 mg/kg max. In western Europe, pig lead is available in various grades with from 99.9%-99.985% purity. Impurities are similar to those found in US and Japanese products.

Lead acetate is usually available as the hydrate, *lead acetate trihydrate*. In the US, it is available in reagent, purified and technical grades. Trace impurities typically found include chloride ion and iron, the concentration of each of which does not exceed 5 mg/kg in the reagent grade product (J. T. Baker Chemical Co., 1976a).

Lead acetate trihydrate is available in the Federal Republic of Germany with the following specifications: 99% minimum purity; nitrate and nitrite (as NO_3), 0.005% max; copper, 20 mg/kg max; iron, 10 mg/kg max; matter insoluble in water, 0.001% max; chloride, 5 mg/kg max; acetic acid content, 32% max; and lead content, 54.5% min. In Japan, lead acetate trihydrate is available with a minimum of 99% purity. Impurities include copper, 20 mg/kg max; iron, 20 mg/kg max; and chloride, 10 mg/kg max.

Lead carbonate is available in the US as a commercial reagent grade with a minimum purity of 99.0%. Impurities typically present include: nitrate and nitrite (as NO_3), 0.005% max; zinc, 30 mg/kg max; chloride, 20 mg/kg max; cadmium, 20 mg/kg max; and iron, 20 mg/kg max (J.T. Baker Chemical Co., 1976b). Lead carbonate available in Japan has a minimum purity of 99.0%. It may contain the following impurities: water, 1% max; matter soluble in water, 0.5% max; and matter insoluble in acetic acid, 0.1% max.

Reagent grade *lead chloride* has a minimum purity of 99.0%. Typical impurities are sulphate, 0.01% max; copper, 50 mg/kg max; nitrate, 0.005% max; and iron, 10 mg/kg max (J. T. Baker Chemical Co., 1976c). In Japan, lead chloride is produced in two grades, with 99.5% purity or 99.0% purity.

Lead naphthenate available in the US contains 24% lead and 67% max. nonvolatile matter or 16% lead and 60% max. nonvolatile matter (National Paint & Coatings Association, 1973).

Lead nitrate is available commercially in the US in technical and reagent grades. Impurities typically present in the reagent grade include copper, iron and chloride (J. T. Baker Chemical Co., 1975). Lead nitrate available in western Europe has the following specifications: minimum purity, 98.0%; insoluble matter, 0.1% max; copper, 100 mg/kg max; silver, 250 mg/kg max; iron, 10 mg/kg max; and mercury, 10 mg/kg max. In Japan, lead nitrate is available with a minimum purity of 99.0% and containing 5 mg/kg max.iron and 3 mg/kg max.copper.

Lead oxide used in storage battery plates in the US exists in two crystalline forms, the yellow orthorhombic and the red tetragonal forms. Both 100% tetragonal and mixed crystalline products contain 15-30% lead by weight. High purity must be maintained in the manufacturing process because tellurium, nickel, antimony and copper reduce negative plate end-of-charge voltage; however, small amounts of iron ($\leqslant$200 mg/kg) impurities may be allowed in some types of batteries (Doe, 1978). In western Europe, lead oxide is available in three grades containing 100, 50 and 10 mg/kg maximum total metallic impurities. Lead oxide available in Japan has a minimum purity of 99.5% and contains 20 mg/kg max.cupric oxide and 10 mg/kg max.iron oxide.

No data on the technical products and impurities of *lead phosphate* were available to the Working Group.

Reagent grade *lead subacetate* available commercially in the US has the following specifications: basic lead, 33.0% min; nitrate and nitrite (as NO_3), 0.003% max; chloride, 20 mg/kg max; copper, 20 mg/kg max; iron, 20 mg/kg max; and substances not precipitated by hydrogen sulphide (as SO_4), 0.2% max. (J.T. Baker Chemical Co., 1977). In western Europe, lead subacetate is available with the following specifications: lead, 72% min; acetic acid, 24% min; matter insoluble in water, 1% max; matter insoluble in dilute acetic acid, 0.02% max; chloride, 50 mg/kg max; and iron, 20 mg/kg max.

Lead tetroxide is available in the US for most applications as pigment grades containing 85, 95, 97 or 98% active ingredient; the remainder is usually lead oxide, PbO (Dunn, 1973a). One supplier offers a technical grade (composition unknown) and a 99.999% active grade (Atomergic Chemetals Company, undated). Other grades available include an orange mineral grade (Dunn, 1973a) and a ceramic grade, but no information on their composition was available. In the Federal Republic of Germany, refined lead tetroxide is available containing a minimum of 99.97% active ingredient (Metallgesellschaft Aktiengesellschaft, 1979).

Tetraethyllead and *tetramethyllead* are used as active ingredients in motor and aviation gasoline antiknock mixes; these also contain a number of other components, including scavenging agents [typically, 18.81% by weight 1,2-dichloroethane (see IARC, 1980) and 18% by weight ethylene dibromide (see IARC, 1977)], a dye, a solvent (usually kerosene or toluene), an antioxidant and sometimes a diluent. Tetraethyllead and tetramethyllead available in Japan have lead contents of 60.06% by weight and 77.5% by weight, respectively.

2. Production, Use, Occurrence and Analysis

2.1 Production and use

LEAD

(a) Production

Lead is one of the oldest metals known to man; artifacts have been discovered that date from 3000 B.C. It was mined in considerable quantities by the Greeks and Romans and has continued to be of commercial significance throughout modern history (Mellor, 1947).

Lead is recovered from naturally-occurring sulphide ores that usually contain 1-6% lead. Zinc and other metal sulphides are often associated with lead sulphide. Lead ore is beneficiated at mine sites by standard crushing, grinding and flotation techniques, resulting in concentrates that contain 55-70% lead. The concentrate is sintered, resulting in the formation of lead oxide, which is reduced in the sinter to produce molten lead bullion and refired to eliminate impurities.

In North America, lead was mined and smelted as early as 1621. Annual US production was about 909 thousand kg from 1801 through 1810 and increased to about 2.7 million kg from 1831 to 1840. Production from scrap metal was first reported in the US in 1907, when it amounted to 23.6 million kg. In 1976, when world mine production of lead amounted to 3.4 billion kg, US production accounted for 550 million kg (US Bureau of Mines, 1978); US imports (ore and refined metal) were 208 million kg in 1976, 318 million kg in 1977 and 284 million kg in 1978, and exports (lead materials) were 5.3 million kg in 1976, 9.0 million kg in 1977 and 8 million kg in 1978 (Lead Industries Association, Inc., 1978; US Bureau of Mines, 1980). The US lead mining industry comprises about 30 mines in 15 states and six smelters in four states which reduce lead concentrates to lead bullion.

Lead was first produced commercially in Japan in 1920; two companies currently produce it. In 1977, production amounted to 221.4 million kg, imports were 25.6 million kg, and exports amounted to 7.9 million kg.

There are about 26 producers of lead in western Europe; production in 1976 amounted to 1.3 billion kg and that in 1977 to 1.4 billion kg. Production of refined lead in the European Economic Community in 1978 was 1.7 billion kg. Production figures in 1978 for refined lead are available for the following countries (in million kg): USA, 773.7; USSR (not refined), 640;   Federal Republic of Germany, 305; UK, 247.4; Australia, 239.3; Japan, 228.4; France, 208.2; Canada, 194.1; Mexico, 159.3; Belgium and Luxembourg, 104.2; Spain, 87.8; Peru, 74.6; Italy, 55.8; Sweden, 45.3; The Netherlands, 31.9 and Austria, 15.9 (Metallgesellschaft Aktiengesellschaft, 1979).

(b)   Use

In the US in 1977 lead metal was used as follows: 57% for storage batteries (30% for oxides and 27% for posts and grids), 15% as an intermediate for tetraalkyl leads (e.g., tetraethyl- and tetramethyllead) used as antiknock additives for motor fuels, 5% for red lead (lead tetroxide) and lead oxide (lead monoxide), 4% for ammunition and 4% for solder. The other 15% was used in pigment colours, weights and ballast, sheet metal, brass and bronze, cable covering, calking, type metal, bearings, annealing, galvanizing, plating and other miscellaneous uses (Lead Industries Association, Inc., 1978).

In 1978, 1.24 billion kg were used in the European Economic Community. The use pattern in 1977 was as follows: lead products (as metal, except in batteries and alloys), 390 million kg; batteries, 430 million kg; alloys, 77 million kg; and chemical products, 300 million kg.

LEAD ACETATE AND LEAD ACETATE TRIHYDRATE

(a)   Production

Lead acetate is currently made by dissolving lead oxide in strong acetic acid. The commercial product, lead acetate trihydrate, is manufactured by dissolving lead oxide in hot dilute acetic acid solution (Thompson, 1967).

Lead acetate was first produced commercially in the US in 1944 (US Tariff Commission, 1946). In 1977, three US companies reported production of an undisclosed amount (see preamble, p. 20   ) (US International Trade Commission, 1978). US imports in 1978 were 112.7 kg (US Bureau of the Census, 1979).

Lead acetate was first produced commercially as the trihydrate in Japan before 1940, and three companies produce it currently, by the reaction of lead oxide with gaseous acetic acid. Production in 1972 was about 350 thousand kg, which had declined to 200 thousand kg by 1977.

Available information indicated that it is also produced by one company in Austria, by three in the Federal Republic of Germany, by one in France, by three in Italy and by four companies in Spain and four in the UK, although it may be produced elsewhere as well.

(b) Use

Lead acetate trihydrate is used in the US as an intermediate in the manufacture of other lead salts, such as basic lead carbonate and lead chromate. It is also used as a mordant in cotton dyes, as a drier in paints, and in the lead coating of metals. Dilute solutions have been used in medicine as poultices and washes for treatment of poison ivy inflammation (Thompson, 1967; van Thoor, 1968). It was used as an astringent in lotions but has largely been replaced by other drugs (Modell, 1977). Small amounts of the chemical have been used in explosives. Lead acetate in concentrations up to 3% is used as a colour additive in hair dyes; it darkens the hair gradually by the slow formation of lead sulphide (Marzulli et al., 1978; Searle & Harnden, 1979). In the US, the closing date for the provisional listing of lead acetate for use in hair dyes has been extended from 1 March to 30 June 1980.

In Japan, lead acetate trihydrate is used primarily as a scouring agent in the removal of gold and silver from their ores.

LEAD CARBONATE

(a) Production

Lead carbonate was first prepared by Becquerel in 1852; he allowed a concentrated solution of sodium and calcium carbonates to act for seven years on a lead plate wrapped with platinum wire (Mellor, 1947). It can be prepared more rapidly by passing carbon dioxide through a cold, dilute solution of lead acetate or by adding a soluble lead compound to ammonium carbonate solution (Thompson, 1967).

Lead carbonate itself has very limited industrial use (Thompson, 1967); however, one basic lead carbonate, lead dihydroxydicarbonate [$2PbCO_3.Pb(OH)_2$], containing 62-66% lead carbonate, is used commercially. It is produced by rotating a charge of lead oxide in a cylinder and spraying it with acetic acid solution; carbon dioxide from flue gas is introduced, and the basic lead carbonate is formed. It is also made by oxidizing a lead oxide slurry and introducing flue gas to carbonate the product (Dunn, 1973b).

Basic lead carbonate has been produced commercially since the early seventeenth century. US production reached a peak of 154 million kg per year in the early twentieth century, when approximately 40 plants manufactured it (Dunn, 1973b). In 1976, US production of basic lead carbonate was 1.48 million kg (US Bureau of Mines, 1978); US imports in 1978 were 178 thousand kg (US Bureau of the Census, 1979). Separate export data are not reported.

In Japan, basic lead carbonate is produced commercially by one company by oxidation of lead (in the presence of lead acetate) to lead hydroxide, followed by the addition of carbon dioxide. Production of basic lead carbonate began in Japan before 1940; it was 1.24 million kg in 1973 but had declined to 625 thousand kg by 1977. Japanese imports of basic lead carbonate are insignificant, and export data are not available.

Available information indicated that basic lead carbonate is also produced by 10 companies in the Federal Republic of Germany, three in The Netherlands, two in Spain and two in the UK and one in Portugal and in Switzerland, although it may be produced elsewhere as well.

(b) Use

In 1973, use of basic lead carbonate in the US was as follows: miscellaneous uses, 66%; paints, 33.5%; and ceramics, 0.5% (US Bureau of Mines, 1978). It is used as a white hiding pigment for linseed oil paints (Dunn, 1973b), in ceramic glazes and in putty. It is also used in cements and in basic lead carbonate paper.

In Japan, 536 thousand kg basic lead carbonate were used in 1977; the pattern is estimated to be as follows: ceramics, 37%; paints, 36% and miscellaneous uses [including use as a stabilizer for polyvinyl chloride resin (see IARC, 1979)], 27%.

LEAD CHLORIDE

(a) Production

Lead chloride has been known since the Middle Ages. It was prepared in 1656 by addition of hydrochloric acid to a solution of lead in nitric acid (Mellor, 1947). It is prepared commercially by treating an aqueous solution of a lead salt with a soluble chloride or with hydrochloric acid or by reacting lead oxide or basic lead carbonate with hydrochloric acid (Thompson, 1967).

At present, lead chloride is believed to be produced in the US by only one manufacturer of reagent grade chemicals in an undisclosed amount (see preamble, p. 20). Data on US imports and exports are not reported.

In Japan, only nominal quantities of lead chloride are produced for use as a reagent.

Available information indicates that it is also produced by one company in the Federal Republic of Germany, three in Italy, one in The Netherlands and four in the UK, although it may be produced elsewhere as well.

(b) Use

Lead chloride can be used to make basic lead chlorides such as Pattison's lead white, an artists' pigment (Thompson, 1967), other pigments and lead oxychloride and as an ingredient in solder and flux (Windholz, 1976). It has been used as a laboratory reagent for drying alcohol.

LEAD NAPHTHENATE

(a)   Production

Lead naphthenate is prepared commercially by the reaction of naphthenic acid with lead oxide (Whitaker, 1965). Commercial production in the US was first reported in 1944 (US Tariff Commission, 1946). In 1969, US production of lead naphthenate was 8.2 million kg; in 1977, eight US companies reported total production of 2.2 million kg (US International Trade Commission, 1978). Separate US imports and exports data are not reported.

In Japan, where there are currently eleven producers, total annual production of lead naphthenate has been approximately 300 thousand kg in recent years.

There are approximately 20 producers of lead naphthenate in western Europe. Three of these producers are in Austria, where lead naphthenate has been produced since about 1930; production in that country is declining, with amounts of less than one million kg produced per year. In Italy, where there are four producers, production is less than one million kg per year, and there are no imports or exports. In the UK, where commercial production started between 1900 and 1910, there are presently four producing companies. Annual production is in the range of 1 - 5 million kg and is believed to be dropping. Imports and exports are both less than one million kg per year.

No information was available on whether it is also produced elsewhere.

(b)   Use

Lead naphthenate is used almost exclusively as a paint drier in the US. It has been widely used as an extreme pressure agent in lubricants (Jolly, 1967). In Austria, 90% of the lead naphthenate is used in heavy lubricating oils and greases, and 10% is used as a paint drier.

LEAD NITRATE

(a)   Production

Lead nitrate was prepared in 1595 by Libavius by the reaction of pulverized lead with nitric acid (Mellor, 1947). It is prepared commercially by dissolving lead or lead monoxide in nitric acid and cooling (van Thoor, 1968).

Commercial production of lead nitrate in the US was first reported in 1943 (US Bureau of the Census, 1947). It is currently produced in the US by three companies, but separate production data are not reported. US imports of lead nitrate in 1978 were 480 thousand kg (US Bureau of the Census, 1979). Separate export data are not available.

There are two commercial producers of lead nitrate in Japan and four companies which produce it as an intermediate. Production began prior to 1940 and has been constant for the past few years, with a level of 300 thousand kg in 1977. Separate data on imports and exports are not available.

Lead nitrate is produced by five companies in the UK. Only one of these is believed to be a commercial producer; the remaining companies produce it as an intermediate. Production is over 100 million kg per year, and exports are between 50 and 100 million kg annually. Available information indicates that lead nitrate is also produced by one company in Austria, in France and in Switzerland, by two companies in Belgium, four companies in the Federal Republic of Germany and five companies in Italy, although it may be produced elsewhere as well.

(b) Use

Lead nitrate is used as a mordant in dyeing and printing cotton (van Thoor, 1968). It is also used in the manufacture of matches and pyrotechnics. Lead nitrate can be used as a chemical reagent and as an intermediate in the production of lead chromate (chrome yellow) (Gloger, 1968; Thompson, 1967). In Japan, it is reportedly used as a defoaming agent for optical glass.

LEAD OXIDE

(a) Production

Lead oxide has been known since the first century A.D. Impure lead oxide was prepared by Dioscorides from a plumbiferous silver, from lead, and from a plumbiferous sand (Mellor, 1947). It is produced commercially for chemical uses by air oxidation of lead at high temperatures (above $500^\circ C$), followed by quick cooling below $300^\circ C$ to avoid formation of undesired oxides.

It is believed that there are currently nine US producers of lead oxide. US production in 1976 was 120 million kg; imports in 1978 were 20 million kg, primarily from Mexico (US Bureau of the Census, 1979). Separate export data are not reported.

In Japan, where there are currently five producers, lead oxide has been produced commercially since before 1940. Production was 35.4 million kg in 1973, but had declined to 28.6 million kg by 1977. In 1977, combined imports of lead oxide and lead tetroxide were 178 thousand kg. Separate data on Japanese exports are not available.

There are about 17 producers of lead oxide in western Europe. Largest amounts are used in Italy, where 50-100 million kg are used annually. Annual consumption in Benelux, the Federal Republic of Germany, France, Spain and the UK is from 10-50 million kg each; 1-5 million kg are used annually in Austria and in Scandinavia; and less than 1 million kg are used in Switzerland. Between 5-10 million kg are imported annually into the Federal Republic of Germany and Italy; 1-5 million kg into Benelux, France and Scandinavia; and less than 1 million kg into Austria, Spain, Switzerland and the UK. France is the greatest exporter, with 10-50 million kg annually; Benelux, the Federal Republic of Germany and the UK each export 5-10 million kg; Austria exports 1-5 million kg; and Italy, Scandinavia, Spain and Switzerland each export less than 1 million kg.

No information was available on whether it is also produced elsewhere.

(b) Use

In the US in 1976, 111 million kg lead oxide were used, as follows: miscellaneous uses (including storage batteries and oil refining), 64%; ceramics, 26%; paints, 7%; and rubber, 3% (US Bureau of Mines, 1978).

The major use of lead oxide is as a partially oxidized powder, containing about 60-80% lead oxide, for the preparation of storage battery plates. The next most important use is in ceramic industries for the manufacture of certain glasses, glazes and vitreous enamels. Lead content in glasses imparts greater brilliance, resonance and toughness. In paints, lead oxide is used as a drier; it is also used as an activator in rubber compounding (Thompson, 1967).

Miscellaneous uses of lead oxide include the preparation of plumbite solution for the conversion of thiols to disulphides in oil refining and as the usual starting material for the manufacture of other lead chemicals (e.g., chrome pigments, basic lead carbonate, basic lead sulphate); it has also been used in insecticides (Thompson, 1967).

In Japan in 1977, 28.5 million kg lead oxide were used, as follows: glass, 54%; stabilizers for polyvinylchloride resins (see IARC, 1979), 35%; pigments, 3%; paint driers, 2%; miscellaneous (including rubber processing), 6%.

LEAD PHOSPHATE

(a) Production

Lead phosphate was prepared in 1816 by digesting lead hydrophosphate with aqueous ammonia (Mellor, 1947). It can be prepared commercially by the reaction of lead acetate with sodium orthophosphate (Thompson, 1967).

There is one producer in the Federal Republic of Germany and one in Italy.

No evidence was found that lead phosphate is presently being produced in commercial quantities in the US or Japan; however, it may be produced elsewhere.

(b) Use

Lead phosphate is believed to be used as a stabilizer in styrene and casein plastics. It may also be used in small amounts for special glasses (van Wazer, 1968).

It has been produced in Japan in small quantities for use as a reagent.

LEAD SUBACETATE

(a) Production

Lead subacetate was prepared in 1912 by saturating a lead acetate solution with lead oxide (White & Patterson, 1912). It is made commercially by dissolving lead oxide and lead hydroxide in aqueous solutions of lead acetate (Thompson, 1967).

Commercial production of lead subacetate was first reported in the US in 1947 (US Tariff Commission, 1949). In 1977, only one US company, which specializes in reagent chemicals, reported production of an undisclosed amount (see preamble, p. 20) (US International Trade Commission, 1978). Data on US exports and imports are not available.

Available information indicated that lead subacetate is also produced by one company in Italy and one in Switzerland and by two companies in the Federal Republic of Germany and two in the UK, although it may be produced elsewhere as well.

(b) Use

Lead subacetate is used primarily as an analytical reagent. It is reportedly used (as Hanes' dry lead) to remove colourants in sugar analysis and to decolour solutions of other organic substances. It can be used as an astringent in lotions (Modell, 1977).

LEAD TETROXIDE

(a) Production

The Egyptions, Greeks and Romans were involved in the early production and use of lead tetroxide: in 77 A.D., Pliny reported the use of lead tetroxide by Micias in 320 B.C. The principal technique for manufacture was the roasting of white lead (basic lead carbonate) (Dunn, 1973b).

Two different manufacturing techniques are currently employed, each of which yields a different grade of product, furnace red lead or fumed red lead. The first involves calcining either lead oxide or a combination of lead oxide and finely divided lead particles at 450-470°C. Fumed red lead is produced by first atomizing molten metallic lead into finely divided particles and then instantaneously heating to 1800°C (Dunn, 1973b).

There are two producers of lead tetroxide in the US; total production in 1976 was 18 million kg (US Bureau of Mines, 1978). In 1976, US imports were 800 thousand kg (US Bureau of Mines, 1978); and in 1979, import levels are believed to have been about 1 million kg. In 1977, approximately 1-15 million kg were exported.

Available information indicates that there are six producers in Spain, four in France, three each in the Federal Republic of Germany and Italy, two each in Portugal and the UK and one each in the Netherlands and Switzerland, although it may be produced elsewhere as well.

(b) Use

Of the 17 million kg of lead tetroxide shipped in the US in 1976, 35% was used in pigments for corrosion-inhibiting primers and paints, and 65% was used in miscellaneous applications, of which use in lead storage batteries is the most significant (US Bureau of Mines, 1978). Other miscellaneous applications include the production of ceramics and glass, pigments and oxidizing agents (van Thoor, 1968).

TETRAETHYLLEAD AND TETRAMETHYLLEAD

(a) Production

Tetraethyllead was prepared in 1853 by the reaction of a sodium-lead alloy with ethyl iodide (Shapiro & Frey, 1967). It is manufactured commercially principally by alkylation of a sodium-lead alloy with ethyl chloride. however, one US company manufactures it by the electrolysis of ethylmagnesium chloride in an ether solution with excess ethyl chloride and lead pellets.

Tetramethyllead was prepared in 1862 by the reaction of a sodium-lead alloy with methyl iodide (Prager *et al.*, 1922). It is manufactured commercially by the same processes that are used to make tetraethyllead, except that methylated compounds are substituted for the ethylated ones.

Commercial production of tetraethyllead in the US was first reported in 1923 (US Tariff Commission, 1925). US production reached a peak of 266 million kg in 1964 (US Tariff Commission, 1965) but by 1977 had fallen to 148 million kg (US International Trade Commission, 1978). US imports of tetraethyllead in 1978 were 17 thousand kg; 85% came from Canada and 15% from Israel (US Bureau of the Census, 1979).

Commercial production of tetramethyllead in the US was first reported in 1960 (US Tariff Commission, 1961); and in 1977, 54 million kg were produced (US International Trade Commission, 1978). In 1974, 13.8 thousand kg were imported, all from the Federal Republic of Germany.

Tetramethyl- and tetraethyllead are not exported as such from the US; however, anti-knock mixes for petrols are exported, which may contain either tetraethyllead, tetramethyl-lead, physical mixtures of these two lead alkyl compounds and various reaction product mixtures produced by catalytic equilibration between varying amounts of tetraethyllead and tetramethyllead. In 1977, about 42 million kg of 100% lead alkyls were exported as components of such antiknock mixes, assuming that the reported exports of antiknock mixes had a lead alkyl content of 61.48% by weight. Details are given in Table 3.

Approximately 85% of the world production capacity for tetraethyllead and tetra-methyllead is represented by two US companies and one UK company. The Federal Republic of Germany, France, Greece and Mexico each have one producer; there are two producers in Canada and three in Italy. It may also be produced elsewhere.

Neither tetraethyl- nor tetramethyllead is produced in Japan; imports in 1973, primarily from the US, of tetraethyllead were 1.8 million kg and those of tetramethyllead, 1.1 million kg. In 1977, imports had declined to 352 and 297 thousand kg, respectively.

(b) Use

Tetraethyl- and tetramethyllead are used primarily as components of formulated anti-knock mixes for motor petrol. In 1969-1970, US consumption of all tetraalkyllead compounds reached a peak of 312 million kg. Use decreased in 1971, as unleaded and low-lead fuels were produced for vehicles equipped with low-compression engines. Between 1974 and 1978, consumption declined significantly after the US Environmental Protection Agency issued regulations requiring a gradual reduction in the lead content of petrol. In 1978, US consumption of 100% pure tetraethyllead in antiknock mixes is estimated to have been 157 million kg.

Tetraethyllead has also been used as an intermediate in the production of organo-mercury fungicides (Shapiro & Frey, 1967).

Table 3. US exports of tetraethyllead compounds in 1977[a]

Country of destination	Quantity[b] (thousand kg)
Venezuela	7070
The Netherlands	5464
Indonesia	5263
Australia	4875
Spain	4778
Brazil	4488
Taiwan	2832
Mexico	2052
Peru	1739
Netherlands Antilles	1593
Republic of Korea	1427
New Zealand	1592
Republic of the Philippines	1256
Thailand	1185
Finland	1015
Singapore	1003
Federal Republic of Germany	961
Canary Islands	818
Hong Kong	815
Israel	568
Argentina	534
Egypt	500
Other countries	3217
TOTAL	54733[c]

[a] US Bureau of the Census, 1978

[b] Calculated 100% lead alkyl content, assuming that the reported exports of anti-knock mixes had a lead alkyl content of 61.48% by weight

[c] Data may not add up to reported total because of rounding off

2.2 Regulatory status (see also preamble, p. 21)

(a) General

The WHO International standard (WHO, 1971) and WHO European standard (WHO, 1970) for lead in drinking-water are 0.1 mg/l. In the US (US Environmental Protection Agency, 1976) and in the European Economic Community (EEC, 1975a), the maximum contaminant level for lead has been established at 0.05 mg/l. In the European Community, a limit of 0.05 mg/l is set for the characteristics of surface water intended for the abstraction of drinking-water (EEC, 1975b). In Japan, the content of lead in drinking-water must be no more than 0.1 mg/l (Ministry of Health & Welfare, 1978).

Effluent limitation guidelines have been established for lead in the US; these require that any process waste water discharged from primary lead and copper smelting facilities not contain a concentration of lead exceeding a maximum daily limit of 1.0 mg/l or an average daily limit of 0.5 mg/l for 30 consecutive days (US Environmental Protection Agency, 1977a). Similarly, pretreatment standards have been set that limit the concentration of lead which may be introduced into a publicly owned waste-treatment works by plants producing lead oxide. The maximum total lead permitted in any one day is 2.0 mg/l, and the average of daily values for 30 consecutive days shall not exceed 1 mg/l (US Environmental Protection Agency, 1977b).

An ambient air quality standard limiting the concentration of lead in air to 1.5 $\mu g/m^3$, as an arithmetic mean averaged over a calendar quarter, has been established in the US (US Environmental Protection Agency, 1978).

A permissible exposure limit at work of 50 $\mu g/m^3$ averaged over an 8-hour period, and a blood lead level of 500 $\mu g/l$ above which removal from exposure is necessary, have also been set in the US (US Occupational Safety & Health Administration, 1979).

In the Federal Republic of Germany, the recommendation of the MAK Committee is 0.1 mg/m^3 (Senatskommission, 1977). The time-weighted average allowable concentrations for lead as inorganic fumes and dusts are 0.15 mg/m^3 in the German Democratic Republic, 0.1 mg/m^3 in Sweden and 0.05 mg/m^3 in Czechoslovakia. The maximum ceiling concentration allowed in the USSR is 0.01 mg/m^3 (Winell, 1975).

Objects for consumer use, particularly if accessible to children, are banned as hazardous products in the US if they contain more than 0.06% lead by weight in the surface paint or other similar surface coatings.

In Japan, the acceptable level of lead in tinned juices and soft drinks is 0.4 mg/l. The Codex Alimentarius Committee of the Food and Agricultural Organization has considered a tolerance of 0.3 mg/kg for tinned fruits and vegetables (Tuna Research Foundation, 1974).

The FAO/WHO Expert Committee on Food Additives established in 1972 a 'provisional tolerable weekly intake' of 3 mg of lead per person for adults, equivalent to 0.05 mg/kg bw, when ingested orally (FAO/WHO, 1972).

Regulations to limit the lead content in petrol have been passed in a number of countries. In the US, the present limit is 0.8 g/gallon (211 mg/l) and is to be reduced to 0.5 g/gallon (132 mg/l) in 1980. In the European Communities, a Council Directive of 1978 (EEC, 1978) limits the level to 0.15-0.4 g/l.

Biological limits in terms of blood lead were also established in the European Community in 1977 (EEC, 1977): median levels for the general population must not exceed 200 μg/l, and those for individuals 350 μg/l, above which action is required to reduce exposure.

Maximum permitted levels for lead in animal feed in the European Community varies from 5 mg/kg in complete feeds to 40 mg/kg in green fodder (EEC, 1974, 1976).

(b) Specific compounds

Permissible levels of tetraethyllead in the working environment have been established in various countries. In the US and the Federal Republic of Germany, it is required that an employee's exposure to tetraethyl- and tetramethyllead at no time exceed 0.075 mg/m^3 (measured as lead) (Senatskommission, 1977; US Occupational Safety & Health Administration, 1979). The 8-hour time-weighted average maximum concentrations for tetraethyllead (measured as lead) are 0.075 mg/m^3 in the Federal Republic of Germany and Sweden and 0.05 mg/m^3 in the German Democratic Republic; the maximum allowable concentration in the USSR is 0.005 mg/m^3 (Winell, 1975).

2.3 Occurrence [1]

(a) Natural environment

Isotopes of lead with the following atomic weights occur in nature: 204.0 (1.5%), 206.0 (23.6%), 207.0 (22.6%) and 208.0 (52.3%). Lead is the final radioactive disintegration product of uranium and thorium. It occurs naturally mainly in the forms of galena, galenite and lead sulphide in the US, Australia, Mexico, Bolivia, Upper Silesia and Spain. Lead also occurs as basic lead carbonate in cerussite (white lead ore), as lead sulphate in anglesite and lanarkite, as the monoxide in massicot and as basic lead chloride in matlockite. Large quantities of lead vanadate are found as vanadinite in southern Africa. Lead occurs naturally in the earth's crust in a concentration of about 13 mg/kg (UNEP/WHO, 1977). It has been suggested (Patterson, 1965) that the lead concentration in the biosphere has increased sub-

---

[1] Lead, and lead compounds calculated as lead, unless otherwise specified

stantially over a period of several millenia as a result of human technology.

(b) Air

Atmospheric concentrations of lead range from 0.0001-0.001 $\mu g/m^3$ in areas remote from civilization. It has been estimated from geochemical data that the concentration of lead of natural origin in air is about 0.0006 $\mu g/m^3$ (UNEP/WHO, 1977). Natural concentrations result from airborne dust, containing on the average 10-15 $\mu g/g$ lead, and from gases diffusing from the earth's crust (National Academy of Sciences, 1972).

Atmospheric concentrations of lead from seven rural sites in the UK in 1974 ranged from 27-200 ng/kg (33-245 ng/m^3) (Cawse, 1975); concentrations in European air ranged from 0.4-7.4 $\mu g/m^3$; and the average annual concentration for 10 sites in Tokyo was 0.65 $\mu g/m^3$ (Fishbein, 1976). Lead concentrations in air decrease with distance from urban centres: average urban concentrations have been reported to be 1.1 $\mu g/m^3$, non-urban (near cities), 0.21 $\mu g/m^3$; and remote areas, 0.02 $\mu g/m^3$ (National Academy of Sciences, 1972). Analysis of air samples collected in the US between 1965 and 1974 from 92 urban and 16 non-urban sites showed that composite lead concentrations in air were highest (1.1 $\mu g/m^3$) in 1971 but had declined to 0.84 $\mu g/m^3$ by 1973. A downtown Los Angeles sampling site had the highest concentration (4-5 μ/m^3); in 1971 concentrations began to decrease, to reach 2.0 $\mu g/m^3$ in 1974. The decreases were attributed to the lower lead content of petrol sold in recent years (Faoro & McMullen, 1977).

About 98% of the total emissions of lead (mostly as inorganic lead) to the atmosphere in the US are from the combustion of leaded petrol. Concentrations in ambient air are closely related to the density of vehicular traffic: lead concentrations measured along a major highway in Los Angeles during the morning rush hour were as high as 54.3 $\mu g/m^3$ (National Academy of Sciences, 1972).

The highest sources of lead emissions into the atmosphere next to the combustion of leaded petrol are lead smelting and solid waste disposal (Faoro & McMullen, 1977; National Academy of Sciences, 1972). Lead concentrations in air samples taken at two primary lead smelters in the US ranged from 6.67-2990 $\mu g/m^3$ (Constant et al., 1977). Several solid waste disposal practices may be responsible for lead emissions: lead wastes are remelted in secondary smelters; and non-recycled, lead-containing consumer products such as cable scrap, battery casings, products painted with lead pigments and bottle caps are burned in municipal incinerators (UNEP/WHO, 1977).

The burning of coal, and to a lesser extent, oil, are minor sources of atmospheric lead emissions in the US (UNEP/WHO, 1977). However, the global contribution to atmospheric lead from the burning of coal is reported to be approximately equivalent to that of burning petrol (Fishbein, 1976).

Harrison & Perry (1977) have reviewed the occurrence of organic lead compounds in urban air. Air samples taken at filling stations reportedly contained levels of organic lead ranging from 0.21-1.54 μg lead/m^3, primarily as a result of the evaporative loss of petrol containing lead additives. Organic lead levels were reported to be 1.9-2.2 μg/m^3 in an underground parking garage, where the accumulation of evaporative losses and the exhausts of cars starting with cold engines might be expected to give rise to elevated lead levels.

Ambient urban air concentrations of organic lead measured in the US have been found to vary from 0.006-0.3 μg/m^3. Measured levels of organic lead in Stockholm, Sweden, varied from 0.4-3.37 μg/m^3, with daily levels of tetraalkyllead ranging from 0.22-0.59 μg/m^3. Measurements taken on London streets revealed organic lead concentrations ranging from 0.04-0.11 μg/m^3 (Harrison & Perry, 1977).

(c) Cigarette smoke

Lead concentrations in several brands of US cigarettes in 1957 were in the range of 21-84 μg per cigarette, with 1.0-3.3 μg per cigarette transferred to mainstream smoke (smoke which is inhaled). These concentrations are believed to have resulted from residues of the insecticide lead arsenate once used heavily in tobacco fields. More recent findings of the occurrence of lead in cigarette smoke report average lead levels ranging from 10.4 to 12.15 μg per cigarette and 0.48 μg of lead per cigarette in total smoke. It is believed that 2% of the lead in cigarettes is transferred to mainstream smoke and that the direct inhalation intake of lead from smoking 20 cigarettes per day could be as high as 5 μg (UNEP/WHO, 1977).

(d) Occupational exposure

The National Institute for Occupational Safety & Health (1978) in the US has studied the industrial operations in which occupational exposure to lead occurs (Table 4).

The principal types of primary industries with occupational exposure to lead are lead mining, smelting and refining, storage battery manufacture, welding and steel cutting and printing (UNEP/WHO, 1977). Highest exposures to lead occur in the smelting and refining of lead. Molten lead and lead alloys are brought to high temperatures, resulting in the vaporization of lead. In three US primary lead smelters, mean lead concentrations in air were reported to be 80-4470 μg/m^3.

Table 4. Occupational exposure to lead in selected industrial operations utilizing lead [a]

| Operation | Average lead concentrations | | | |
| | Air (mg/m³) | | Urine (mg/l) | |
	Average	Max	Average	Max
Metallizing :	-	-	-	-
Paint spraying: red lead	1.8	3.5	-	-
Brush painting: red lead	-	-	0.26	0.35
Paint sanding, scraping	0.32	-	0.30	0.48
Paint mixing	1.75	5.8	0.17	0.29
Painting	-	-	0.09	0.16
Paint spraying: chrome yellow	3.9	-	0.10	-
Leaded iron pouring	19.5	-	-	-
Bearing bronze pouring	1.86	3.4	0.54	0.82
Bearing bronze grinding	0.84	-	0.33	-
Bronze pouring	0.34	1.56	0.20	0.34
Bronze grinding	0.47	1.24	0.17	0.34
Storage-battery manufacturing:				
Mixing	0.73	3.8	0.70	1.00
Pasting	0.75	2.1	0.26	0.48
Grouping	0.50	4.0	0.22	0.68
Separating	0.15	0.41	0.15	0.27
Casting	0.26	0.65	0.19	0.31
Lead smelting, refining	0.35	1.45	0.35	0.88
Lead casting	0.12	0.35	0.14	0.37
Lead burning	0.57	1.5	0.26	0.37
Homogenizing	3	-	-	-
Painted-steel burning	-	-	0.41	0.50
Lead powder mixing	2.2	10.2	0.22	0.32
Lead sanding, grinding	4.2	7.4	0.26	-
Wire patenting	0.29	0.60	0.12	0.21
Steel tempering	0.13	0.22	0.10	0.21
Printing:				
Stereotyping	0.26	0.51	0.15	0.22
Linotyping	0.07	0.24	0.08	0.14
Soldering, tinning	0.25	0.62	0.15	0.23
Lead sawing	0.25	-	-	-
Lead-glass working	0.01	0.02	0.05	0.10
Petrol-tank cleaning	-	-	0.07	0.14

[a]From National Institute for Occupational Safety & Health, 1978

Exposure to airborne lead also occurs in secondary smelters and foundries: in one foundry using molten lead, atmospheric concentrations ranged from 280-290 $\mu g/m^3$ (UNEP/WHO, 1977). In a foundry in Lawrence, Massachusetts, airborne lead dust concentrations ranged from 139-394 $\mu g/m^3$ for workers involved in melting, pouring and grinding operations (Hollett, 1976). Of 20 smelter and foundry workers studied in a Finnish secondary lead smelter, 16 had blood-lead concentrations equal to or greater than 700 $\mu g/l$ (UNEP/WHO, 1977).

The electric storage battery manufacturing industry is a source of occupational exposure to lead oxide dust; mean airborne concentrations of lead range from 50-5400 $\mu g/m^3$ (UNEP/WHO, 1977).

Lead dust concentrations in the houses of lead workers are significantly higher than those in the houses of non-lead workers. It has been suggested that the lead dust enters the houses from work clothing (Bureau of National Affairs, Inc., 1977; O'Tuama et al., 1979).

Exposure to lead fumes occurs during high-temperature (>500°C) operations such as welding or spray-coating of metals with molten lead (Key et al., 1977). The average lead concentration in the breathing zone of welders of structural steel has been found to be 1200 $\mu g/m^3$. Welding of zinc silicate-coated steel can give rise to lead concentrations in air greater than 150 $\mu g/m^3$, and the welding of galvanized steel creates air concentrations of 400-500 $\mu g/m^3$. Blood-lead levels in welders have been reported to be as high as 700 $\mu g/l$ (UNEP/WHO, 1977).

Recovery of scrap metal during the dismantling of ships involves cutting steel coated with lead-based paint with electric torches, resulting in exposure to lead fumes. Air samples taken near the breathing zone of shipbreakers show lead concentrations as high as 2700 $\mu g/m^3$ (UNEP/WHO, 1977).

Lead oxide dust is dispersed during the smelting of type in the printing industry. Print shops in Japan have been reported to have airborne lead levels of 30-360 $\mu g/m^3$ (UNEP/WHO, 1977).

Potential exposure to tetramethyl- and tetraethyllead, used as petrol ingredients, may occur during synthesis, handling, transport or mixing with petrol; petrol additive workers and storage tank cleaners may be exposed (Key et al., 1977). Average concentrations of organic lead compounds in the air of a plant manufacturing alkyllead compounds have been reported to be 179 $\mu g/m^3$ in the tetramethyllead synthesis operation and 120 $\mu g/m^3$ in the tetraethyllead operation (UNEP/WHO, 1977). De Silva & Donnan (1977) reported mean venous blood-lead levels of 182 $\mu g/l$ in petrol station workers, as compared with 109 $\mu g/l$ in a control group.

(e)   Water

The global mean lead content of lakes and rivers has been estimated to be 1-10 µg/l; analyses of groundwater have revealed concentrations varying from 1-60 µg/l. Coastal sea-waters reportedly contain 0.08-0.4 µg/l, and central Atlantic waters contain an average of 0.05 µg/l. Sea-water below 1000 m in the Pacific and Atlantic Oceans and the Mediterranean Sea contains 0.03-0.04 µg/l (UNEP/WHO, 1977).

A study of raw (untreated) and finished (treated for distribution) water in the US revealed lead levels ranging from 1-139 µg/l in finished water, with a mean of 33.9 µg/l, and from 2-140 µg/l in raw water, with a mean of 23 µg/l. Tap-water from 969 water systems in the US contained an average lead concentration of 13.1 µg/l, with a maximum concentration of 64 µg/l (Safe Drinking Water Committee, 1977).

Comparison of finished water and tap-water in two US cities using lead piping, where the water was slightly acidic and chlorination was the only treatment process used, showed that the majority of tap-water samples contained more than 50 µg/l lead. Further studies found lead concentrations at the tap which ranged from 13-1510 µg/l, with an overall mean of 30 µg/l; in every one of 383 households samples, the lead concentration was higher at the tap than at the treatment plant. Lead appears to enter drinking-water chiefly in the distribution system, including household plumbing, where lead is picked up from the pipes (Safe Drinking Water Committee, 1977).

Lead can enter fresh-water streams from municipal sewage treatment plant discharges. Sargent (1975) found 15 µg/l in Cayuga Creek, New York, attributable to industrial wastes discharged by the municipal sewage treatment plant.

Lead has been found in waste-waters from metal finishing plants, in concentrations ranging from >0.5-200 µg/l, and in raw textile waste as a result of dyes used during the finishing process (Allen *et al.*, 1976; Pfaender *et al.*, 1977). It has been estimated that the annual discharge of lead into waters along a part of the southern California coast are as follows: from municipal waste-water, 161 thousand kg; from dry aerial fallout, 240 thousand kg; from storm runoff, 90 thousand kg; and from electrical power plant cooling water discharges, 800 kg (Young *et al.*, 1977).

Lead concentrations in drinking-water have been observed to increase following storms, as a result of the entry of metals into urban watersheds from surface runoff and urban storm-water collection systems (Pfaender *et al.*, 1977).

(f) Sediments

Average lead concentrations measured by five US laboratories in near-shore marine sediments were 23-51 mg/kg dry weight (average, 37 mg/kg) (Heit, 1977). Lead concentrations in sediments from the San Francisco Bay ranged from 0-47.3 mg/kg (Bradford, 1976). Lead concentrations in the sediments of the estuary and Gulf of St Lawrence in Canada varied from 9-66 μg/g, with an average concentration of 21 μg/g (Lohring, 1978). Deep marine sediments commonly contain levels of 100-200 mg/kg lead (UNEP/WHO, 1977).

Sediments of an Idaho lake contained concentrations ranging from 100-4700 mg/kg; higher lead values occurred in sediments of lakes closer to mining waste discharge sites. Background sedimentary lead concentrations were reported to be less than 300 mg/kg as measured in lake sediments that did not receive mining wastes (Rabe & Bauer, 1977).

(g) Soil

The lead contents of soils remove from human activity are similar to those found in rocks, with an average range of 5-25 mg/kg. Some organic matter is rich in chelating components which bind lead, either promoting its movement out of the soil or fixing it, depending on the solubility of the complex (UNEP/WHO, 1977).

Soils receive an average of 1 μg/cm^2 lead per year from precipitation and 0.2 μg/cm^2 per year from dustfall as well as from mining and from fallout from industrial operations and motor vehicles. In the dust of 77 US cities, the average lead concentrations at residential and commercial sites were 1636 mg/kg and 2413 mg/kg, respectively. Surface soils in US city parks were found to contain lead at the following average levels: San Diego, 194 mg/kg; San Francisco, 560 mg/kg; Los Angeles, 3357 mg/kg (National Academy of Sciences, 1972).

The lead content of the top 5 m of soil along a highway was found to be reduced by about 65-75% when the sampling site was moved from 8 to 32 m away from the highway, which had traffic densities ranging from 7500 to 48,000 cars per day (National Academy of Sciences, 1972).

Davies (1978) found lead concentrations ranging from 10-680 mg/kg, with a mean of 163 mg/kg, in garden soils in the UK. The sources of lead were identified as fallout from industries (such as smelters), power stations and vehicle exhausts. Levels of lead in soil as high as 1014 mg/kg were found associated with the nearby presence of a battery factory.

(h) Plants

Lead occurs naturally in all plants. The normal concentration in leaves and twigs of woody plants is 2.5 mg/kg on a dry weight basis. Some trees apparently have the capacity to accumulate high concentrations of lead; the tips of larches, firs and white pines were found to contain 100 mg/kg on a dry weight basis when grown in lead mining areas where the soil concentration of lead was 20,000 mg/kg. Cereals are believed to contain levels of lead in the range of 0.1-1.0 mg/kg by weight; the usual concentration of lead in pasture grasses has been found to be 1.0 mg/kg dry weight (UNEP/WHO, 1977).

Lead in air increases the concentration of lead in leafy parts of plants near highways but does not affect the other portions of the plant (National Academy of Sciences, 1972).

(i) Food

Lead has been found in virtually all foods, from both primitive and industrial societies, although concentrations are highly variable. The natural content of lead in food should be less than 1 mg/kg fresh weight, and most of the lead present in food is from industrial sources (National Academy of Sciences, 1972).

The following concentrations of lead have been reported in foods (on a fresh weight basis): condiments, 0-1.5 mg/kg; fish and seafood, 0.2-2.5 mg/kg; meats and eggs, 0-0.37 mg/kg; grains, 0-1.39 mg/kg; vegetables, 0-1.3 mg/kg. Lead concentrations in wine have been found to range from 60-255 μg/l, with average concentrations of 130-190 μg/l. A mean concentration of 299 μg/l has also been reported (UNEP/WHO, 1977).

Lead has also been found in milk. Milk taken directly from cows contained 9 μg/l, but concentrations are higher in processed milk; an average of 40 μg/l was reported for whole bulk milk, and values ranging from 20-40 μg/l were reported for local market milk in the US.

Davies (1978) reported finding lead in radishes (1.1-56.7 mg/kg dry weight) and in potatoes (1.91-3.91 mg/kg dry weight) grown in soils containing lead, although the concentrations in the plants did not correlate with the levels of lead in the soil.

Fruits and vegetables grown in areas exposed to smelter emissions may be appreciably contaminated with lead: the total daily ingestion of lead with food by people living near a smelter ranged from 670-2640 μg (UNEP/WHO, 1977).

Watkins *et al.* (1976) reported the presence of lead in food wrappings: concentrations ranged from 1400 mg/kg in an ice-cream bar wrapping to 28,700 mg/kg in a bread wrapping.

Evaporated milk has been reported to contain an average lead concentration of 202 μg/l; apparently the lead solder in the seams and caps of tins containing milk and other foods contributes to the lead content (UNEP/WHO, 1977). During 1977, 1978 and 1979, tinned food contamination was monitored by Joint FAO/WHO Collaborating Centres in 15 countries for the period 1971-1975. The following levels were found: tinned fruit, 0.01-14.0 mg/kg; tinned fruit juices, including concentrates, 0.01-3.1 mg/kg; tinned vegetables, 0.01-38.6 mg/kg; and tinned milks, 0.05-0.2 mg/kg (WHO, 1979). Tinned tuna fish has been reported to contain an average lead concentration of 0.08 mg/kg (Tuna Research Foundation, 1974). Concentrations of lead in tinned tuna fish may exceed the natural concentrations by up to 4000 times due to contamination *via* the soldered cans (Settle & Patterson, 1980). Fox & Boylen (1978) found lead in concentrations ranging from 0.1-3600 mg/kg in pet-food ingredients.

Average total dietary intake of lead has been estimated to range from 100-500 μg/day. Children under 3 years of age with only dietary exposure are believed to take in 130 μg lead daily (National Academy of Sciences, 1972).

(j)   Animals

Cattle and dogs may be exposed to lead by licking lead-based paints and a variety of discarded lead-containing products (e.g., used motor oil, discarded oil filters, storage batteries), and by ingesting forage or crops near highways or contaminated by industrial lead operations (National Academy of Sciences, 1972).

The principal source of exposure to lead for ducks and other waterfowl is spent lead shot that is ingested by the birds in search of gravel. The occurrence of lead in the fresh livers of birds of 28 different species with no known other lead exposure was found to range from 0.3-7.0 mg/kg. Lead concentrations in apparently healthy pheasants were 0.22-0.27 mg/kg blood, 0.09-0.84 mg/kg liver and 0.11-0.27 mg/kg kidney (National Academy of Sciences, 1972).

(k)   Marine organisms

Concentrations of lead in freshwater fish have been reported to range from 0.16-0.24 mg/kg, with 12 mg/kg in liver, 5.7 mg/kg in gills and 1.4 mg/kg in muscle (National Academy of Sciences, 1972).

Manly & George (1977) found lead in the soft tissue of freshwater mussels in the Thames River, with mean concentrations ranging from 9.8-42.5 mg/kg (dry weight). The higher levels were found in mussels taken from urban sites along the river; public sewage effluent, industrial effluent and motor vehicle exhaust were cited as the apparent sources of lead.

Shellfish in general have been reported to contain an average of 0.31 mg/kg, soft shell clams an average of 0.7 mg/kg and northern quahog clams an average of 0.52 mg/kg lead on a wet weight basis. Oysters have been found to contain 0.47 mg/kg and accumulate lead taken up from the sea water (National Academy of Sciences, 1972).

Fresh tuna fish muscle was reported to contain 0.3 mg/kg lead (Settle & Patterson, 1980).

(l)   Human tissues and secretions

The total lead content of the body may reach more than 200 mg in men aged 60-70 years, but is lower for women. About 95% of the total body lead occurs in bone tissue, where lead has a strong tendency to localize and accumulate. The skeleton appears to be a repository for lead, which reflects long-term, cumulative exposure, whereas the body fluids and soft tissues equilibrate it reasonably fast and reflect current and recent exposure (UNEP/WHO, 1977).

In two studies, lead concentrations in human breast milk were reported as 12 μg/l and <5 μg/l (UNEP/WHO, 1977).

The majority of studies of blood lead concentrations in adults have reported levels for occupationally unexposed, rural and urban populations that range from 100-250 μg/l. Populations in northern Italy and France have somewhat higher mean concentrations, ranging from 240-350 μg/l; lower levels have been reported in Swedish women (85 μg/l), Finnish women (79 μg/l in rural areas and 97 μg/l in urban areas) and children from rural western Ireland (<130 μg/l). In a survey of children in the Federal Republic of Germany, a mean blood-lead level of 33 μg/l was found for the first year of life; levels increased each year and reached a mean of 115 μg/l at the age of 6-8 years. Children aged 1-5 in rural US counties had an average level of 228 μg/l blood lead. Many urban children display elevated levels, with some values exceeding 590 μg/l. The blood levels of 80-100% of children living in a city with a large smelter in Texas were >400 μg/l (UNEP/WHO, 1977).

Children of lead smelter employees have elevated (>300 μg/l) blood lead levels (Bureau of National Affairs, Inc., 1977); children of lead-acid battery workers also have elevated blood lead levels, suggesting exposure to lead from contaminated work clothing of parents (O'Tuama *et al.*, 1979).

Johnson *et al.* (1975) compared the urinary lead concentrations of several groups of people in Houston, Texas. For non-exposed controls, mean urinary lead concentrations ranged from 19.0-27.8 μg/l; the same groups also had lead in the hair at levels ranging from 6.0-29.7 mg/kg and in the faeces, from 2.2-2.7 mg/kg. The exposed groups, policemen on foot patrol, garage attendants and females living near a motorway, exhibited mean urinary lead concentrations of 24.8-32.0 μg/l, concentrations in hair ranging from 7.4-47.6 mg/kg, and concentrations in faeces between 2.4-2.9 mg/kg.

(m) Other exposure

Infants and young children are exposed to lead contained in paints: children often lick, chew or eat objects covered with lead-based paints. One survey reported that in 75% of cases, children with blood lead levels of 600 μg/l or more were exposed in their houses to at least one surface on which the paint contained more than 1% lead. Children are also exposed to lead in coloured newsprint: inks used in coloured magazine illustrations contain 1140-3170 mg/kg (UNEP/WHO, 1977).

High concentrations of lead occur in illicitly distilled whisky in the US. Condensers used in homemade stills are often discarded automobile radiators containing substantial amounts of lead in the soldered joints. Concentrations of lead in the whisky frequently exceed 10 mg/l (UNEP/WHO, 1977).

Other sources of exposure to lead for the general population are the use of discarded storage battery casings for fuel and the use of lead wire core wicks in candles. Facial cosmetics in Oriental countries can contain up to 67% lead and have been identified as a source of lead poisoning in Japan, India and Pakistan (UNEP/WHO, 1977).

2.4 Analysis (see also preamble, p. 21)

Methods of analysis for lead and its compounds have been reviewed (Mack, 1975; Minear & Murray, 1973; Pierce *et al.*, 1976; Schuller & Egan, 1976; UNEP/WHO, 1977). Greifer *et al.* (1972) reviewed and evaluated the analytical methods for determining levels of lead in formulations such as paint and building materials; and Harrison & Perry (1977) have described methods for determining tetraalkyllead compounds in air.

Pierce *et al.* (1976) and Delves (1977) reviewed analytical methods for determining lead in blood. The accuracy of the various methods for analysing lead in biological materials was found to be unsatisfactory in a number of interlaboratory comparison programmes (UNEP/WHO, 1977). Practical considerations regarding sampling and analytical methods for lead in biological materials have been summarized by UNEP/WHO (1977), together with a discussion of ancillary biological indices of lead exposure, such as measurements of erythrocyte δ-aminolevulinic acid synthetase activity, erythrocyte protoporphyrin concentration and urinary excretion of protoporphyrin precursors and metabolites.

Typical methods of analysis for determining levels of lead in environmental samples are summarized in Table 5. Abbreviations are: AAS, atomic absorption spectrometry; AES, atomic emission spectrometry; FAAS, flameless atomic absorption spectrometry; GC, gas chromatography; ICP-AES, inductively coupled plasma-atomic emission spectrometry; NAA, neutron activation analysis ; and X-RF, X-ray fluorescence.

Table 5. Analytical methods for lead and lead compounds

Sample matrix	Sample preparation	Assay procedure	Limit of detection or sensitivity	Reference
Inorganic and total lead				
Air	Collect on filter; wet ash with nitric acid; dilute solution with water	AAS	Range of analysis: 0.128-0.399 mg/m^3	National Institute for Occupational Safety & Health (1976)
	Particulate lead: collect on filter; wet ash with nitric, sulphuric and perchloric acids	Spectrophotometry	0.0002 mg/m^3	American Society for Testing & Materials (1977)
	Non-particulate (organic) lead compounds: collect on filter; dissolve in acidified potassium iodide solution ; remove excess iodide with sodium sulphite; treat with citric acid; add ammoniacal buffer; extract with chloroform solution of ciphenylthiocarbazone			
	Collect on filter; wet with sodium chloride solution; ash at 440°C; mix with graphite; press into graphite electrode	AES	0.00002 mg/m^3	Delespaul et al. (1977)
	Collect on filter; irradiate	NAA		Shani & Cohen (1977)

Table 5 (contd)

Sample matrix	Sample preparation	Assay procedure	Limit of detection or sensitivity	Reference
Water	Preserve sample with nitric acid; add buffer and aqueous ammonium pyrrolidine-dithiocarbamate; extract with methyl isobutyl ketone; aspirate into spectrometer	AAS	0.6 mg/m^3	Timperley (1977)
	Collect lead cations on chelating resin (Chelex-100); filter; irradiate	X-RF		Holyńska (1974)
Sea water	Filter; vacuum-pull through chelate-ion exchange matrix; elute with nitric acid	ICP-AES	0.001 mg/l	Kerfoot & Crawford (1977)
Soil	Centrifuge with hydrochloric acid or dry ash at 500°C; add nitric acid or wet ash with nitric acid or with nitric and hydrochloric or with nitric and hydrofluoric acids	AAS		Harrison & Laxen (1977)
Rocks, soils, stream sediment	Wet ash with potassium chlorate and hydrochloric acid; extract into methyl isobutyl ketone with ascorbic acid and potassium iodide	AAS	0.2 mg/kg	Viets (1978)
Plants	Dry ash; mix with aluminium oxide, calcium carbonate and potassium carbonate	Anodic excitation spectrography	1 mg/kg	Parle & Fleming (1977)
Food	Wet ash with nitric, sulphuric and perchloric acids and hydrogen peroxide; complex with chelating agent; extract with solvent	AAS		Schuller & Egan (1976)
Milk	Solubilize with quaternary ammonium hydroxide	FAAS	0.005 mg/l	Barlow (1977)

Table 5 (contd)

Sample matrix	Sample preparation	Assay procedure	Limit of detection or sensitivity	Reference
Animal tissue				
Drosophila	Wet ash with nitric acid and hydrogen peroxide; dilute with nitric acid	FAAS	2.0 mg/kg	Wallace & Koirtyohann (1974)
Clams and oysters	Dry ash at 475°C; dissolve in dilute nitric acid; extract as complex with diethylammonium dithiocarbamate; extract with butyl acetate	AAS	0.06 mg/l	Capar (1977)
Fish	Dry ash; extract in methyl isobutyl ketone with ammonium pyrrolidine dithiocarbamate; partition in aqueous acid solution	FAAS	0.005 ng	Okuno *et al.* (1978)
Human tissue samples				
Brain, heart, liver, lung, spleen	Lyophilize; solubilize with nitric acid; neutralize with sodium hydroxide and sodium bicarbonate; extract lead as pyrrolidine dithiocarbamate complex	AAS	0.14 mg/kg (wet weight)	Farris *et al.* (1978)
Kidney, liver, lung	Homogenize with water; pipette into microsampling cup	AAS	0.01 mg/kg (wet tissue)	Jackson *et al.* (1978)
Hair	Wet ash with acid	AAS	0.4 mg/kg	Johnson *et al.* (1974)
Faeces	Wet ash with perchloric and nitric acids; centrifuge; pipette into graphite furnace	FAAS	0.07 mg/kg	Johnson *et al.* (1974)
Blood	Dilute with water; add nitric acid; inject into graphite furnace	FAAS		Watanabe *et al.* (1977)

Table 5 (contd)

Sample matrix	Sample preparation	Assay procedure	Limit of detection or sensitivity	Reference
Blood (contd)	Wet ash with nitric, perchloric and sulphuric acids ; add ammonium hydroxide and ammonium pyrrolidine dithiocarbamate; extract with methyl isobutyl ketone	AAS		Watanabe *et al.* (1977)
Urine	Dilute with hydrochloric acid	FAAS	0.0046 mg/l	Johnson *et al.* (1974)
Tetraalkylleads				
Air	Trap from air on OV-1 at -80°C; heat to drive off compounds	GC AAS	0.1 μg	Chau *et al.* (1976)
	Trap from air on porous polymer beads; heat to drive compounds into burner	AAS	10-20 ng (as lead)	Coker (1978)
	Pass air through solution of iodine monochloride in hydrochloric acid; extract as dithiozonates; decompose by shaking with nitric acid - hydrogen peroxide solution	FAAS	7 ng (as lead)	Hancock & Slater (1975)

3. Biological Data Relevant to the Evaluation

of Carcinogenic Risk to Humans

Summaries of the scientific literature on lead carcinogenesis in experimental animals and humans have been compiled by Sunderman (1971, 1977) and by Moore & Meredith (1979).

3.1 Carcinogenicity studies in animals

(a) Oral administration

Mouse: Lead subacetate was administered to 2 groups of 50 male and female Swiss mice at dosages of 0.1 and 1.0% in the diet; the 1.0% level was decreased to 0.5% during the fourth month of the experiment because of excessive toxicity. Within 2 years, 7 mice that were receiving 0.1% lead subacetate developed renal tumours (3 adenomas and 4 carcinomas). Most of the mice that received the 1.0/0.5% dose died early in the experiment, and only 1 renal tumour (carcinoma) was found. No renal tumours were seen in 50 control mice. The incidences of extrarenal tumours were similar in control and treated mice (Van Esch & Kroes, 1969).

Rat: Fairhall & Miller (1941) reported kidney changes (enlargement of cells, vesiculation of nuclei and accumulation of brown granules) but no tumours in 104 male rats fed diets containing 0.1% *lead arsenate*[1] (49 rats) or *lead carbonate* (55 rats) for 2 years.

In a lifetime carcinogenesis study, male and female Wistar rats were fed *lead arsenate*[1] in the diet at levels of 463 or 1850 mg/kg diet. The test rats were nursed by mothers that received the same diet during lactation. The incidences of malignant tumours were 11/98 in controls *versus* 1/28 and 6/78 in treated rats at the high- and low-dosage levels, respectively. A renal cortical adenoma and a bile-duct carcinoma were found in the group fed 1850 mg/kg diet lead arsenate (see also monograph on arsenic) (Kroes *et al.*, 1974).

Male Wistar rats were fed 1% *lead acetate* in the diet for 1 year. Of 16/20 rats that survived for 320 days or more 15 developed kidney tumours, 14 of which were renal carcinomas. No untreated control group was studied (Boyland *et al.*, 1962).

---

[1] Data on the chemical and physical properties, production, use and occurrence of lead arsenate are given in the monograph on arsenic.

A group of 126 male and female Wistar rats received a diet containing *lead acetate*, such that each rat received 3 mg/day for 2 months and then 4 mg/day for 16 months. Renal adenomas were found in 55 rats and renal carcinomas in 17. Leydig-cell tumours of the testis were found in 23/94 male rats. No renal tumours were seen in 32 control rats, which received the same diet without added lead acetate (Zawirska & Medras, 1968) [The Working Group noted that the incidence of Leydig-cell tumours in controls was unspecified].

Groups of 47 male and 47 female Wistar rats, 30 weeks old, were fed a diet to which *lead acetate* was added in a dosage of 3 mg/rat per day for periods of 60-504 days. In treated rats, 12 renal adenomas, 10 cerebral gliomas, 17 pituitary adenomas, 11 thyroid adenomas, 5 parathyroid adenomas, 15 adrenal adenomas, 11 prostatic adenomas and 8 mammary adenomas were found. No tumours were found in 31 male and 31 female controls (Zawirska & Medras, 1972) [The Working Group noted the absence of neoplasms and lack of survival data for control rats].

Two groups of male and female Wistar rats were fed diets containing 0.1% or 1.0% *lead subacetate* for periods of 29 or 24 months, respectively. Two control groups of 24-30 rats were fed the same diets without addition of lead subacetate. The incidences of renal tumours were 11/32 (including 3 carcinomas) in rats that received 0.1% lead subacetate and 13/24 (including 6 carcinomas) in rats that received 1% lead subacetate. No renal tumours were observed in the control groups (Van Esch *et al.*, 1962).

A group of 40 Wistar rats were fed a diet supplemented with 0.5-1.0% *lead subacetate.* Controls received the same diet without added lead. Selected rats in both groups were killed at 6-week intervals for 92 weeks; renal tumours were found from about 6 months. Most tumours were renal adenomas or papillary adenomas, but a few were adenocarcinomas, hypernephromas or undifferentiated carcinomas. The numbers of tumours were not specified. Eosinophilic intranuclear inclusions appeared consistently in the cortical tubular epithelium of the kidneys, where tumours subsequently developed in treated rats. No primary renal tumours were found in animals in the control group (Shakerin & Paloucek, 1965). In an extension of this experiment, a group of 40 male Wistar rats were fed a diet containing 1% *lead subacetate* plus 0.06% 2-acetylaminofluorene. 'A greater incidence of hepatic and renal carcinomas with metastasis to the lungs' was found, as compared with groups fed 2-acetylaminofluorene or lead subacetate alone (Shakerin *et al.*, 1965).

A group of 24 male Charles River CD rats were fed a basal synthetic diet containing 0.5-1.0% *lead subacetate* and 1.6% (w/w) indole. All rats died or were killed by 74 weeks. Renal adenocarcinomas were found in 11 rats, renal cystomas in 22 rats, and renal adenomas in 19 rats. Renal tumorigenesis was not significantly affected by addition of 2-acetylamino-fluorene and linseed oil to the therapeutic regimen. Two brain tumours (gliomas) were found in 24 rats that received lead subacetate and indole, 4 brain tumours (gliomas) in 50 rats that received lead subacetate, linseed oil and indole and 11 brain tumours (8 gliomas and 3 other tumours) in 74 rats that received a combination of lead subacetate, indole, 2-acetylamino-fluorene and linseed oil. No control group was tested (Hass *et al.*, 1967) [Although the authors mentioned that the combined regime favoured early appearance of cerebral gliomas and increased their incidence, the apparent increase in incidence of gliomas was not statistically significant].

Oyasu *et al.* (1970) continued the investigations initially reported by Shakerin *et al.* (1965) and Hass *et al.* (1967) of the carcinogenicity of *lead subacetate* and 2-acetylamino-fluorene fed to male rats singly or in combination. Of 17 male Sprague-Dawley rats fed a diet containing 1% lead subacetate alone, 13 developed renal cortical tumours (adenomas or carcinomas) and 2 developed cerebral gliomas. In 285 male and female control rats that received the same diet without added lead subacetate, only one cerebral glioma was found. Of 41 rats fed a diet containing 1% lead subacetate plus 1.6% indole, 25 developed renal cortical tumours, one developed a bladder tumour and 3 developed cerebral gliomas. The incidence of renal tumours in the control rats was not stated. Combined exposure of rats to 2-acetylaminofluorene and lead subacetate did not increase the incidence of gliomas or renal cortical tumours, compared with that in rats given the lead salt only [The Working Group noted that the survival time in control rats was 50-60 weeks, which was similar to the mean survival time in treated groups].

Mao & Molnar (1967) reported renal adenomas or carcinomas composed of solid, papillary or acinar-glandular structures in 31/40 male Wistar rats subjected to long-term feeding of a diet that containined 1% *lead subacetate*. One renal sarcoma was found in 20 control rats.

A diet containing 1.5% *lead subacetate* was administered to 10 male Wistar rats for 48 weeks. All rats developed renal tumours, comprising 6 adenomas and 4 carcinomas; no extrarenal tumours were found. No untreated controls were tested (Ito *et al.*, 1971).

Lead subacetate was administered to male Wistar rats at a dietary concentration of 1.5%. No renal tumours developed in 13 rats that ingested lead subacetate for 23 weeks, whereas 9 renal tumours developed in 11 rats that ingested it for 48.5 weeks. Unilateral nephrectomy possibly increased the susceptibility of rats to lead-induced renal neoplasia, since 2 tumours of non-resected kidneys were found in 11 rats that ingested lead subacetate for 23 weeks following unilateral nephrectomy. The 11 renal tumours in treated rats were

7 adenomas and 4 carcinomas. No untreated control rats were used (Ito, 1973).

Lead nitrate was administered to 52 male Long-Evans rats in drinking-water, as 25 µg/l lead, from weaning until death. Longevity of lead-treated rats did not differ significantly from that of controls. Tumours (type and location unspecified) were found in 7 or 43 treated rats that were autopsied, which did not differ significantly from the tumour incidence (10/50) in controls (Schroeder *et al.*, 1970) [The Working Group noted the very low dose used].

Lead powder suspended in corn oil was administered to male and female Fischer 344 rats by stomach tube (10 mg twice a month for 12 months). Control rats were given 0.5 ml of corn oil by stomach tube according to the same schedule. One lymphoma and 4 leukaemias were found in 5/47 lead-treated rats; this did not differ significantly from the incidence of 3 lymphomas in 29 controls. No other neoplasms were reported in treated or control rats (Furst *et al.*, 1976).

Hamster: Two groups, each of 22 male and 24 female golden hamsters, were fed diets containing 0.1 and 0.5% *lead subacetate* for up to 2 years. Pleomorphic cells and intranuclear inclusion bodies were found in the proximal renal tubules, but no neoplasms were observed. No renal tumours were found in a control group of 22 males and 23 females. The overall incidences of other tumours and hyperplasias in the 2 lead subacetate groups and in the control group were 25/46, 18/46 and 36/45, respectively (Van Esch & Kroes, 1969).

(b) Skin application

Mouse: Lead naphthenate was applied as a 20% solution in benzene to the skin of 59 male Schofield mice once or twice weekly for 12 months (total dose, 6 ml). The test substance was a complex mixture of lead salts of aromatic and carboxylic acids obtained during the manufacture of hydrocarbon distillates. The lead napthenate treatment did not evoke neoplasia in mouse skin, but it induced kidney damage. Four mice developed renal adenomas, and 1 mouse developed a renal carcinoma (Baldwin *et al.*, 1964)   [Although indicative of a carcinogenic effect of lead naphthenate on the kidney, these results cannot be evaluated, since no control mice were painted with the benzene vehicle alone].

(c) Inhalation and/or intratracheal administration

Hamster: Four groups of 15 male and 15 female Syrian golden hamsters were given 10 weekly intratracheal injections of *lead oxide* (1 mg/animal), benzo[a]pyrene (1 mg/animal), benzo[a]pyrene mixed with lead oxide (1 mg of each compound/animal) or vehicle (isotonic saline solution plus 0.5% carboxymethylcellulose, 0.2 ml/rat). Another group of 30 hamsters served as untreated controls. Atypical epithelial proliferation, 11 adenomas and 1 adenocarcinoma were observed in lungs of hamsters that received benzo[a]pyrene mixed with lead oxide. No lung neoplasms were found in animals in the other three groups or in untreated controls. The authors concluded that lead oxide exerted a co-carcinogenic effect with benzo[a]pyrene in hamster lungs (Kobayashi & Okamoto, 1974) [The Working Group noted that the lead acetate may have been a carrier for benzo[a]pyrene].

(d) Subcutaneous and/or intramuscular administration

Mouse: *Tetraethyllead* dissolved in tricaprylin was injected subcutaneously into male and female Swiss mice on 1 to 4 occasions between birth and 21 days. After a single injection of 2 mg on the first day of life, all of 69 mice died before weaning. Total doses of 1.2 mg in 4 divided doses killed 92% of mice before weaning, and total doses of 0.6 mg given in 4 divided doses killed 20% of the mice. Of 41 female mice that survived for 36 weeks after treatment with 0.6 mg tetraethyllead, 5 developed malignant lymphomas between 36 and 51 weeks. Of 48 female control mice that received injections of tricaprylin alone, none developed lymphomas. Lymphomas developed in 1 of 26 males that received a total dose of 0.6 mg tetraethyllead and in 1 of 39 control males (Epstein & Mantel, 1968) [The Working Group noted the low incidence of lymphomas in animals of one sex only and concluded that a further study is warranted in order to confirm or refute these results].

Rat: A group of 270 albino rats (strain and sex unspecified) received weekly s.c. injections of 20 mg *lead phosphate* according to several dosage schedules; total doses ranged from 40-760 mg/rat during treatment periods of up to 16 months. Forty untreated rats served as controls. Nineteen of 29 rats that survived for 10 or more months from the start of treatment developed renal tumours; these rats had received total doses of 120-680 mg/rat. The tumours included adenomas, papillomas, cystadenomas and 3 carcinomas of the renal cortex (Zollinger, 1953).

Lead phosphate was administered to 80 albino rats by weekly or fortnightly s.c. injections of 20 mg for 18 months. Rats that survived until the end of the treatment had received a total dosage of 1.3 g. Renal adenomas developed in 29 rats, the first after 354 days; no malignant tumours were found. No renal adenomas were found in 20 untreated controls (Balo *et al.*, 1965).

In a study reported as an abstract, repeated s.c. injections of *lead subacetate* in Sprague-Dawley rats induced renal cortical adenomas and carcinomas and local sarcomas (Coogan *et al.*, 1972) [The Working Group noted the incomplete reporting of the experiment].

Lead powder suspended in trioctanoin was administered intramuscularly to 25 male and 25 female Fischer rats as 9 monthly injections of 10 mg, then 3 monthly injections of 5 mg. An equal number of vehicle controls were used. One treated female developed a fibrosarcoma at the site of implantation of the metal powder; the lymphoma rate was the same in treated as in control animals (Furst *et al.*, 1976).

(e) Intraperitoneal administration

Mouse: Groups of 20 male and female strain A/Strong mice were given i.p. injections of *lead subacetate* 3 times weely for 5 weeks (total doses, 30, 75 and 150 mg/kg bw); the experiment was terminated after 30 weeks. A group of 20 control mice received i.p. injections of the vehicle (tricaprylin) 3 times weekly for 8 weeks. The incidences of lung adenomas in treated groups were 6/17, 5/12 and 11/15 *versus* 8/18 in controls, and the average numbers of lung adenomas per mouse were 0.35 ± 0.09, 0.50 ± 0.14 and 1.47 ± 0.38, respectively, compared with 0.50 ± 0.12 in controls. The average number of pulmonary adenomas per mouse was significantly increased with the highest dose of lead ($P<0.05$) (Stoner *et al.*, 1976).

Rat: In a study reported as an abstract, repeated i.p. injections of *lead subacetate* in Sprague-Dawley rats induced renal cortical adenomas and carcinomas (Coogan *et al.*, 1972) [The Working Group noted the incomplete reporting of the experiment].

(f) Other experimental systems

Combined subcutaneous and intraperitoneal injections: *Lead phosphate* was administered to 3 groups of 24 male Chester Beatty *rats* by repeated s.c. and subsequent i.p. injections according to a complex dosage schedule. No renal tumours were found in 23 rats that survived more than 200 days with a total dosage of 29 mg lead phosphate. In contrast, renal tumours were found in 14/23 surviving rats with a total dosage of 145 mg lead phosphate and in 2/3 surviving rats with a total dosage of 450 mg lead phosphate. Renal tumours included adenomas, adenocarcinomas and one undifferentiated malignant tumour. Two renal tumours were found in 2/24 untreated control rats (1 undifferentiated malignant tumour and 1 transitional-cell carcinoma) (Roe *et al.*, 1965).

3.2 Other relevant biological data

(a) Experimental systems

Toxic effects

A detailed review of the pathological effects of lead has been made by Goyer & Rhyne (1973).

Soluble lead salts are more toxic than insoluble salts; rabbits and guinea-pigs are more susceptible than rats and mice. The i.p. LD_{50} in rats of lead oxide was 400 mg/kg bw (371 as lead) and that of lead tetroxide, 220 mg/kg bw (20 as lead); the oral LD_{50} of lead chloride in guinea-pigs was 2000 mg/kg bw (1490 as lead) (Luckey & Venugopal, 1977). In rats, the i.p. LD_{50} of lead acetate is 215 mg/kg bw per day for 2 days and that of lead nitrate is 66 mg/kg bw per day for 2 days (Adler & Adler, 1977).

Administration of 100 mg/kg diet lead acetate to young dogs has been found to cause anaemia, enlargement of the liver, kidney and brain associated with alterations of serum enzymes, fatty metamorphosis of the liver and formation of nuclear inclusion bodies and necrosis in renal proximal tubule cells (Stowe et al., 1973).

Lead exposure has also been found to produce karyomegaly in proximal tubule cells of rats exposed to 5 mg/l lead acetate in utero and in drinking-water for 9 months (Fowler et al., 1980). Suckling rats whose mothers were fed a diet containing 4.5% lead acetate during the suckling period displayed pronounced growth retardation and retardation of new cell formation in the cerebellum, ataxia, paraplegia and cerebellar vascular damage. This effect was not associated with statistically significant changes in DNA, RNA or protein concentrations in the cerebellum or cerebral cortex (Michaelson, 1973).

Similar findings were reported in suckling mice whose mothers received a diet containing 1% lead carbonate ; they developed an encephalopathy characterized by broad-based gait and ataxia associated with intercapillary fibrosis and astrocytosis (Rosenblum & Johnson, 1968).

Baboons exposed to about 100 mg/kg lead carbonate for 4-8 doses by intratracheal injection developed seizures, cerebral oedema and focal brain necrosis (Hopkins & Dayan, 1974).

Leucocytosis has been reported in female mice 4 days after i.p. injection of 100-200 mg/kg bw lead acetate (Hogan & Adams, 1979).

Mice exposed to 130 or 1300 mg/l lead acetate in drinking water showed decreased β-lymphocyte responsiveness and humoral antibody titres (Koller & Kovacic, 1974; Koller & Brauner, 1977). Similar findings were obtained by Luster et al. (1978) in rats exposed to 25 or 50 mg/l lead acetate in drinking-water for 35-45 days.

The i.v. LD_{50} for tetraethyllead in rats is about 15 mg/kg bw ; a minimum lethal i.p. dose in rats is 10 mg/kg (Luckey & Venugopal, 1977). In rats, the LD_{50} of tetramethyl-lead is about 110 mg/kg bw by oral administration (Cremer & Callaway, 1961).

Effects on reproduction and prenatal toxicity

Three groups, each of 15 NMRI mice, received a single i.v. injection of 40 mg/kg bw lead chloride on day 3, day 4 or day 6 of pregnancy. Attachment of the blastocyst was observed on day 5 in 6/15 treated animals (controls, 12/15); invasion of the trophoblast was seen on day 6 in 1/15 treated animals (controls, 16/17); and formation of the primitive streak was seen on day 8 in 6/15 treated animals (controls, 7/7). The authors concluded that all three developmental stages studied were affected by the action of lead, and that invasion of the trophoblast was the most susceptible (Wide & Nilsson, 1977).

I.v. treatment of prairie voles (*Microtus ochrogaster*) with 32 mg/kg bw lead acetate on days 7-10 of pregnancy gave rise to exencephaly in 5 pups of 3/16 litters; spina bifida was also seen. No abnormalities were found with doses of 8 or 16 mg/kg bw. Five of eight pregnant animals treated with 64 mg/kg bw had total litter resorption (Kruckenberg et al., 1976).

Golden hamsters treated intravenously with 50 mg/kg bw of various lead salts (nitrate, chloride, acetate) on day 7, 8 or 9 of pregnancy produced fetuses (evaluated between days 12-15 of gestation) with various abnormalities; the most frequent were tail abnormalities, but anophthalmia, fused ribs, spina bifida and exencephaly were also seen. The 7- or 8-day old embryos appeared to be the most susceptible. Fetomortality was 10-18% with those dosages that resulted in the most extensive teratogenic effect; no control data were given. The dose caused little or no effect in the maternal organism (Ferm & Carpenter, 1967).

The organ and phase specificity of the teratogenic effect of lead in golden hamsters were confirmed in further studies: with i.v. doses of 25 or 50 mg/kg bw lead nitrate   on days 8 or 9 of pregnancy, only malformations of the sacral and tail region and a few   cases of rib fusion were observed. The authors discussed the possibility that lead interferes with a specific enzymic event during development (Ferm & Ferm, 1971).

It was reported in an abstract that in golden hamsters administered 50 mg/kg bw lead nitrate intravenously on day 8 of pregnancy, hyperplasia and disorientation of neuroepithelial cells of the dorsal region of the caudal neural tube were observed in embryos on day 9. Haematomas and extensive necroses occurred throughout the dorsal region of the compressed neural tube on day 10 of gestation. The sacral neural tube displayed overgrowths of neural tissue, resulting in the abnormal formation and development of the sacral vertebrae (Carpenter & Ferm, 1974).

The teratogenic effect of i.v. injections of a combination of cadmium sulphate (2 mg/kg bw) and lead acetate (25 or 50 mg/kg bw) represents an example of a complex interaction of teratogenic agents. While the frequency and severity of clefts in lip or palate caused by cadmium (19/96; controls, 0/131) was reduced by the simultaneous administration of lead (8/122 with 25 mg/kg bw Pb; 0/86 with 50 mg/kg bw Pb; 0/98 with Pb only), the posterior tail malformations caused by lead (40/98 with 50 mg/kg bw Pb) appeared to be potentiated in the presence of Cd (65/86 with the combination; 0/96 with 2 mg/kg bw Cd only). In addition, sympodia, a severe malformation of the lower extremities, was observed in fetuses exposed to the combination (12/86) but was never seen with exposure to lead only. Resorption rates under these conditions were: 7%, controls; 27%, 2 mg/kg bw Cd; 38%, 50 mg/kg bw Pb; and 46%, combination of Cd and 50 mg/kg bw Pb (Ferm, 1969). The occurrence of 'sirenomelia' (fusion of the hind limbs) in the offspring of golden hamsters exposed intravenously on day 7.5 of pregnancy to 2 mg/kg bw cadmium chloride plus 25 mg/kg bw lead nitrate was confirmed in an abstract by Hilbelink et al. (1976).

Simonsen Sprague-Dawley rats received a single dose of 25-70 mg/kg bw lead nitrate intravenously on days 8-17 of pregnancy. With 50 and 70 mg/kg bw, malformations of the urogenital and intestinal tracts and abnormalities of the posterior extremities were produced when the doses were given on day 9 of pregnancy. Lead was increasingly fetolethal when given on days 10-15 of pregnancy, but no malformations were produced. Hydrocephalus and haemorrhage of the central nervous system occurred with treatment on day 16 of pregnancy. Fetal mortality declined sharply when treatment was after day 16. Only 10% of newborn exposed to 50 mg/kg bw lead in utero on day 9 of gestation were alive on postnatal day 4, even when they were placed with untreated foster-mothers (McClain & Becker, 1975).

C57Bl mice (50 animals per group) were fed diets containing 0, 0.125, 0.25 or 0.5% lead given as lead acetate over the entire period of pregnancy; and fetuses and corpora lutea were evaluated on days 16-18 of pregnancy. The following results were obtained in the 4 groups, respectively: pregnant females, 26, 28, 11, 8; corpora lutea, 352, 381, 138, 92; live embryos per pregnant mouse, 8.3, 8.3, 8.3, 7.5; dead embryos per pregnant mouse, 1.2, 1.5, 1.9, 2.4; loss before implantation per pregnant mouse, 4.0, 3.9, 2.4, 1.6; mean weight of fetuses on day 18 of gestation, 978, 922, 850, 793 mg. No gross malformations were observed in the lead-exposed fetuses (Jacquet et al., 1975).

Female C57Bl mice were mated and kept on diets containing 0, 0.125, 0.25 or 0.5% lead; and δ-aminolaevulinic acid dehydratase activity (ALA-D) and porphyrin contents were measured in the fetuses on the 16th, 17th or 18th day of gestation. The following results were obtained in the 4 groups, respectively: 16th day of gestation - μg DNA/embryo, 440, 503, 324, 330; ng porphyrins/embryo, 60, 86, 87, 120; mU ALA-D/embryo, 1.9, 1.4, 1.4, 1.4; 17th day of gestation - μg DNA/embryo, 657, 566, 627, 470; ng porphyrins/embryo, 117, 194, 284, 340: mU ALA-D/embryo, 3.3, 1.6, 0.9, 0.9. No data on blood ALA-D levels were given (Jacquet et al., 1977a).

Pregnant C57Bl mice, fed normal or calcium-deficient diets, received an i.p. injection of 15 or 35 mg/kg bw lead acetate on day 8, 9, 10 or 12 of gestation. In those receiving the normal diet, injection of lead significantly increased postimplantation mortality and the rate of skeletal anomalies among the fetuses ($P \leqslant 0.05$). The malformations were specifically located in the anterior part of the axial skeleton and consisted essentially of the fusion of 2 or more cervical vertebrae. Fetal mortality was highest when mice were injected on day 9 of pregnancy, and malformations were induced predominantly after injection on day 8 or 9. In the calcium-deficient group, all these effects were increased ($P \leqslant 0.01$), and fetuses suffered loss of weight and delayed ossification (Jacquet & Gerber, 1979).

It was reported in an abstract that histological examinations of the brains of rats exposed to 400 or 750 mg lead acetate daily during (i) gestation and nursing, (ii) gestation, nursing and post-weaning, or (iii) post-weaning only revealed various degrees of dendritic spine loss, abnormalities in pyramidal and stellate cells and a significant difference in spine count between controls and those exposed to 750 mg/day, with all intervals of exposure (Murray et al., 1977).

Thirty Wistar rats were treated with 25 mg/kg bw lead acetate as a single i.p. injection on the 9th day of pregnancy. On day 21 of pregnancy, 8 litters were found to be totally resorbed. Only 34 living and 10 dead fetuses could be recovered from the remaining 22 rats. Two of the fetuses showed abnormally shaped heads (meningocele), and various defects were observed in 7 other fetuses (anophthalmia, tooth defects). No data on controls were given (Zegarska et al., 1974).

Two of 3 cows fed 5 mg/kg bw lead acetate on days 22-90, 45-90 or 51-120 of pregnancy gave birth to normal calves. The other died from lead poisoning, but at the time of death it had a normally developing fetus (Shupe et al., 1967).

Twelve sheep were exposed to finely powdered metallic lead in their diet (doses, 0.5-16 mg/kg bw) during the entire period of pregnancy; blood levels were about 0.4 mg/l, without resulting in death. Nine animals served as controls. The rate of lambing was 18% in the exposed (27% abortions) and 100% in the unexposed sheep (no abortions). No malformations were reported. The authors concluded that chronic lead poisoning in sheep caused abortion, miscarriage and transitory sterility (Sharma & Buck, 1976).

Lead-chelate complexes (1:1 molar ratio of lead nitrate with ethylenediaminetetra-acetic acid; nitrilotriacetic acid; iminodiacetic acid; and penicillamine) given by i.v. injection at a dose of 50 mg/kg bw lead nitrate to Charles River CD rats on day 9, 11 or 16 of pregnancy either reduced or equalled, but did not enhance, overall embryo- or feto-toxicity of lead, although some of them had been shown to increase the lead content in the fetus under certain experimental conditions (McClain & Siekierka, 1975a).

Pregnant rats were exposed for 21 days (entire pregnancy period) to lead aerosols (3 mg Pb/m^3), carbon monoxide (CO) (500 ppm) or to a combination. Activities of ALA-D in maternal:fetal blood on day 21 of pregnancy (untreated controls = 100:100%) were 13.9:23.1% (3 mg Pb/m^3); 121.2:114.5% (500 ppm CO); 11.1:75.1% (3 mg Pb/m^3 + 500 ppm CO). The authors concluded that the mode of inhibition by lead of ALA-D differs in fetuses and adults (Prigge & Greve, 1977).

Lead nitrate was administered in drinking-water to groups of 4 female Sprague-Dawley rats at doses of 0, 0.1, 1 or 10 mg/l for 3 weeks before mating, during pregnancy and for 3 weeks after delivery. The animals were sacrificed 21 days after delivery, and blood and tissues of adults and offspring were analysed for ALA-D. A pronounced decrease in enzyme activity was found in the blood and some decrease in the kidneys of offspring of the group treated with 10 mg/l: no clear-cut decrease was observed in maternal blood or kidneys. Lead concentrations in the blood of mothers and newborn were significantly increased only with the highest dose. The authors concluded that the developing organism of the rat was more susceptible to the biological action of lead than was the organism of the adult animal. The 'no-effect' level of lead was suggested from these studies to be about 1 mg/l (Hubermont et al., 1976).

Female Sprague-Dawley rats, 90 days of age, were kept for lifespan on a diet containing 1% lead (as lead acetate). When they reached 220 g bw they were mated with normal males; their offspring were kept on the same diet, and when the females reached 200 g bw, they were mated as follows: control female to control male (CF:CM); control female to lead-treated male (CF:PbM); lead-treated female to control male (PbF:CM); lead-treated female to lead-treated male (PbF:PbM). The following results were obtained: number of (first) pregnancies: 22 CF-CM, 24 CF-PbM, 35 PbF-CM, 16 PbF-PbM; off-spring/litter: 11.9, 10.1, 8.8, 7.8; birthweight of newborn in g: 6.7, 5.9, 5.4, 4.8; survival rate in %: 90, 74, 53, 30. No malformed fetuses were observed in any of P_1, F_1 or F_2 offspring from lead-intoxicated rats (Stowe & Goyer, 1971).

In rats, lead can be transferred from the mother to the fetus at various stages of gestation; transport is rapid, so that the fetus is in equilibrium with the mother 24 hours after injection. Significant amounts of lead are transferred via the milk to nursing rats even a week after a single administration. The lead was found to be concentrated more in the head than in other parts of the body (Green & Gruener, 1974).

Postnatal manifestations (such as on physical development, learning ability and neuro-logical behaviour) of lesions induced by lead prenatally in rats and lambs have been reported by a number of authors (Brady et al., 1975; Carson et al., 1974; Grant et al., 1976; Tesh & Pritchard, 1977; Van Gelder et al., 1973) [It is questionable to what extent these animal studies actually provide models for changes observed in children after lead exposure in utero].

Groups of 9 male and 9 female rats, 21 days of age, were given diets containing 64 or 512 mg/kg diet lead (as lead acetate) ad libitum. They were first mated at the age of 90-110 days; the litters of four consecutive pregnancies were studied and, in addition, the first litter of the second generation. No significant reduction in birthweight was observed with 64 or with 512 mg/kg lead. No decrease in weight gain was found during the first 15 post-natal days in any of the litters studied. When compared with newborn of a control series (0.56 mg/kg dry weight), 4.2-4.7 mg/kg lead were found in newborn from animals fed 64 mg/kg diet, and 22.3-27.0 mg/kg in newborn of rats fed 512 mg/kg diet. Essentially the same concentration of lead was found in the 15-day old rats, suggesting lead uptake from the milk (Morris et al., 1938).

In a three-generation experiment, Long-Evans BLU:(LE) rats and Charles River CD mice received 25 mg/l lead as a soluble salt in the drinking-water and a diet containing 0.20 mg/kg lead per wet weight of diet. With these doses, the interval between litters in the F1 generation of mice was 48 days (controls, 30 days), and the average litter size was 12 animals (controls, 11). In the treated group of 72 offspring of the first generation, 69 runts were observed (0 in the control group of 209 animals), and 2/8 litters were born dead. No maternal mortality was reported with the doses applied. In the F2 generation, only 23 offspring were obtained (248 in controls), and the experiment was discontinued before the F3 generation. In rats, no change was observed in the interval between litters, but the average litter size was 9.1 (controls, 11.4) in the F1 generation. The male:female ratio of the offspring was normal in the F2 and F3 generations. In the F1 generation, 2/19 litters were born dead (0/10 in controls), 40/173 young rats were runts (0 in 114 controls), and the dose was lethal to 2 mothers (0 in controls). In the F2 generation, 1/32 litters was born dead, 26 runts were observed among 311 rats, 35 young animals died, and 3 animals failed to breed (1 runt in 113 controls of 10 litters with no mortalities). In the F3 generation 4/22 rats (6 litters) were runts, one animal failed to breed, and 1/6 litter was born dead. No maternal deaths occurred in the F2 and F3 generations (Schroeder & Mitchener, 1971).

Simonsen Sprague-Dawley rats were given 7.5, 15 or 30 mg/kg bw tetraethyllead or 40, 80, 112 or 160 mg/kg bw tetramethyllead orally on 3 consecutive days (9, 10, 11 or 12, 13, 14) of organogenesis. Doses up to those lethal to some mother animals were 'essentially nonteratogenic' to offspring (McClain & Becker, 1972).

CD-1 random-bred albino mice and COBS random-bred albino rats were treated on days 5-15 (mice) or 6-16 (rats) of pregnancy with oral doses of 7.14, 71.4 or 714 mg/kg bw lead acetate (3.9, 39, 390 mg/kg bw lead) or 0.01, 0.1, 1 or 10 mg/kg bw tetraethyllead. No teratogenic effects were observed. While the dose of 71.4 mg/kg bw lead acetate had no toxic action in maternal animals, 714 mg/kg bw resulted in hypoactivity, severe diarrhoea and sharply reduced body weights, forcing discontinuation of the treatment after 3 doses; several of the treated animals died. Symptoms of maternal toxicity were also observed with 10 mg/kg bw tetraethyllead; the maternal LD_{50} was approximately 65 mg/kg bw in mice and 53 mg/kg bw in rats. An increase in fetal resorptions occurred in both species after exposure to 714 mg/kg bw lead acetate or 1 mg/kg bw tetraethyllead. The authors concluded that no teratogenic response is produced in rats and mice following exposure *in utero* to maximum tolerated doses of either lead acetate or tetraethyllead, although embryo-lethality is observed at levels resulting in severe maternal toxicity (Kennedy *et al.*, 1975).

Absorption, distribution and excretion

Absorption of lead from the gastrointestinal tract of rats varied greatly with chemical form; lead carbonate showed a 12-fold greater absorption coefficient than metallic lead (Barltrop & Meek, 1975). Absorption of lead from the gut declined steadily from 83% in 16-day-old to 16% in 89-day-old rats (Forbes & Reina, 1972). Similar effects have been observed in monkeys: young individuals retained 64.5% of an administered oral dose of lead, while only 3.2% was retained by mature adults (Willes *et al.*, 1977). Factors known to influence absorption of lead in rats are dietary calcium level (Mahaffey-Six & Goyer, 1970; Meredith *et al.*, 1977), iron (Conrad & Barton, 1978; Mahaffey-Six & Goyer, 1972) and lipid levels (Barltrop & Meek, 1975). Skin absorption of 0.24 M lead acetate or naphthenate solutions has also been observed in rats (Rastogi & Clausen, 1976).

Tissue distribution studies of lead in rats and dogs exposed by inhalation to lethal doses of tetraethyl- or tetramethyllead revealed lead levels of 7-100 mg/kg tissue in lung, brain, liver, kidney, spleen and heart (Davis *et al.*, 1963).

Charles River CD rats received an infusion of ^{210}Pb-lead nitrate (75 cpm/μg) on day 18 of pregnancy. Lead nitrate was given either separately or as a 1:1 molar lead:chelate complex (IDA - iminodiacetic acid disodium salt; NTA - nitrilotriacetic acid disodium salt; PEN - penicillamine; EDTA - ethylenediaminetetraacetic acid disodium salt). Fetal lead content was much greater than maternal blood concentrations with Pb-NTA, Pb-PEN and Pb-EDTA. In a similar experiment, 50 mg/kg bw ^{210}Pb-lead nitrate (25 cpm/μg) were injected intravenously into rats on day 16 of pregnancy. Four hours after administration, 4-5 times more radioactivity was found in the fetuses with Pb-NTA and Pb-PEN than with non-chelated lead; no difference was found with Pb-IDA or Pb-EDTA. A further increase in the amount of radioactivity was observed during the first 24 hrs with Pb and with Pb-IDA, but not with the other three chelates, which were apparently cleared rapidly from maternal blood (McClain & Siekierka, 1975b).

The mobilization of lead during pregnancy was studied in 4 groups of Sprague-Dawley rats: (i) controls; (ii) females receiving 1 mg/l lead as lead nitrate in drinking-water for 150 days before mating, over pregnancy and for 3 weeks after delivery; (iii) females receiving 1 mg/l lead for 150 days before mating, but discontinued on day 1 of pregnancy; and (iv) females receiving 1 mg/l lead for 150 days, but discontinued 50 days before mating. On day 21 after delivery, mothers and offspring were sacrificed and Pb concentrations and free porphyrins were measured in blood (FEP) and various tissues (FTP). The following results were obtained for the 4 groups, respectively: μg/l lead in blood - mothers, 30, 18, 11, 49; offspring, 20, 9, 6, 36; ng lead per mg protein in brain - mothers, 0.5, 0.2, 0.2, 0.7; offspring, 0.02, 0.02, 0.02, 0.23; ng FPT per mg protein in brain - mothers, 1.0, 0.7, 0.9, 1.6; offspring, 0.8, 0.7, 0.8, 1.1. It was concluded from the data that lead stored in the organism can be mobilized during pregnancy (Buchet et al., 1977).

Inhalation studies on rats exposed to a ^{210}Pb-dibenzoylmethane petrol aerosol for 30-45 minutes showed that, 6 days after inhalation, less than 1% of the lead was retained in lung and that 40% had been eliminated in faeces, 15% in urine, 40% fixed in the skeleton and 4-5% in soft tissue (Boudene et al., 1977). Studies by Morgan & Holmes (1978) using rats exposed to ^{203}Pb-tetraethyllead for 40-60 minutes showed that less than 2% of the administered dose remained in the lungs at 124 hours. Mean total deposition of lead was calculated to be 30.5%.

Injection of 25 μCi ^{210}Pb into adult rats resulted in a lead half-life in bone of 64-109 days (Torvik et al., 1974). After i.v. injection of ^{203}Pb-lead chloride to rats, 20% of the dose was found initially in the kidney; subsequent long-term deposition of 25-30% occurred in bone (Morgan et al., 1977). Suckling rats excrete less injected ^{203}Pb than adults, with a higher concentration in the liver than in kidney; after 192 hours, the percentage of lead retained in brain was 8 times higher in sucklings than in adults (Bayley & Brown, 1974; Momcilovic & Kostial, 1974). Studies on dogs using ^{210}Pb showed that 56-75% of the lead was excreted in the faeces, and most of the retained lead was present in the skeleton (Hursh, 1973; Lloyd et al., 1975). In rats, 6.7-8.5% of ^{210}Pb-lead nitrate administered intravenously was excreted in the bile within 24 hours; biliary excretion thus plays an important role in the enterohepatic circulation of lead (Cikrt, 1972; Cikry & Tichy, 1975). Studies on the renal handling of lead in dogs, using ^{203}Pb, showed that plasma lead is filtered and re-absorbed but that there is no evidence of tubular secretion of lead (Vander et al., 1977).

Effects on intermediary metabolism

Mitrochondrial swelling in renal proximal tubule cells associated with inhibition of mitrochondrial respiratory function and haembiosynthetic pathway enzymes is seen with doses of 50 and 250 mg/l lead acetate given to rats in drinking-water for 9 months (Fowler *et al.*, 1980).

Exposure to lead *in vivo* has also been found to inhibit oxidative and phosphorylative activities of kidney mitochondria from rats fed 1% lead acetate in the diet (Goyer & Krall, 1969); and both nicotinamide adenine trinucleotide (NAD)-linked and succinate-mediated respiration are inhibited with 50-250 mg/l dose levels in drinking-water after 9 months (Fowler *et al.*, 1980). Decreased hepatic cytochrome P-450 levels are seen in rats injected intravenously with 5 mg/kg bw lead chloride, with associated decreases in microsomal oxidative demethylation and hydroxylation enzyme activities (Alvares *et al.*, 1972).

Similar findings were observed for microsomal monooxygenase enzyme systems in mice injected intraperitoneally with 100 mg/kg bw lead acetate; decreased hepatic levels of glutathione were also observed (Dalvi & Robbins, 1978).

These biochemical effects were not observed in monkeys given 20 mg/kg bw lead acetate in drinking-water for 30 days (Allen *et al.*, 1974). The effects on microsomal drug metabolizing capacity are due in part to the inhibiting effects of lead on the haembiosynthetic pathway *in vivo* (Buchet *et al.*, 1976; Fowler *et al.*, 1980).

Injection of 5 mg/kg bw lead into mice produces a 45-fold increase in DNA synthesis in the kidney (Choie & Richter, 1974a). This effect was found to be preceded by a general increase in synthesis of RNA and protein (Choie & Richter, 1974b). I.p. injection of 10 mg/kg bw lead chloride into rats caused a 2-fold increase in renal synthesis of DNA and RNA; RNA synthesis in liver and lung was also increased 2-fold, but DNA synthesis was decreased (Stevenson *et al.*, 1977). Nuclear inclusion body formation has been observed in kidneys of rabbits (Hass *et al.*, 1964), rats (Fowler *et al.*, 1980; Goyer *et al.*, 1970), monkeys (Allen *et al.*, 1974) and dogs (Stowe *et al.*, 1973).

Mutagenicity and other short-term tests

The genetic effects of lead have been reviewed by Léonard & Gerber (1973) and by Damstra (1977).

Lead (as the divalent ion) reacted readily with phosphate groups and nitrogenous bases of purified DNA, giving rise to stable complexes (Luckey & Venugopal, 1977; Sissoëff *et al.*, 1976).

Lead chloride (4 mM) decreased the fidelity and rate of synthesis of avian myeloblastosis virus DNA polymerase-mediated DNA synthesis (Sirover & Loeb, 1976).

In systems containing *Escherichia coli* RNA polymerase and either calf-thymus DNA or T4 DNA, lead chloride stimulated chain initiation of RNA synthesis at a concentration (0.1 mM) which inhibited overall RNA synthesis (Hoffman & Niyogi, 1977).

Lead acetate was inactive in the following short-term tests: (i) *Salmonella*/microsome assay for point mutations (Rosenkranz & Poirier, 1979; Simmon, 1979a); (ii) *E. coli* $polA^+$/$polA^-$ assay for DNA-modifying effects (Rozenkranz & Poirier, 1979) and *Saccharomyces cerevisiae* D3 assay for mitotic recombination (Simmon, 1979b); and (iii) i.p. host-mediated assay, using adult male Swiss-Webster mice and *S. typhimurium* strains TA1530, TA1535 and TA1538 and *S. cerevisiae* D3 (Simmon *et al.*, 1979).

Lead acetate and lead chloride were inactive in a *rec* assay using *Bacillus subtilis* (Nishioka, 1975). In a similar assay, lead acetate, lead chloride, lead oxide and lead tetroxide were found to be inactive (Kada *et al.*, 1980). Lead chloride was not mutagenic in the *Salmonella*/microsome test nor in plate or fluctuation tests using *E. coli* WP2 (Nestmann *et al.*, 1979).

Lead acetate (20-30 mM) caused mitotic abnormalities (e.g., bridge formation, chromatid breakage) in root-tip cells of *Allium cepa* (Mukherji & Maitra, 1976). Lead chloride (0.1 mM) was weakly mutagenic to rice seeds, causing chlorophyll mutations (Reddy & Vaidyanath, 1978).

There are conflicting reports on the effects of lead salts on mammalian chromosomes *in vitro* and *in vivo*. The chromosomes of Chinese hamster cells treated in culture with 1 mM lead acetate contained more achromatic lesions than controls, but there were no significant increases in structural chromosome aberrations or mitotic abnormalities (Bauchinger & Schmid, 1972).

With 10^3 -10 mM lead acetate and 48- and 72-hr human leucocyte cultures, Schmid *et al.* (1972) found no significant increases in frequency or type of structural chromosome damage over the levels found in sodium acetate-treated or untreated cultures. However, Beek & Obe (1974) found a significant increase in achromatic lesions and chromatid and isochromatid breaks in human leucocytes treated for 24 hrs with 10^2 mM lead acetate and cultured for a total of 72 hrs, but no excess of these lesions in cells treated and cultured for 51 hrs. Lead acetate (10^{-2} mM) did not increase the frequency of sister chromatid exchanges in these cells (Beek & Obe, 1975).

Stella *et al.* (1978) found a significant increase in chromatid gaps and a slight increase in chromosome fragments in human lymphocytes cultured for 72 hrs and treated with 1 mM lead acetate during the last 24 hrs. There was no excess chromosomal damage in human lymphocytes (48-hr and 72-hr cultures) treated with lead acetate at doses of 0.1 and 1 mM (Deknudt & Deminatti, 1978). Lead acetate (1-2.5 g/l medium) induced morphological transformation of Syrian hamster secondary embryo cells: cells derived from transformed colonies produced fibrosarcomas when injected subcutaneously into Syrian hamsters or nude mice (DiPaolo *et al.*, 1978).

Lead acetate did not induce heritable dominant lethal effects in mice (Kennedy & Arnold, 1971). Varma *et al.* (1974) reported that dominant lethal effects were induced in mice fed 2% aqueous lead subacetate in their drinking-water for 28 days [This claim is difficult to interpret because of the heterogeneity of the data and the inadequacy of the statistical evaluation].

BALB/C mice were given lead acetate in their drinking-water at concentrations ranging from 0.1-1000 mg/l (expressed as lead) for 9 months (equivalent to a total intake of 3.3 mg - 31 kg/kg bw). Neither the survival nor the fertility of treated mice differed significantly from those in control mice given 0.5% acetic acid in their drinking-water. There was no excess of chromosomal damage in bone-marrow cells or in spermatocytes of treated mice (Léonard *et al.*, 1973).

Chromosomes from bone-marrow cells cultured for 4 days after removal from mice fed for 2 weeks with 10,000 mg/kg diet lead acetate showed an excess of gaps and breaks (usually involving single chromatids) and of fragments (Muro & Goyer, 1969). However, Jacquet *et al.* (1977b) found no excess of severe chromosome or chromatid aberrations in bone-marrow cells (examined directly) of mice fed for 1-3 months with 2500-10,000 mg/kg diet lead (as lead acetate). Significant increases in chromatid gaps were seen only in mice fed the highest levels of lead acetate, when blood lead concentrations reached about 800 μg/l. No increase in the number of micronuclei was observed in polychromatic erythrocytes after 2 i.p. injections of 25 mg/kg bw lead.

An increase in the number of bone-marrow cells containing chromatid gaps, fragments, deletions and translocations (usually involving single chromatids) was observed in rats (5 males, 3 females) that received 1% lead acetate in their drinking-water for 30 days (Teodorescu & Calugaru, 1972).

There was no significant excess of chromosome damage in cultured leucocytes obtained from 9 cows accidentally intoxicated with a mixture of heavy metals and shown to have toxic levels of lead in liver and kidneys (Léonard et al., 1974).

Cynomolgus monkeys (Macaca irus) were given 0, 1.5, 6 or 15 mg lead acetate orally on 6 days a week for 16 months; another group given 6 mg were maintained on a low-calcium diet. Chromosome analysis of 48-hr cultured lymphocytes taken after 3, 10 and 16 months' treatment showed that dicentrics, rings, translocations and exchanges were significantly increased only in the group given the low-calcium diet, whereas chromatid gaps and fragments increased with time in all lead-treated groups. Blood levels ranged from 100-1340 μg/l during these experiments (Deknudt et al., 1977a).

Tetraethyllead did not promote a dominant lethal effect in mice (Kennedy & Arnold, 1971).

(b) Humans

Most non-occupational exposure (in water, surface coatings, pigments, air, etc) is to inorganic lead compounds.

Toxicity

A detailed review of the pathological effects of lead was made by Goyer & Rhyne (1973). Damstra (1977) reviewed the toxicological effects.

Encephalopathy in adults due to lead has been described in numerous reports. Major signs and symptoms are dullness, restlessness, irritability, loss of memory and inability to concentrate, with delirium, convulsions, paralysis and coma at later stages of intoxication. The symptoms of encephalopathy in infants and small children are similar to those seen in adults. Blood lead levels in exposed children with brain dysfunction were always higher than 400 μg/l (Horn Rummo et al., 1979; Irwig et al., 1978; Pueschel et al., 1972; Valciukas et al., 1978; Whitfield et al., 1972).

Impairment of reproduction in men exposed occupationally to lead has been reported in several papers. Lancranjan et al. (1975) found increased frequency of asthenospermia, hypospermia and teratospermia in 16 workers with lead poisoning (blood lead level, 745 ± 260 μg/l) and in 29 with moderately increased absorption (blood lead level, 528 ± 210 μg/l), but not in 50 with 'normal' absorption (blood lead level, 230 ± 150 μg/l).

In a WHO (1977) document it was concluded that prolonged exposure to lead leading to a blood level of more than 700 μg/l may give rise to chronic, irreversible nephropathy. Little is known about dose-effect relationships or about time-effect relationships for lead-induced chronic interstitial nephritis. Renal effects of lead in exposed workers have been associated with aminoaciduria (Goyer et al., 1972) and with decreased urinary kallikrein activity (Boscolo et al., 1978).

Exposure to inorganic lead inhibits the haem biosynthetic pathway in humans, with corresponding increases in zinc protoporphyrin, inhibition of δ-aminolaevulinic acid dehydratase in blood and increases in blood and urinary δ-aminolaevulinic acid (Lilis et al., 1978; Meredith et al., 1978). In 5 people with blood lead values greater than 500 μg/l and changes in haem biosynthesis, only minimal changes were observed in hepatic cytochrome P-450-mediated drug metabolizing reactions (Fischbein et al., 1977). The haem biosynthetic pathway is inhibited to a greater extent in women than in men after lead exposure (Roels et al., 1975; Stuik, 1974). When standardized for total internal lead burden, only elevated zinc protoporphyrin was found to show a statistical difference (Alessio et al., 1977). Exposure to tetraethyllead, resulting in blood lead levels in 4 men of 600-925 μg/l, inhibited δ-aminolaevulinic acid dehydratase in blood but did not enhance excretion of δ-aminolaevulinic acid or that of coproporphyrin (Beattie et al., 1972).

Acute exposure to tetraethyllead produced renal and hepatic damage in 1/2 adolescents with blood lead levels of 1200-1400 μg/l (Robinson, 1978). Other signs of lead toxicity involve encephalopathy, peripheral neuropathy and muscular weakness, following exposure to either tetraethyllead (Forycki et al., 1977; Hansen & Sharp, 1978; Robinson, 1978) or inorganic lead (Irwig et al., 1978; Whitfield et al., 1972) in patients with blood levels over 400 μg/l.

Effects on reproduction and prenatal toxicity

In 1860, Paul first published his observations on the toxic effects of lead in the conceptus. Since that time, a voluminous literature has accumulated, showing that this heavy metal can exert toxic effects on conception, pregnancy and the fetus. Selected references only can be summarized here. A review of the literature on lead poisoning during pregnancy and a case report are given by Angle & McIntire (1964). The literature on fetal hazards from environmental pollution with lead (and mercury and other non-essential trace metals) (Scanlon, 1972) and the effects of lead on women (Rom, 1976) have also been reviewed.

Current water lead levels were measured in the houses that had been occupied during the first year of life by 77 mentally retarded children aged 2-6 years and 77 non-retarded matched controls, and in the houses occupied by their mothers during pregnancy. The water lead content was significantly higher for the retarded group, and the probability of mental retardation was significantly increased when water lead exceeded 800 μg/l. Blood lead levels were also significantly higher in the retarded group. It was concluded that lead contamination of water may be one factor in the multifactorial etiology of mental retardation and that every effort should be made to reduce the lead content of drinking-water (Beattie et al., 1975) [The Working Group noted that the current water lead levels may not have reflected those encountered by the children in utero or in the first year of life].

Blood lead concentrations were measured retrospectively in the blood contained on cards used for testing for phenylketonuria in the first two weeks of life taken from a group of 77 children with mental retardation of unknown etiology and 77 controls; 24 pairs were evaluated. There was a highly significant trend towards higher blood lead concentrations in mentally retarded children. Water lead concentrations in the maternal home during pregnancy correlated with blood lead concentrations in the mentally retarded children (Moore et al., 1977).

Placental lead levels were studied in a series of Birmingham births classified as still-birth, neonatal death or survival beyond one week. There was an appreciable range of lead levels even in normal births (0.15-3.56 mg/kg), but average results showed a pronounced excess of lead in those who failed to survive either birth or the neonatal period. There was no association between placental lead content and impaired birthweight among survivors. The possibility was discussed that under conditions of impaired fetal health in late pregnancy the placenta may concentrate lead (Wibberley et al., 1977).

It was mentioned in an abstract that no significant correlation was found between the lead content of water samples collected from houses in 48 areas of South Wales and the frequency of central nervous system malformation rates (Morton & Elwood, 1974).

A series of papers deals with a possible embryotoxic hazard produced by a Swedish smelter which emits into the environment a number of potentially genotoxic substances, such as lead, arsenic and sulphur dioxide. A significant reduction of birthweight was found in the offspring of employees and of the inhabitants of two small industrial areas near the smelter (3391 ± 526g in 323 offspring of employees versus 3460 ± 554g in 2700 controls living in Umeå; P<0.05). Later pregnancies were particularly affected. Moreover, a higher frequency of spontaneous abortion was noted in women working at the smelter during or before pregnancy (11.3% of first pregnancies and 15.1% of all pregnancies) or living close to the smelter (10.1% of first pregnancies and 11% of all pregnancies), when compared with those living further away (5.1% of first pregnancies and 7.6% of all pregnancies). The abortion frequency was increased when both parents were employed at the smelter (19.4% of all pregnancies versus 13.5% when the mother only was working at the smelter). The frequency of malformations was significantly increased in the offspring of women who had worked at the smelter during pregnancy, but not in the offspring of women living near the smelter (Nordstrom *et al.*, 1978a, b, 1979a, b) [It is not possible to determine the specific environmental factor(s) associated with the observed effects. The contribution of effects due to exposure of men cannot be excluded for all the data given].

Absorption, distribution, excretion and metabolism

Early literature on the lead content of human fetuses was reviewed by Hansmann & Perry (1940).

Adult men absorbed about 10% of an ingested dose of ^{204}Pb- or ^{207}Pb-lead nitrate (Rabinowitz *et al.*, 1973, 1976). When ^{203}Pb-lead chloride was administered to 10 adult men, 5 had a mean absorption of about 11.5%; the others had higher but more widely varied absorption (Blake, 1976). In infants, a mean of 41.5% of ingested lead was observed; individual absorption was related inversely to dietary calcium level (Ziegler *et al.*, 1978). Inhalation of ^{203}Pb-tetraethyllead exhaust by 7 subjects resulted in 35-40% deposition in the lungs (Chamberlain *et al.*, 1975a,b).

Tissue distribution studies of lead in men fatally poisoned by tetraethyllead revealed lead levels of 7-240 mg/kg tissue in lung, brain, liver and kidney (Davis *et al.*, 1963).

The concentration of trace metals was measured in maternal and cord blood and in placental tissue of 25 maternal/fetal pairs from 8 different areas in the US. Mean values of lead found were 333 μg/l in maternal blood, 318 μg/l in cord blood and 373 μg/kg in placental tissue (Creason *et al.*, 1976).

It was reported in an abstract that lead concentrations were measured by atomic absorption spectrometry in 50 embryos and fetuses, ranging in gestational age from 31-261 days, from normal pregnancies terminated by legal abortions; the mothers were not known to have experienced undue lead exposure during pregnancy. Lead was detected in 66% of the first trimester specimens, without relationship to age, at concentrations of 0.38-2.0 mg/kg wet weight; lead was found in 77% of liver samples (0.84 - 4.04 mg/kg wet weight) and 30% of kidney samples (0.9 - 2.3 mg/kg) but in only 2 (15%) brain samples (Chaube *et al.*, 1972).

The transplacental transfer of lead was studied in 70 pregnant women living in rural areas of Belgium exposed to different lead contents in drinking-water. The concentrations of lead in maternal blood samples ranged from 51-263 μg/l whole blood, those in blood samples from the offspring from 29-249 μg/l and those in the placentas from 43-280 μg/kg tissue. Lead concentrations in maternal and cord blood were also compiled for two groups of women, one of which were exposed to water lead levels of <50 μg/l (mean lead content, 11.8 μg/l) and the other to levels >50 μg/l (mean lead content, 247.4 μg/l). The differences between the two groups, in mean lead concentrations, were $\triangle$ = 32 μg/l for maternal and $\triangle$ = 33 μg/l for umbilical blood.   Significant correlations were found between lead content of water and lead concentration in both maternal and newborn blood levels.   An increase in lead concentration of water from 50 to 500 μg/l was found to increase blood lead concentrations in mothers and newborns by about 30 μg/l (Hubermont *et al.*, 1978).

Concentrations of lead in ribs and vertebrae of 26 stillbirths were 5.7 mg/kg wet weight in ribs (range, 0.4 - 24.2) and 2.9 mg/kg (range, 0.2 - 13.2) in vertebrae. Necropsy samples from 6 infants (6 weeks to 10 months of age) who died in traffic accidents or of infections showed bone lead levels ranging from 0.2 to 0.6 mg/kg wet weight.   The mean values in stillbirths thus appear to be 5 - 10 times greater than normal (Bryce-Smith *et al.*, 1977).

Exact blood and urine levels in women in the pregestation period and during pregnancy are given in only a few reports.   A case report containing such data was made for a woman exposed occupationally to lead, who gave birth to an apparently normal child (Greenfield, 1957).

Blood lead levels in 294 newborns in the Federal Republic of Germany were 149.8 ± 78.9 μg/l, and those in maternal blood 168.9 ± 85.7 μg/l (correlation constant, r = 0.54). There was also a correlation between the excretion of δ-aminolaevulinic acid in the urine of newborns and their blood lead levels (Haas *et al.*, 1972).   Mean blood lead levels in 315 mature and immature neonates and 198 mothers in the Ruhr district of the Federal Republic of Germany were 129 ± 41 μg/l in newborns and 139 ± 38 μg/l in maternal blood (r = 0.50) (Hower *et al.*, 1976).   Mean blood lead levels in 24 mothers in Connecticut during labour were 132 (range, 100-200) μg/l and those in cord blood 123 (range, 100-200) μg/l (Harris & Holley, 1972).

The lead content of placentas of 18 mothers in Vienna was 74.25 mg/kg and that of 12 mothers from adjacent rural communities was 18.4 mg/kg; for 39% of the urban group the value exceeded the maximum tolerated value by 1.2 mg/kg. Maternal δ-aminolaevulinic acid excretion in urine also differed in the two groups (Maruna *et al.*, 1975).

The median concentration of lead in placentas from 474 Belgian women was 7.5 mg/kg wet weight.   Lead concentration in placenta correlated significantly with that in maternal blood (r = 0.22) (Roels *et al.*, 1978).

No correlation was found between the amount of lead in the placenta and that in the blood of mothers from different environments in the Federal Republic of Germany, as determined by atomic absorption spectrometry.   The blood lead levels of mothers and newborns, however, correlated by an average factor of 1.4 (Schaller *et al.*, 1976).

The mean lead concentration in 541 samples of umbilical cord blood from different parts of Sweden was 76 μg/l. The mean blood lead value in 297 mothers was 87 μg/l. There was a significant correlation between the blood lead levels of the mother and of the infant, as studied in 253 pairs (r = 0.5) (Zetterlund et al., 1977).

Blood lead levels were measured in 122 mothers and their infants, who were resident in a township 3000 m from a lead mine and smelter in Africa, where the annual mean atmospheric lead concentration was 9.6 μg/m^3 and the soil lead concentration 100-9400 mg/kg. Mean blood levels were high: 412 μg/l and 370 μg/l for mothers and infants, respectively, with a significant correlation (r = 0.77, P < 0.001) (Clark, 1977).

In a volunteer who ingested a diet supplemented with ^{204}Pb in addition to the lead absorbed through inhalation of ambient air and tobacco, 76% of the total intake was excreted in the urine, 16% was excreted via the gut and 8% through sweat, hair and nails (Rabinowitz et al., 1973). Renal clearance of lead occurs essentially by glomerular filtration (WHO, 1977).

After absorption, tetraethyllead is distributed throughout various tissues, and particularly in brain; it breaks down into triethyllead and minute amounts of inorganic lead, mainly in the liver. Both products are excreted in the urine within a relatively short period of time (Tsuchiya, 1979).

Mutagenicity and other short-term tests

Cytogenetic studies of people who have been exposed to lead have given conflicting results: nine positive and six negative studies are summarized in Tables 6 and 7, respectively.

3.3 Case reports and epidemiological studies

(a) Case reports

Portal (1961) described the occurrence of a cerebral tumour in a lead worker. This case was reported to illustrate the difficulty of distinguishing between intracranial tumour and lead encephalopathy.

Jecklin (1956) found concentrations of lead to be no higher in the lungs of 5 patients who died from lung cancer than in the lungs of 5 persons who died from other causes; levels of 1-1.8 mg/kg of lung tissue were found in both groups.

Table 6. Cytogenetic investigations of cells from individuals exposed to lead: 9 positive studies

Number of exposed subjects	Number of controls	Cell culture time (hrs)	Urine or blood level (µg/l)	Exposed subjects	Type of damage	Remarks	Reference
8	14	?	620-890 (blood)	Workers in a lead oxide factory	Chromatid and chromosome breaks	Increase in chromosomal damage correlated with increased δ-aminolaevulinic acid excretion	Schwanitz et al. (1970)
10	10	72	600-1000 (blood)	Workers in a chemical factory	Chromatid gaps, breaks	No correlation with blood lead levels	Gath & Thiess (1972)
14	5	48	155-720 (urine)	Workers in a zinc plant, exposed to fumes & dust of cadmium, zinc & lead	Gaps, fragments, exchanges, dicentrics, rings	Thought to be caused by lead, not cadmium or zinc	Deknudt et al. (1973)
105	-	72	116-974 mean, 377 (blood)	Blast-furnace workers, metal grinders, scrap metal processers	'Structural abnormalities', gaps, breaks, hyperploidy	No correlation with δ-aminolaevulinic acid excretion or blood lead levels	Schwanitz et al. (1975)
11 (before and after exposure)	-	68-70	340-640 (blood)	Workers in a lead-acid battery plant and a lead foundry	Gaps, breaks, fragments	No correlation with δ-aminolaevulinic acid dehydratase activity in red cells	Forni et al. (1976)

Table 6 (contd)

Number of exposed subjects	Number of controls	Cell culture time (hrs)	Urine or blood level (μg/l)	Exposed subjects	Type of damage	Remarks	Reference
44	15	72	300-750 (blood)	Individuals in a lead oxide factory	Chromatid and chromosome aberrations	Positive correlation with length of exposure	Garza-Chapa et al. (1977)
23	20	48	440-950 (not given)	Lead-acid battery melters, tin workers	Dicentrics, rings, fragments	Factors other than lead exposure may be required for severe aberrations	Deknudt et al. (1977b)
20	20	46-48	530-1000 (blood)	Ceramic, lead & battery workers	Breaks, fragments	Positive correlation with blood lead levels	Sarto et al. (1978)
26 (4 low, 16 medium, 6 high exposure)	not given	72	225-650 (blood)	Smelter workers	Gaps, chromatid and chromosome aberrations	Positive correlation with blood lead levels	Nordenson et al. (1978)

Table 7. Cytogenetic investigations of cells from individuals exposed to lead: 6 negative studies

Number of exposed subjects	Number of controls	Cell culture time (hrs)	Blood lead level (µg/l)	Exposed subjects	Reference
29	20	46-48	not given, stated to be 20-30% higher than controls	Policemen 'permanently in contact with high levels of automotive exhaust'	Bauchinger et al. (1972)
32	20	46-48	range not given; highest level was 590 mg/l [sic]	Workers in lead manufacturing industry; 3 had acute lead intoxication	Schmid et al. (1972)
35	35	45-48	control, ⟨ 40; exposed, 40-⟩120	Shipyard workers employed as 'burners' cutting metal structures on ships	O'Riordan & Evans (1974)
24	15	48	193 (lead) 4 (cadmium)	Mixed exposure to zinc, lead and cadmium in a zinc-smelting plant; significant increase in chromatid breaks & exchanges. Authors suggest that cadmium was the major cause of this damage	Bauchinger et al. (1976)
9	9	72	400 ± 50, 7 weeks	Volunteers ingested capsules containing lead acetate	Bulsma & DeFrance (1976)
30	20	48	control, 118-132; exposed, 290-330	Children living near a lead smelter	Bauchinger et al. (1977)

Dingwall-Fordyce & Lane (1963) examined causes of death for 184/425 men, 65 years of age or over, who had worked 25 years or more in lead-related industries, and causes of death for 153 men who had died while employed in an accumulator factory where lead was used. The men were grouped into 3 levels of lead exposure: none, negligible (mean urine lead levels within 'normal range') and heavy (mean urine lead levels of 100-250 μg/l). The observed/expected deaths from all malignant neoplasms for these groups were 24/20.1, 25/14.2 and 27/31.0, respectively, showing no excess of overall cancer deaths in the group with highest lead exposure.

Using employment records from 6 'smelters' and 10 lead-acid battery factories, 7032 men employed between 1946 and 1970 for one or more years were identified and followed through 31 December 1970. Vital status was determined from company pension records, Social Security Administration files and other sources; 2% of smelter workers and 5% of battery factory workers were lost to follow-up. Expected numbers of deaths were calculated by applying US male age-specific and cause-specific death rates to the number of person-years observed for each 5-year age group. The ratio of observed to expected deaths (Standardized Mortality Ratio, SMR) was determined and then corrected to account for missing death certificates. The SMR for all causes of death combined was 107 for smelter workers and 99 for battery workers. The authors reported an excess of deaths from all malignant neoplasms in smelter workers (69 observed *versus* 54.95 expected; $P<0.05$, calculated by Chiang's method) but not in battery plant workers (186 observed *versus* 180.34 expected), and a statistically nonsignificant excess of deaths due to cancer of the digestive organs and the respiratory system [The Working Group recalculated the data using Poisson's method and found no statistical significance in any group (Table 8)]. Observed numbers of

Table 8. Expected and observed deaths for selected malignant neoplasms between 1 January 1947 and 31 December 1970 for lead workers[a]

Cause of death (ICD 8th rev. codes)	Smelters			Battery factory workers		
	Observed	Expected	O:E (95% confidence limits)	Observed	Expected	O:E (95% confidence limits)
All malignant neoplasms (140-205)	69	54.95	1.25 (0.97-1.6)	186	180.34	1.0 (0.89-1.2)
Digestive organs (150-159)	25	17.63	1.4 (0.92-2.1)	70	61.48	1.1 (0.89-1.4)
Respiratory organs (160-164)	22	15.76	1.4 (0.88-2.1)	61	49.51	1.2 (0.94-1.6)

[a]From Cooper & Gaffey, 1975

malignant neoplasms were higher than expected, although not significantly so, in the smelter workers, who had higher mean urinary and blood lead levels than battery plant workers (173.2 *versus* 129.7 µg/l in urine; 79.7 *versus* 62.7 µg/l in blood); however, 60% of them had less than 20 years since first employment, a period which may be too short adequately to reflect cancer risk. On the other hand, 64% of the battery workers had more than 20 years since start of employment, and their observed rates were very close to those expected. It was noted that smelter workers were exposed to factors in the working environment other than those to which battery workers were exposed (Cooper & Gaffey, 1975).

Robinson (1976) compared information on health variables for 153 current white male 'wage roll' employees who had had occupational exposure to tetraethyllead for 20 or more years with those for a similar group of workers matched individually for age and years of service who had had no recognized occupational exposure to tetraethyllead or to any other lead compounds. Mean urinary lead levels taken over 8-10 years were 3-4 times higher in subjects than in controls. Information on health was obtained retrospectively, from results of periodic physical examinations and laboratory studies, medical records of absence from work due to illness, and long-term medical histories in the form of cumulative diagnoses. The prevalence of skin cancer among exposed workers was 7/139 (5%), not significantly different from that of non-exposed workers (4/139, 2.9%). There were no cases of cancer other than of the skin in either group [The Working Group noted that workers who left employment for any reason (including illness or retirement) were not included; this study was therefore considered inadequate to determine the carcinogenic risk of exposure to tetra-ethyllead].

In an investigation of workers at a copper smelter, mine and concentrater in Utah, Rencher *et al*. (1977) noted a 3-fold excess risk of lung cancer among the smelter workers as compared with workers in other areas of the plant and with the population of the state. Cumulative exposure indices for sulphur dioxide, arsenic and lead were statistically significantly higher for the lung cancer cases [The relative contributions of the three exposures in relation to lung cancer cannot be established on the basis of the data presented (see also monograph on arsenic, p. 110)].

Three studies have addressed the question of fathers' 'hydrocarbon-related' occupations in relation to childhood cancer; they are considered here since some of these occupations may be associated with exposure to lead compounds. Case-control studies by Fabia & Thuy (1974) and by Hakulinen *et al*. (1976) analysed childhood deaths at under the age of five and incident cancers, respectively: using arbitrary but similar occupational categories, Fabia & Thuy found a positive correlation between 'hydrocarbon-related' occupations and childhood cancers. Hakulinen *et al*. did not confirm this correlation. Kantor *et al*. (1979), using a similar study design, compared 149 incident cases of Wilms' tumour from the Connecticut Tumor Registry for the period 1935 to 1973 with 149 non-cancer controls matched for sex, race and year of birth. They confirmed the association with 'hydrocarbon-related' occupations (24 cases *versus* 10 controls), but noted in addition that 'lead-related' occupations were more prevalent among the fathers of the Wilms' tumour cases (22 cases *versus* 6 controls; P<0.05) [The occupation categories were based on birth certificate statements, and the groupings used by the authors do not necessarily reflect the most appropriate collection of lead-related occupations. It is impossible to assess the lead exposure of the fathers. Moreover, the apparent protective effect of farming (1 case *versus* 8 controls) must be reconsidered in view of the fact that farmers may also be exposed to petrol. In view of these limitations, there is insufficient evidence to suggest that paternal exposure to lead causes Wilms' tumours in offspring].

4. Summary of Data Reported and Evaluation

4.1 Experimental data

Lead acetate, lead subacetate and lead phosphate are carcinogenic to rats and lead subacetate to mice: these compounds induced benign and malignant tumours of the kidney following oral or parenteral administration. Gliomas occurred in rats given lead acetate or lead subacetate by the oral route.

When tetraethyllead was administered by subcutaneous injection to neonatal mice, an increased incidence of lymphomas occurred in female animals only; additional studies are required before an evaluation of the carcinogenicity of this compound can be made.

No evaluation could be made of the carcinogenicity of lead arsenate, lead carbonate, lead oxide, metallic lead powder, lead naphthenate or lead nitrate.

Lead chloride gave positive results in DNA misincorporation tests. Lead acetate induced morphological transformations in Syrian hamster cells. There is no evidence that lead acetate or lead chloride induces mutations or allied effects in bacteria; some chromosomal aberration tests in mammalian systems (either *in vitro* or *in vivo*) have given positive results. There was insufficient evidence to evaluate the mutagenicity of organometallic lead compounds.

Lead salts have been reported to cross the placenta and to induce embryo- and feto-mortality. They also have a teratogenic effect in some animal species. No teratogenic effects have been reported with exposure to organometallic lead compounds.

4.2 Human data

Three epidemiological studies have been made of workers who were exposed to either lead and inorganic lead compounds or to tetraethyllead. One of the two studies on metallic lead workers showed no excess of cancer deaths. The other showed a slight (although not significant) excess of deaths due to cancers of the digestive system and respiratory system among smelter workers but not among workers in a lead-acid battery factory. As 60% of the members of the smelter workers cohort were hired after 1950, further follow-up of this cohort is warranted, in order to determine more reliably if there is an excess risk. In the third study, a slight but not significant increase of skin cancer was observed among workers exposed to tetraethyllead.

Several case-control studies have investigated the possibility that there is a causal link between paternal occupation and childhood cancer. The one study that specifically links lead-related occupations with the occurrence of Wilms' tumour cannot be considered to exhibit a causal link in view of the disputable appropriateness of the occupation sub-categories used.

In nine studies, chromosomal aberrations were found in peripheral lymphocytes of lead-exposed populations whose blood lead levels ranged from 100-1000 μg/l. Negative results were obtained in six studies in which blood lead levels ranged from 40-500 μg/l.

In numerous reports, lead has been shown readily to cross the placenta. Good correlations have been reported between maternal and fetal blood levels. Adverse effects of lead on human reproduction, embryonic and fetal development and postnatal (e.g., mental) development have been reported.

4.3 Evaluation

Experimental and epidemiological data on metallic lead and organic lead compounds were either unavailable or inadequate, and no evaluation of their carcinogenicity was possible.

There is *sufficient evidence* that lead subacetate is carcinogenic to mice and rats and that lead acetate and lead phosphate are carcinogenic to rats. In the absence of adequate human data, it is reasonable, for practical purposes, to regard these compounds as if they presented a carcinogenic risk to humans.

5. References

Adler, M.W. & Adler, C.H. (1977) Toxicity to heavy metals and relationship to seizure thresholds. *Clin. Pharmacol. Ther., 22,* 774-779

Alessio, L., Castoldi, M.R., Buratti, M., Maroni, M. & Bertazzi, P.A. (1977) Behaviour of some indicators of biological effect in female lead workers. *Int. Arch. occup. environ. Health, 40,* 283-292

Allen, F.R., Garrison, A.W. & Taylor, C.E. (1976) *Chemical Analysis of Metal Finishing Wastewaters,* Athens, GA, Environmental Research Laboratory

Allen, J.R., McWey, P.J. & Suomi, S.J. (1974) Pathobiological and behavioral effects of lead intoxication in the infant rhesus monkey. *Environ. Health Perspect., 7,* 239-246

Alvares, A.P., Leigh, S., Cohn, J. & Kappas, A. (1972) Lead and methyl mercury: effects of acute exposure on cytochrome P-450 and the mixed function oxidase system in liver. *J. exp. Med., 135,* 1406-1409

American Society for Testing & Materials (1977) *1977 Annual Book of ASTM Standards, Part 8, Nonferrous Metals - Nickel, Lead, and Tin Alloys, Precious Metals, Primary Metals, Reactive Metals,* Philadelphia, PA, pp. 47-49

Angle, C.R. & McIntire, M.S. (1964) Lead poisoning during pregnancy. *Am. J. Dis. Child., 108,* 436-439

Atomergic Chemetals Company (undated) *Chemetals Catalog,* Carle Place, Long Island, NY, p. 49

J.T. Baker Chemical Co. (1975) *Product Information Bulletin, Lead Nitrate, Technical Flake (lead (II) nitrate),* Phillipsburg, NJ

J.T. Baker Chemical Co. (1976a) *Product Information Bulletin, Lead Acetate,* Phillipsburg, NJ, pp. 1-3

J.T. Baker Chemical Co. (1976b) *Lead Carbonate, Powder, 'Baker Analyzed'* ® *Reagent, Product No. 2300,* Phillipsburg, NJ

J.T. Baker Chemical Co. (1976c) *Lead Chloride, Powder, 'Baker Analyzed'* ® *Reagent, Product No. 2308,* Phillipsburg, NJ

J.T. Baker Chemical Co. (1977) *Lead Sub-Acetate, Powder, 'Baker Analyzed'* ® *Reagent, for Sugar Analysis, Product No. 2290,* Phillipsburg, NJ

Baldwin, R.W., Cunningham, G.J. & Pratt, D. (1964) Carcinogenic action of motor engine oil additives. *Br. J. Cancer, 18,* 503-507

Baló, J., Batjai, A. & Szende, B. (1965) Experimental adenomas of the kidney produced by chronic administration of lead phosphate. *Magyar Onkol., 9,* 144-151

Barlow, P.J. (1977) Micro-determination of lead and cadmium in pasteurized market milks by flameless atomic absorption spectroscopy using a base digest. *J. Dairy Res., 44,* 377-381

Barltrop, D. & Meek, F. (1975) Absorption of different lead compounds. *Postgrad. med. J., 51,* 805-809

Bauchinger, M. & Schmid, E. (1972) Chromosome analysis in Chinese hamster cell cultures after treatment with lead acetate (Ger.). *Mutat. Res., 14,* 95-100

Bauchinger, M., Schmid, E. & Schmidt, D. (1972) Chromosome analysis of policemen with increased blood lead level (Ger.). *Mutat. Res., 16,* 407-412

Bauchinger, M., Schmid, E., Einbrodt, H.J. & Dresp, J. (1976) Chromosome aberrations in lymphocytes after occupational exposure to lead and cadmium. *Mutat. Res., 40,* 57-62

Bauchinger, M., Dresp, J., Schmid, E., Englert, N. & Krause, C. (1977) Chromosome analyses of children after ecological lead exposure. *Mutat. Res., 56,* 75-80

Bayley, M. & Brown, D.R. (1974) Low renal lead excretion in lead treated immature rats. *Pharmacologist, 16,* 207

Beattie, A.D., Moore, M.R. & Goldberg, A. (1972) Tetraethyl-lead poisoning. *Lancet, ii,* 12-15

Beattie, A.D., Moore, M.R., Goldberg, A., Finlayson, M.J.W., Graham, J.F., Mackie, E.M., Main, J.C., McLaren, D.A., Murdoch, R.M. & Stewart, G.T. (1975) Role of chronic low-level lead exposure in the aetiology of mental retardation. *Lancet, i,* 589-592

Beek, B. & Obe, G. (1974) Effect of lead acetate on human leukocyte chromosomes *in vitro. Experientia, 30,* 1006-1007

Beek, B. & Obe, G. (1975) The human leukocyte test system. VI. The use of sister chromatid exchanges as possible indicators for mutagenic activities. *Humangenetik, 29,* 127-134

Blake, K.C.H. (1976) Absorption of [203]Pb from gastrointestinal tract of man. *Environ. Res., 11,* 1-4

Boscolo, P., Porcelli, G., Cecchetti, G., Salimei, E. & Iannaccone, A. (1978) Urinary kallikrein activity of workers exposed to lead. *Br. J. ind. Med., 35,* 226-229

Boudene, C., Malet, D. & Masse, R. (1977) Fate of ^{210}Pb inhaled by rats. *Toxicol. appl. Pharmacol., 41,* 271-276

Boyland, E., Dukes, C.E., Grover, P.L. & Mitchley, B.C.V. (1962) The induction of renal tumours by feeding lead acetate to rats. *Br. J. Cancer, 16,* 283-288

Bradford, W.L. (1976) *Distribution and Movement of Zinc and Other Heavy Metals in South San Francisco Bay, California,* Report No. USGS/WRD/WRI-76104, US Geological Survey, Springfield, VA, National Technical Information Service, pp. 41-42

Brady, K., Herrera, Y. & Zenick, H. (1975) Influence of parental lead exposure on subsequent learning ability of offspring. *Pharmacol. Biochem. Behav., 3,* 561-565

Bryce-Smith, D., Deshpande, R.R., Hughes, J. & Waldron, H.A. (1977) Lead and cadmium levels in stillbirths. *Lancet, i,* 1159

Buchet, J.-P., Roels, H., Hubermont, G. & Lauwerys, R. (1976) Effect of lead on some parameters of the heme biosynthetic pathway in rat tissues *in vivo. Toxicology, 6,* 21-34

Buchet, J.-P., Lauwerys, R., Roels, H. & Hubermont, G. (1977) Mobilization of lead during pregnancy in rats. *Int. Arch. occup. environ. Health, 40,* 33-36

Bulsma, J.B. & De France, H.F. (1976) Cytogenetic investigations in volunteers ingesting inorganic lead. *Int. Arch. occup. environ. Health, 38,* 145-148

Bureau of National Affairs, Inc. (1977) Abnormal blood-lead levels found in children of smelter employees. *Occup. Saf. Health Rep., 6,* 1182-1183

Capar, S.G. (1977) Atomic absorption spectrophotometric determination of lead, cadmium zinc, and copper in clams and oysters: collaborative study. *J. Assoc. off. anal. Chem., 60,* 1400-1407

Carpenter, S.J. & Ferm, V.H. (1974) Embryogenesis of sacral-tail malformations in lead-treated hamsters (Abstract). *Anat. Rec., 178,* 323

Carson, T.L., Van Gelder, G.A., Karas, G.C. & Buck, W.B. (1974) Slowed learning in lambs prenatally exposed to lead. *Arch. environ. Health, 29,* 154-156

Cawse, P.A. (1975) *A Survey of Atmospheric Trace Elements in the UK: Results for 1974,* Environmental and Medical Sciences Division, Harwell, Berks, Atomic Energy Research Establishment

Chamberlain, A.C., Clough, W.S., Heard, M.J., Newton, D., Stott, A.N.B. & Wells, A.C. (1975a) Uptake of lead by inhalation of motor exhaust. *Proc. R. Soc. Lond. B., 192,* 77-110

Chamberlain, A.C., Clough, W.S., Heard, M.J., Newton, D., Stott, A.N.B. & Wells, A.C. (1975b) Uptake of inhaled lead from motor exhaust. *Postgrad. med. J., 51,* 790-794

Chau, Y.K., Wong, P.T.S. & Saitoh, H. (1976) Determination of tetraalkyl lead compounds in the atmosphere. *J. chromatogr. Sci., 14,* 162-164

Chaube, S., Swinyard, C.A. & Nishimura, H. (1972) A quantitative study of human embryonic and fetal lead with considerations of maternal-fetal lead gradients and the effect of lead on human reproduction (Abstract). *Teratology, 5,* 253

Choie, D.D. & Richter, G.W. (1974a) Cell proliferation in mouse kidney induced by lead. I. Synthesis of deoxyribonucleic acid. *Lab. Invest., 30,* 647-651

Choie, D.D. & Richter, G.W. (1974b) Cell proliferation in mouse kidney induced by lead. II. Synthesis of ribonucleic acid and protein. *Lab. Invest., 30,* 652-656

Cikrt, M. (1972) Biliary excretion of ^{203}Hg, ^{64}Cu, ^{52}Mn, and ^{210}Pb in the rat. *Br. J. ind. Med., 29,* 74-80

Cikrt, M. & Tichy, M. (1975) Role of bile in intestinal absorption of ^{203}Pb in rats. *Experientia, 31,* 1320-1321

Clark, A.R.L. (1977) Placental transfer of lead and its effects on the newborn. *Postgrad. med. J., 53,* 674-678

Coker, D.T. (1978) A simple, sensitive technique for personal and environmental sampling and analysis of lead alkyl vapours in air. *Ann. occup. Hyg., 21,* 33-38

Conrad, M.E. & Barton, J.C. (1978) Factors affecting the absorption and excretion of lead in the rat. *Gastroenterology, 74,* 731-740

Constant, P., Marcus, M. & Maxwell, W. (1977) *Sample Fugitive Lead Emissions from Two Primary Lead Smelters,* Report No. EPA-450/3-77-031, Midwest Research Institute for US Environmental Protection Agency, Springfield, VA, National Technical Information Service, pp. 92-98

oK

Coogan, P., Stein, L., Hsu, G. & Hass, G. (1972) The tumorigenic action of lead in rats. *Lab. Invest., 26,* 473

Cooper, W.C. & Gaffey, W.R. (1975) Mortality of lead workers. *J. occup. Med., 17,* 100-107

Creason, J.P., Svendsgaard, D., Bumgarner, J., Pinkerton, C. & Hinners, T. (1976) Maternal-fetal tissue levels of 16 trace elements in 8 selected continental United States communities. *Trace Subst. environ. Health, 10,* 53-62

Cremer, J.E. & Callaway, S. (1961) Further studies on the toxicity of some tetra and trialkyl lead compounds. *Br. J. ind. Med., 18,* 277-282

Dalvi, R.R. & Robbins, T.J. (1978) Comparative studies on the effect of cadmium, cobalt, lead and selenium on hepatic microsomal monooxygenase enzymes and glutathione levels in mice. *J. environ. Pathol. Toxicol., 1,* 601-607

missing   MISSING
Damstra, T. (1977) Toxicological properties of lead. *Environ. Health Perspect., 19,* 297- CA
307   stucko

Davies, B.E. (1978) Plant-available lead and other metals in British garden soils. *Sci. total Environ., 9,* 243-262

Davis, R.K., Horton, A.W., Larson, E.E. & Stemmer, K.L. (1963) Inhalation of tetramethyllead and tetraethyllead. A comparison of the effects in rats and dogs. *Arch. environ. Health, 6,* 473-479

Deknudt, G. & Deminatti, M. (1978) Chromosome studies in human lymphocytes after *in vitro* exposure to metal salts. *Toxicology, 10,* 67-75

Deknudt, G., Léonard, A. & Ivanov, B. (1973) Chromosome aberrations observed in male workers occupationally exposed to lead. *Environ. Physiol. Biochem., 3,* 132-138

Deknudt, G., Colle, A. & Gerber, G.B. (1977a) Chromosomal abnormalities in lymphocytes from monkeys poisoned with lead. *Mutat. Res., 45,* 77-83

Deknudt, G., Manuel, Y. & Gerber, G.B. (1977b) Chromosomal aberrations in workers professionally exposed to lead. *J. Toxicol. environ. Health, 3,* 885-891

Delespaul, I., Peperstraete, H. & Rymen, T. (1977) *Analysis and calibration techniques for measuring airborne particulates and gaseous pollutants.* In: Kirchoff, W.H., ed., *Methods and Standards for Environmental Measurement,* National Bureau of Standards Special Publication 464, Washington DC, US Government Printing Office, pp. 617-623

Delves, H.T. (1977) Analytical techniques for blood-lead measurements. *J. anal. Toxicol., 1,* 261-264

De Silva, P.E. & Donnan, M.B. (1977) Petrol vendors, capillary blood lead levels and contamination. *Med. J. Aust., 1,* 344-347

Dingwall-Fordyce, I. & Lane, R.E. (1963) A follow-up study of lead workers. *Br. J. ind. Med., 20,* 313-315

DiPaolo, J.A., Nelson, R.L. & Casto, B.C. (1978) *In vitro* neoplastic transformation of Syrian hamster cells by lead acetate and its relevance to environmental carcinogenesis. *Br. J. Cancer, 38,* 452-455

Doe, J.B. (1978) *Batteries, secondary (lead-acid).* In: Grayson, M., ed., *Kirk-Othmer Encyclopedia of Chemical Technology,* 3rd ed., Vol 3, New York, NY, John Wiley & Sons, p. 654

Dunn, E.J., Jr (1973a) *Red lead.* In: Patton, T.C., ed., *Pigment Handbook,* Vol. 1, New York, NY, John Wiley & Sons, pp. 837-842

Dunn, E.J., Jr (1973b) *White hiding lead pigments.* In: Patton, T.C., ed., *Pigment Handbook,* Vol. 1, New York, NY, John Wiley & Sons, pp. 65-73

EEC (1974) Council Directive of 17 December 1973 on the fixing of maximum permitted levels for undesirable substances and products in feeding stuffs. *Off. J. Eur. Comm., L. 38,* 31-36

EEC (1975a) Proposal for a Council Directive relating to the quality of water for human consumption. *Off. J. Eur. Comm., C 214,* 2-17

EEC (1975b) Council directive of 16 June 1975 concerning the quality required of surface water intended for the abstraction of drinking water in the Member States. *Off. J. Eur. Comm., L 194,* 26-31

EEC (1976) First Commission Directive of 15 December 1975 amending the Annex to Council Directive 74/63/EEC of 17 December 1973 on the fixing of maximum permitted levels for undesirable substances and products in feeding stuffs. *Off. J. Eur. Comm., L 4,* 24

EEC (1977) Council Directive of 29 March 1977 on biological screening of the population for lead. *Off. J. Eur. Comm., L 105,* 10-17

EEC (1978) Council Directive of 29 June 1978 on the approximation of the laws of the Member States concerning the lead content of petrol. *Off. J. Eur. Comm., L 197,* 19-21

Epstein, S.S. & Mantel, N. (1968) Carcinogenicity of tetraethyllead. *Experientia, 24,* 580-581

Fabia, J. & Thuy, T.D. (1974) Occupation of father at time of birth of children dying of malignant diseases. *Br. J. prev. soc. Med., 28,* 98-100

Fairhall, L.T. & Miller, J.W. (1941) A study of the relative toxicity of the molecular components of lead arsenate. *Publ. Health Rep. (Wash.), 56,* 1610-1625

FAO/WHO (1972) Evaluation of mercury, lead, cadmium and the food additives amaranth, diethylpyrocarbonate, and octyl gallate. *World Health Organ. Food Addit. Ser., No. 4,* 46

Faoro, R.B. & McMullen, T.B. (1977) *National Trends in Trace Metals in Ambient Air - 1965-1974,* EPA-450/1-77-003, US Environmental Protection Agency, Washington DC, US Government Printing Office

Farris, F.F., Poklis, A. & Griesmann, G.E. (1978) Atomic absorption spectroscopic determination of lead extracted from acid-solubilized tissues. *J. Assoc. off. anal. Chem., 61,* 660-663

Ferm, V.H. (1969) The synteratogenic effect of lead and cadmium. *Experientia, 25,* 56-57

Ferm, V.H. & Carpenter, S.J. (1967) Developmental malformations resulting from the administration of lead salts. *Exp. mol. Pathol., 7,* 208-213

Ferm, V.H. & Ferm, D.W. (1971) The specificity of the teratogenic effect of lead in the golden hamster. *Life Sci., 10,* 35-39

Fischbein, A., Alvares, A.P., Anderson, K.E., Sassa, S. & Kappas, A. (1977) Lead intoxication among demolition workers: the effect of lead on the hepatic cytochrome P-450 system in humans. *J. Toxicol. environ. Health, 3,* 431-437

Fishbein, L. (1976) Environmental metallic carcinogens: an overview of exposure levels. *J. Toxicol. environ. Health, 2,* 77-109

Forbes, G.B. & Reina, J.C. (1972) Effect of age on gastrointestinal absorption (Fe, Sr, Pb) in the rat. *J. Nutr., 102,* 647-652

Forni, A., Cambiaghi, G. & Secchi, G.C. (1976) Initial occupational exposure to lead: chromosome and biochemical findings. *Arch. environ. Health, 31,* 73-78

Forycki, Z., Zegarski, W. & Bardzik, J. (1977) Two cases of suicidal tetraethyl lead poisoning. *Bull. Inst. Marit. trop. med. Gdynia, 28,* 179-185

Fowler, B.A., Woods, J.S., McConnell, E.E., Kimmel, C.A. & Grant, L.D. (1980) Chronic low-level lead toxicity in the rat. IV. Morphological and biochemical effects on the kidney. *Toxicol. appl. Pharmacol.* (in press)

Fox, J.G. & Boylen, G.W., Jr (1978) Analysis of lead in animal feed ingredients. *Am. J. vet. Res., 39,* 167-169

Furst, A., Schlauder, M. & Sasmore, D.P. (1976) Tumorigenic activity of lead chromate. *Cancer Res., 36,* 1779-1783

Garza-Chapa, R., Leal-Garza, C.H. & Molina-Ballesteros, G. (1977) Chromosome analysis in subjects exposed professionally to lead contamination. *Arch. invest. Med., 8,* 11-20

Gath, J. & Thiess, A.M. (1972) Chromosome studies in chemical workers (Ger.). *Zbl. Arbeitsmed., 22,* 357-362

Gloger, W.A. (1968) *Pigments (inorganic).* In: Kirk, R.E. & Othmer, D.F., eds, *Encyclopedia of Chemical Technology,* 2nd ed., Vol. 15, New York, NY, John Wiley & Sons, p. 536

Goyer, R.A. & Krall, R. (1969) Ultrastructural transformation in mitochondria isolated from kidneys of normal and lead-intoxicated rats. *J. Cell Biol., 41,* 393-400

Goyer, R.A. & Rhyne, B.C. (1973) Pathological effects of lead. *Int. Rev. exp. Pathol., 12,* 1-77

Goyer, R.A., Leonard, D.L., Moore, J.F., Rhyne, B. & Krigman, M.R. (1970) Lead dosage and the role of the intranuclear inclusion body: an experimental study. *Arch. environ. Health, 20,* 705-711

Goyer, R.A., Tsuchiya, K., Leonard, D.L. & Kahyo, H. (1972) Aminoaciduria in Japanese workers in the lead and cadmium industries. *Am. J. clin. Pathol., 57,* 635-642

Grant, L.D., Kimmel, C.A., Martinez-Vargas, C.M. & West, G.L. (1976) Assessment of developmental toxicity associated with chronic lead exposure. *Environ. Health Perspect., 17,* 290

Green, M. & Gruener, N. (1974) Transfer of lead *via* placenta and milk. *Res. Commun. chem. Pathol. Pharmacol., 8,* 735-738

Greenfield, I. (1957) Lead poisoning. X. Effects of lead absorption on the products of conception. *New York State J. Med., 57,* 4032-4034

Greifer, B., Heinrich, K., Durst, R. & Menis, O. (1972) *Experimental Evaluation of Analytical Methods for Determining Lead in Paint and Building Materials,* NBS Report 10 674, Washington DC, National Bureau of Standards

Haas, T., Wieck, A.G., Schaller, K.H., Mache, K. & Valentin, H. (1972) The usual lead load in newborn infants and their mothers (Ger.). *Zbl. Bakt. Hyg. 1 Abt. B, 155,* 341-349

Hakulinen, T., Salonen, T. & Teppo, L. (1976) Cancer in the offspring of fathers in hydro-carbon-related occupations. *Br. J. prev. soc. Med., 30,* 138-140

Hancock, S. & Slater, A. (1975) A specific method for the determination of trace concentrations of tetramethyl- and tetraethyllead vapours in air. *Analyst, 100,* 422-429

Hansen, K.S. & Sharp, F.R. (1978) Gasoline sniffing, lead poisoning and myoclonus. *J. Am. med. Assoc., 240,* 1375-1376

Hansmann, G.H. & Perry, M.C. (1940) Lead absorption and intoxication in man unasso-ciated with occupations or industrial hazards. *Arch. Pathol., 30,* 226-239

Harris, P. & Holley, M.R. (1972) Lead levels in cord blood. *Pediatrics, 49,* 606-608

Harrison, R.M. & Laxen, D.P.H. (1977) A comparative study of methods for the analysis of total lead in soils. *Water Air Soil Pollut., 8,* 387-392

Harrison, R.M. & Perry, R. (1977) The analysis of tetraalkyl lead compounds and their significance as urban air pollutants. *Atmos. Environ., 11,* 847-852

Hass, G.M., Brown, D.V.L., Eisenstein, R. & Hemmens, A. (1964) Relations between lead poisoning in rabbit and man. *Am. J. Pathol., 45,* 691-727

Hass, G.M., McDonald, J.H., Oyasu, R., Battifora, H.A. & Paloucek, J.T. (1967) *Renal neoplasia induced by combinations of dietary lead subacetate and N-2-fluorenyl-acetamide.* In: King, J.S. Jr, ed., *Renal Neoplasia,* Boston, Little-Brown Co., pp. 377-412

Hawley, G.G.,ed. (1977) *The Condensed Chemical Dictionary,* 9th ed., New York, Van Nostrand-Reinhold, p. 506

Heit, M. (1977) An interlaboratory comparison of trace element analyses of a near shore marine sediment. *Environmental Quality (US Energy Research and Development Administration Health and Safety Laboratory) (Oct),* Washington DC, National Technical Information Service, pp. I-25 - I-37

Hilbelink, D.R., Kaplan, S. & Long, S.Y. (1976) Morphological analysis of cadmium and lead induced sirenomelia in golden hamster (Abstract). *Teratology, 13,* **24A/25A**

Hoffman, D.J. & Niyogi, S.K. (1977) Metal mutagens and carcinogens affect RNA synthesis rates in a distinct manner. *Science, 198,* 513-514

Hogan, G.R. & Adams, D.P. (1979) Lead-induced leukocytosis in female mice. *Arch. Toxicol., 41,* 295-300

Hollett, B.A. (1976) *Health Hazard Evaluation Determination, Report No. 75-182-334, New England Foundry, Lawrence, Massachusetts,* National Institute for Occupational Safety & Health, Springfield, VA, National Technical Information Service

Holyńska, B. (1974) *The Use of Chelating Ion Exchanger in Conjunction with Radioiso-tope X-Ray Spectrometry for Determination of Trace Amounts of Metals in Water,* Cracow, Poland, International Atomic Energy Agency

Hopkins, A.P. & Dayan, A.D. (1974) The pathology of experimental lead encephalopathy in the baboon *(Papio anubis)*. *Br. J. ind. Med., 31,* 128-133

Horn Rummo, J., Routh, D.K., Rummo, N.J. & Brown, J.F. (1979) Behavioral and neurological effects of symptomatic and asymptomatic lead exposure in children. *Arch. environ. Health, 34,* 120-124

Hower, J., Prinz, B. & Gono, E. (1976) The importance of lead pollution for pregnant women and the newborn in the Ruhr area. II. Communication (Ger.). *Zbl. Bakt. Hyg. 1 Abt. B, 162,* 70-76

Hubermont, G., Buchet, J.-P., Roels, H. & Lauwerys, R. (1976) Effect of short-term administration of lead to pregnant rats. *Toxicology, 5,* 379-384

Hubermont, G., Buchet, J.P., Roels, H. & Lauwerys, R. (1978) Placental transfer of lead, mercury and cadmium in women living in a rural area. *Int. Arch. occup. environ. Health, 41,* 117-124

Hursh, J.B. (1973) Retention of ^{210}Pb in beagle dogs. *Health Phys., 25,* 29-35

IARC (1972) *IARC Monographs on the Evaluation of Carcinogenic Risk of Chemicals to Man,* Vol. 1, pp. 40-50

IARC (1973) *IARC Monographs on the Evaluation of Carcinogenic Risk of Chemicals to Man,* Vol. 2, *Some Inorganic and Organometallic Compounds,* pp. 150-160

IARC (1977) *IARC Monographs on the Evaluation of the Carcinogenic Risk of Chemicals to Man,* Vol. 15, *Some Fumigants, the Herbicides 2,4-D and 2,4,5-T, Chlorinated Dibenzodioxins and Miscellaneous Industrial Chemicals,* pp. 195-209

IARC (1979) *IARC Monographs on the Evaluation of the Carcinogenic Risk of Chemicals to Humans,* Vol. 19, *Some Monomers, Plastics and Synthetic Elastomers, and Acrolein,* pp. 402-411

IARC (1980) *IARC Monographs on the Evaluation of the Carcinogenic Risk of Chemicals to Humans,* Vol. 20, *Some Halogenated Hydrocarbons,* pp. 429-448

Irwig, L.M., Rocks, P., Harrison, W.O., Webster, I. & Andrew, M. (1978) Lead and morbidity: a dose-response relationship. *Lancet, ii,* 4-7

Ito, N. (1973) Experimental studies on tumors of the urinary system of rats induced by chemical carcinogens. *Acta pathol. jpn., 23,* 87-109

Ito, N., Hiasa, Y., Kamamoto, Y., Makiura, S., Sugihara, S., Marugami, M. & Okajima, E.M. (1971) Histopathological analysis of kidney tumors in rats induced by chemical carcinogens. *Gann, 62,* 435-444

Jackson, K.W., Marczak, E. & Mitchell, D.G. (1978) Rapid determination of lead in biological tissues by microsampling-cup atomic absorption spectrometry. *Anal. chem. Acta, 97,* 37-42

Jacquet, P. & Gerber, G.B. (1979) Teratogenic effects of lead in the mouse. *Biomedicine, 30,* 223-229

Jacquet, P., Léonard, A. & Gerber, G.B. (1975) Embryonic death in mouse due to lead exposure. *Experientia, 31,* 1312-1313

Jacquet, P., Gerber, G.B. & Maes, J. (1977a) Biochemical studies in embryos after exposure of pregnant mice to dietary lead. *Bull environ. Contam. Toxicol., 18,* 271-277

Jacquet, P., Léonard, A. & Gerber, G.B. (1977b) Cytogenetic investigations on mice treated with lead. *J. Toxicol. environ. Health, 2,* 619-624

Jecklin, L. (1956) Lead dust and lung cancer (Ger.). *Schweiz. med. Wschr., 86,* 891-892

Johnson, D.E., Tillery, J.B., Hosenfeld, J.M. & Register, J.W. (1974) *Development of Analytic Techniques to Measure Human Exposure to Fuel Additives,* Report No. EPA-650/1-74-003, Southwest Research Institute for US Environmental Protection Agency, Springfield, VA, National Technical Information Service

Johnson, D.E., Tillery, J.B. & Prevost, R.J. (1975) Trace metals in occupationally and non-occupationally exposed individuals. *Environ. Health Perspect., 10,* 151-158

Jolly, S.E. (1967) *Naphthenic acids.* In: Kirk, R.E. & Othmer, D.F., eds, *Encyclopedia of Chemical Technology,* 2nd ed., Vol. 13, New York, NY, John Wiley & Sons, pp. 732-733

Kada, T., Hirano, K. & Shirasu, Y. (1980) Screening of environmental chemical mutagens by the *rec*-assay system with *Bacillus subtilis. Chem. Mutagens, 6* (in press)

Kantor, A.F., Curnen, M.G. McC., Meigs, J.W. & Flannery, J.T. (1979) Occupations of fathers of patients with Wilms's tumour. *J. Epidemiol. Community Health, 33,* 253-256

Kennedy, G.L. & Arnold, D.W. (1971) Absence of mutagenic effects after treatment of mice with lead compounds. *Environ. Mutagen Soc. Newsl., 5,* 37

Kennedy, G.L., Arnold, D.W. & Calandra, J.C. (1975) Teratogenic evaluation of lead compounds in mice and rats. *Food Cosmet. Toxicol., 13,* 629-632

Kerfoot, W.B. & Crawford, R.L. (1977) Rapid multielement analysis of trace metals in seawater by a laminate membrane adsorptive disc for inductively coupled plasma atomic emission spectroscopy. *Int. Classif. Patents Inf. Newsl., 2,* 289-300

Key, M.M., Henschel, A.F., Butler, J., Ligo, R.N. & Tabershaw, I.R., eds (1977) *Occupational Diseases. A Guide to their Recognition,* revised ed., US Department of Health, Education , & Welfare, National Institute for Occupational Safety & Health, Washington DC, US Government Printing Office, pp. 361-366

Kobayashi, N. & Okamoto, T. (1974) Effects of lead oxide on the induction of lung tumors in Syrian hamsters. *J. natl Cancer Inst., 52,* 1605-1610

Koller, L.D. & Brauner, J.A. (1977) Decreased B-lymphocyte response after exposure to lead and cadmium. *Toxicol. appl. Pharmacol., 42,* 621-624

Koller, L.D. & Kovacic, S. (1974) Decreased antibody formation in mice exposed to lead. *Nature, 250,* 148-150

Kroes, R., Van Logten, M.J., Berkvens, J.M., de Vries, T. & van Esch, G.J. (1974) Study on the carcinogenicity of lead arsenate and sodium arsenate and on the possible synergistic effect of diethylnitrosamine. *Food Cosmet. Toxicol., 12,* 671-679

Kruckenberg, S.M., Dennis, S.M., Leipold, H.W., Oehme, F.W. & Cook, J.E. (1976) Teratogenicity of lead acetate in *Microtus ochrogaster* (prairie voles). *Vet. Toxicol., 18,* 58-60

Lancranjan, I., Popescu, H.I., Găvănescu, O., Klepsch, I. & Serbănescu, M. (1975) Reproductive ability of workmen occupationally exposed to lead. *Arch. environ. Health, 30,* 396-401

Lead Industries Association, Inc. (1978) *Annual Review 1977 US Lead Industry,* New York, NY

Léonard, A. & Gerber, G.B. (1973) Genetic hazards of lead poisoning (Fr.). *Ann. Gembloux, 79,* 109-119

Léonard, A., Linden, G. & Gerber, G.B. (1973) *Study in the mouse of genetic and cytogenetic effects of lead contamination* (Fr.). In: *Proceedings of the International Symposium on Environmental Health Aspects of Lead,* Luxembourg, Commission of the European Communities, pp. 303-309

Léonard, A., Deknudt, G. & Debackere, M. (1974) Cytogenetic investigations on leucocytes of cattle intoxicated with heavy metals. *Toxicology, 2,* 269-273

Lilis, R., Eisinger, J., Blumberg, W., Fischbein, A. & Selikoff, I.J. (1978) Hemoglobin, serum iron, and zinc protoporphyrin in lead-exposed workers. *Environ. Health. Perspect., 25,* 97-102

Lloyd, R.D., Mays, C.W., Atherton, D.R. & Bruenger, F.W. (1975) ^{210}Pb studies in beagles. *Health Phys., 28,* 575-583

Lohring, D.H. (1978) Geochemistry of zinc, copper, and lead in the sediments of the estuary and Gulf of St Lawrence. *Can. J. Earth Sci., 15*(5), 757-772

Luckey, T.D. & Venugopal, B. (1977) *Metal Toxicity in Mammals,* Vol. 2, New York, NY, Plenum Press, pp. 185-195

Luster, M.I., Faith, R.E. & Kimmel, C.A. (1978) Depression of humoral immunity in rats following chronic developmental lead exposure. *J. environ. Pathol. Toxicol., 1,* 397-402

Mack, D.A. (1975) *Environmental Measurements of Air and Water Quality,* LBL 3818, Lawrence Berkeley Laboratory for US Energy Research & Development Administration, Berkeley, CA

Mahaffey-Six, K. & Goyer, R.A. (1970) Experimental enhancement of lead toxicity by low dietary calcium. *J. lab. clin. Med., 76,* 933-942

Mahaffey-Six, K. & Goyer, R.A. (1972) The influence of iron deficiency on tissue content and toxicity of ingested lead in the rat. *J. lab. clin. Med., 79,* 128-136

Manly, R. & George, W.O. (1977) The occurrence of some heavy metals in populations of the freshwater mussel *Anodonta anatina* (L.) from the river Thames. *Environ. Pollut., 14,* 139-154

Mao, P. & Molnar, J.J. (1967) The fine structure and histochemistry of lead-induced renal tumors in rats. *Am. J. Pathol., 50,* 571-603

Maruna, R.F.L., Maruna, H., Altmann, P., Georgiades, E. & Michalica, W. (1975) Placental lead content and urinary δ-aminolaevulinic acid excretion in mothers and their new-borns as an indicator of various exposures to lead (Ger.). *Wiener Med. Wochenschr., 125,* 678-681

Marzulli, F.N., Watlington, P.M. & Maibach, H.I. (1978) Exploratory skin penetration findings relating to the use of lead acetate hair dyes. Hair as a test tissue for monitoring uptake of systemic lead. *Curr. Probl. Dermatol., 7,* 196-204

McClain, R.M. & Becker, B.A. (1972) Effects of organolead compounds on rat embryonic and fetal development. *Toxicol. appl. Pharmacol., 21,* 265-274

McClain, R.M. & Becker, B.A. (1975) Teratogenicity, fetal toxicity, and placental transfer of lead nitrate in rats. *Toxicol. appl. Pharmacol., 31,* 72-82

McClain, R.M. & Siekierka, J.J. (1975a) The effects of various chelating agents on the teratogenicity of lead nitrate in rats. *Toxicol. appl. Pharmacol., 31,* 434-442

McClain, R.M. & Siekierka, J.J. (1975b) The placental transfer of lead-chelate complexes in the rat. *Toxicol. appl. Pharmacol., 31,* 443-451

Mellor, J.W. (1947) *A Comprehensive Treatise on Inorganic and Theoretical Chemistry,* Vol. 7, Chap. 47, *Lead,* London, Longmans, Green & Co., pp. 484-486, 638-639, 643, 706-707, 721-722, 829-830, 839, 856-857, 872, 876-886

Meredith, P.A., Moore, M.R. & Goldberg, A. (1977) The effect of calcium on lead absorption in rats. *Biochem. J., 166,* 531-537

Meredith, P.A., Moore, M.R., Campbell, B.C., Thompson, G.G. & Goldberg, A. (1978) Delta-aminolaevulinic acid metabolism in normal and lead-exposed humans. *Toxicology, 9,* 1-9

Metallgesellschaft Aktiengesesellschaft (1979) *Metallstatistik 1968-1978,* Vol. 66, Frankfurt

Michaelson, I.A. (1973) Effects of inorganic lead on RNA, DNA and protein content in the developing neonatal rat brain. *Toxicol. appl. Pharmacol., 26,* 539-548

Minear, R.A. & Murray, B.B. (1973) *Methods of trace metals analysis in aquatic systems.* In: Singer, P.C., ed., *Trace Metals and Metal-Organic Interaction in Natural Waters,* Ann Arbor, MI, Ann Arbor Science Publishers Inc., pp. 1-41

Ministry of Health & Welfare (1978) *Drinking Water Standards,* Tokyo

Modell, W., ed. (1977) *Drugs in Current Use and New Drugs,* New York, Springer, p. 74

Momcilovic, B. & Kostial, K. (1974) Kinetics of lead retention and distribution in suckling and adult rats. *Environ. Res., 8,* 214-220

Moore, M.R. & Meredith, P.A. (1979) The carcinogenicity of lead. *Arch. Toxicol., 42,* 87-94

Moore, M.R., Meredith, P.A. & Goldberg, A. (1977) A retrospective analysis of blood-lead in mentally retarded children. *Lancet, i,* 717-719

Morgan, A. & Holmes, A. (1978) The fate of lead in petrol-engine exhaust particulates inhaled by the rat. *Environ. Res., 15,* 44-56

Morgan, A., Holmes, A. & Evans, J.C. (1977) Retention, distribution and excretion of lead by the rat after intravenous injection. *Br. J. ind. Med., 34,* 37-42

Morris, H.P., Laug, E.P., Morris, H.J. & Grant, R.L. (1938) The growth and reproduction of rats fed diets containing lead acetate and arsenic trioxide and the lead and arsenic content of newborn and suckling rats. *J. Pharmacol. exp. Ther., 64,* 420-445

Morton, M.S. & Elwood, P.C. (1974) CNS malformations and trace elements in water (Abstract). *Teratology, 10,* 318

Mukherji, S. & Maitra, P. (1976) Toxic effects of lead on growth and metabolism of germinating rice (*Oryza sativa* L.) seeds and on mitosis of onion (*Allium cepa* L.) root tip cells. *Indian J. exp. Biol., 14,* 519-521

Muro, L.A. & Goyer, R.A. (1969) Chromosome damage in experimental lead poisoning. *Arch. Pathol., 87,* 660-663

Murray, H.M., Zenick, H. & Padich, R. (1977) The effects of lead exposure on the developing rat parietal cortex (Abstract). *Anat. Rec., 187,* 662

National Academy of Sciences (1972)   *Biologic Effects of Atmospheric Pollutants. Lead. Airborne Lead in Perspective*, Division of Medical Sciences and National Research Council, Washington DC, pp. 5-84, 131-144, 178-191, 226-248

National Institute for Occupational Safety & Health (1976) *NIOSH Analytical Methods for Set O*, PB-262 402/1 ST, Springfield, VA, National Technical Information Service

National Institute for Occupational Safety & Health (1978) *Criteria for a Recommended Standard - Occupational Exposure to Inorganic Lead, Revised Criteria - 1978*, US Department of Health, Education, & Welfare, Washington DC, US Government Printing Office, pp. IV-1 - IV-4, X-3 - X-17

National Paint & Coatings Association (1973) *Raw Materials Index*, Chemical Specialities Section, Washington DC, pp. 10-12

Nestmann, E.R., Matula, T.I., Douglas, G.R., Bora, K.C. & Kowbel, D.J. (1979) Detection of the mutagenic activity of lead chromate using a battery of microbial tests. *Mutat. Res., 66*, 357-365

Nishioka, H. (1975) Mutagenic activities of metal compounds in bacteria. *Mutat. Res., 31*, 185-189

Nordenson, I., Beckman, G., Beckman, L. & Nordström, S. (1978) Occupational and environmental risks in and around a smelter in northern Sweden. IV. Chromosomal aberrations in workers exposed to lead. *Hereditas, 88*, 263-267

Nordström, S., Beckman, L. & Nordenson, I. (1978a) Occupational and environmental risks in and around a smelter in northern Sweden. I. Variations in birth weight. *Hereditas, 88*, 43-46

Nordström, S., Beckman, L. & Nordenson, I. (1978b) Occupational and environmental risks in and around a smelter in northern Sweden. III. Frequencies of spontaneous abortion. *Hereditas, 88*, 51-54

Nordström, S., Beckman, L. & Nordenson, I. (1979a) Occupational and environmental risks in and around a smelter in northern Sweden. V. Spontaneous abortion among female employees and decreased birth weight in their offspring. *Hereditas, 90*, 291-296

Nordström, S., Beckman, L. & Nordenson, I. (1979b) Occupational and environmental risks in and around a smelter in northern Sweden. VI. Congenital malformations. *Hereditas, 90*, 297-302

Okuno, I., Whitehead, J.A. & White, R.E. (1978) Flameless atomic absorption spectroscopic determination of heavy metals in whole-fish samples. *J. Assoc. off. anal. Chem., 61*, 664-667

O'Riordan, M.L. & Evans, H.J. (1974) Absence of significant chromosome damage in males occupationally exposed to lead. *Nature, 247*, 50-53

O'Tuama, L.A., Rogers, J.F. & Rogan, W. (1979) Lead absorption by children of battery workers. *J. Am. med. Assoc., 241*, 1893

Oyasu, R., Battifora, H.A., Clasen, R.A., McDonald, J.H. & Hass, G.M. (1970) Induction of cerebral gliomas in rats with dietary lead subacetate and 2-acetylaminofluorene. *Cancer Res., 30*, 1248-1261

Parle, P.J. & Fleming, G.A. (1977) A spectrographic method for the determination of some heavy metals and boron in plant ash. *Irish J. agric. Res., 16*, 49-55

Patterson, C.C. (1965) Contaminated and natural lead environments of man. *Arch. environ. Health, 11*, 344-364

Pfaender, F.K., Shuman, M.S., Dempsey, H. & Harden, C.W. (1977) *Monitoring Heavy Metals and Pesticides in the Cape Fear River Basin of North Carolina*, Raleigh, NC, Water Resources Research Institute of the University of North Carolina, pp. 8-17, 85-94

Pierce, J.O., Koirtyohann, S.R., Clevenger, T.E. & Lichte, F.E. (1976) *The Determination of Lead in Blood. A Review and Critique of the State of the Art, 1975*, New York, NY, International Lead Zinc Research Organization, Inc., pp. 10-32

Portal, R.W. (1961) Cerebral tumour in a lead worker. *Br. J. ind. Med., 18*, 153-156

Prager, B., Jacobson, P., Schmidt, P. & Stern, D., eds (1922) *Beilstein's Handbuch der Organischen Chemie*, 4th ed., Vol. 4, Syst. No. 431-433, p. 639

Prigge, E. & Greve, J. (1977) Effects of lead inhalation exposures alone and in combination with carbon monoxide in nonpregnant and pregnant rats and fetuses. II. Effects of δ-aminolevulinic acid dehydratase activity, hematocrit and body weight. *Zbl. Bakt. Hyg., 1. Abt. B, 165*, 294-304

Pueschel, S.M., Kopito, L. & Schwachman, H. (1972) Children with an increased lead burden. A screening and follow up study. *J. Am. med. Assoc., 222*, 462-466

Rabe, F.W. & Bauer, S.B. (1977) Heavy metals in lakes of the Coeur d'Alene river valley, Idaho. *Northwest Sci., 51*, 183-197

Rabinowitz, M.B., Wetherill, G.W. & Kopple, J.D. (1973) Lead metabolism in the normal human: stable isotope studies. *Science, 182*, 725-727

Rabinowitz, M.B., Wetherill, G.W. & Kopple, J.D. (1976) Kinetic analysis of lead metabolism in healthy humans. *J. clin. Invest., 58*, 260-270

Rastogi, S.C. & Clausen, J. (1976) Absorption of lead through the skin. *Toxicology, 6*, 371-376

Reddy, T.P. & Vaidyanath, K. (1978) Synergistic interaction of gamma-rays and some metallic salts in the induction of chlorophyll mutations in rice. *Mutat. Res., 52*, 361-365

Rencher, A.C., Carter, M.W. & McKee, D.W. (1977) A retrospective epidemiological study of mortality at a large western copper smelter. *J. occup. Med., 19*, 754-758

Robinson, R.O. (1978) Tetraethyl lead poisoning from gasoline sniffing. *J. Am. med. Assoc., 240*, 1373-1374

Robinson, T.R. (1976) The health of long service tetraethyl lead workers. *J. occup. Med., 18*, 31-40

Roe, F.J.C., Boyland, E., Dukes, C.E. & Mitchley, B.C.V. (1965) Failure of testosterone or xanthopterin to influence the induction of renal neoplasms by lead in rats. *Br. J. Cancer, 19*, 860-866

Roels, H.A., Lauwerys, R.R., Buchet, J.-P. & Vrelust, M.-T. (1975) Response of free erythrocyte porphyrin and urinary δ-aminolevulinic acid in men and women moderately exposed to lead. *Int. Arch. Arbeitsmed., 34*, 97-108

Roels, H., Hubermont, G., Buchet, J.-P. & Lauwerys, R. (1978) Placental transfer of lead, mercury, cadmium, and carbon monoxide in women. III. Factors influencing the accumulation of heavy metals in the placenta and the relationship between metal concentration in the placenta and in maternal and cord blood. *Environ. Res., 16*, 236-247

Rom, W.N., (1976) Effects of lead on the female and reproduction: a review. *Mt Sinai J. Med., 43,* 542-552

Rosenblum, W.I. & Johnson, M.G. (1968) Neuropathologic changes produced in suckling mice by adding lead to the maternal diet. *Arch. Pathol., 85,* 640-648

Rosenkranz, H.S. & Poirier, L.A. (1979) Evaluation of the mutagenicity and DNA-modifying activity of carcinogens and noncarcinogens in microbial systems. *J. natl Cancer Inst., 62,* 873-892

Safe Drinking Water Committee (1977) *Drinking Water and Health*, Advisory Center on Toxicology, Assembly of Life Sciences, National Research Council, Washington DC, National Academy of Sciences, pp. 254-261

Sargent, D.H. (1975) *Water Pollution Investigation: Buffalo River*, EPA-905/9-74-010, Versar, Inc. for US Environmental Protection Agency, Springfield, VA, National Technical Information Service, pp. 4-5, 46-55

Sarto, F., Stella, M. & Acqua, A. (1978) Cytogenetic studies in twenty workers occupationally exposed to lead (Ital.). *Med. Lav., 69,* 172-180

Scanlon, J. (1972) Human fetal hazards from environmental pollution with certain non-essential trace elements. *Clin. Pediatr., 11,* 135-141

Schaller, K.H., Schiele, R., Weltle, D., Krause, C. & Valentin, H. (1976) The blood lead level of mothers and their newborns and the amount of lead in the tissue of human placenta in relation to the environment (Ger.). *Int. Arch. occup. environ. Health., 37,* 265-276

Schmid, E., Bauchinger, M., Pietruck, S. & Hall, G. (1972) Cytogenetic action of lead in human peripheral lymphocytes *in vitro* and *in vivo* (Ger.). *Mutat. Res., 16,* 401-406

Schroeder, H.A. & Mitchener, M. (1971) Toxic effects of trace elements on the reproduction of mice and rats. *Arch. environ. Health, 23,* 102-106

Schroeder, H.A., Mitchener, M. & Nason, A.P. (1970) Zirconium, niobium, antimony, vanadium and lead in rats: life term studies. *J. Nutr., 100,* 59-68

Schuller, P.L. & Egan, H. (1976) *Cadmium, Lead, Mercury, and Methylmercury Compounds: a Review of Methods of Trace Analysis and Sampling with Special Reference to Food*, Rome, Food & Agriculture Organization of the United Nations, pp. 29-57

Schwanitz, G., Lehnert, G. & Gebhart, E. (1970) Chromosome damage after occupational exposure to lead (Ger.). *Dtsch. med. Wschr., 95*, 1636-1641

Schwanitz, G., Gebhart, E., Rott, H.-D., Schaller, K.-H., Essing, H.-G., Lauer, O. & Prestele, H. (1975) Chromosome investigations in subjects with occupational lead exposure (Ger.). *Dtsch. med. Wochenschr., 100*, 1007-1011

Searle, C.E. & Harnden, D.G. (1979) Lead in hair-dye preparations. *Lancet, ii,* 1070

Senatskommission (1977) *Maximale Arbeitsplatzkonzentrationen, 1977*, Part. 13, Bonn, Deutsche Forschungsgemeinschaft, p. 16

Settle, D.M. & Patterson, C.C. (1980) Lead in albacore: guide to lead pollution in Americans. *Science, 207,* 1167-1176

Shakerin, M. & Paloucek, J. (1965) Intranuclear inclusions and renal tumors in rats fed lead subacetate. *Lab. Invest., 14,* 592

Shakerin, M., Paloucek, J., Oyasu, R. & Hass, G.M. (1965) Carcinogenesis in rats due to dietary 2AAF and lead subacetate. *Fed. Proc., 24,* 684

Shani, G. & Cohen, D. (1977) Measurement of Al, Si, Fe and Pb concentration in the air using 14 MeV neutron activation analysis. *Int. J. appl. Radiat. Isot., 28,* 672-673

Shapiro, H. & Frey, F.W. (1967) *Lead compounds (organic)*. In: Kirk, R.E. & Othmer, D.F., eds, *Encyclopedia of Chemical Technology*, 2nd ed., Vol. 12, New York, NY, John Wiley & Sons, pp. 282-299

Sharma, R.M. & Buck, W.B. (1976) Effects of chronic lead exposure on pregnant sheep and their progeny. *Vet. Toxicol., 18,* 186-188

Shupe, J.L., Binns, W., James, L.F. & Keeler, R.F. (1967) Lupine, a cause of crooked calf disease. *J. Am. vet. med. Assoc., 151,* 198-203

Simmon, V.F. (1979a) *In vitro* mutagenicity assays of chemical carcinogens and related compounds with *Salmonella typhimurium*. *J. natl Cancer Inst., 62,* 893-899

Simmon, V.F. (1979b) *In vitro* assays for recombinogenic activity of chemical carcinogens and related compounds with *Saccharomyces cerevisiae D3*. *J. natl Cancer Inst.,*
62, 901-909

Simmon, V.F., Rosenkranz, H.S., Zeiger, E. & Poirier, L.A. (1979) Mutagenic activity of
chemical carcinogens and related compounds in the intraperitoneal host-mediated assay.
J. natl Cancer Inst., 62, 911-918

Sirover, M.A. & Loeb, L.A. (1976) Infidelity of DNA synthesis *in vitro:* screening for potential metal mutagens or carcinogens. *Science, 194,* 1434-1436

Sissoëff, I., Grisvard, J. & Guillé, E. (1976) Studies on metal ions - DNA interactions:
specific behaviour of reiterative DNA sequences. *Prog. Biophys. mol. Biol., 31,* 165-199

Stella, M., Rossi, R., Martinucci, G.B., Rossi, G. & Bonfante, A. (1978) BUdR as a tracer of
the possible mutagenic activity of Pb^{++} in human lymphocyte cultures. *Biochem. exp.*
Biol., 14, 221-231

Stevenson, A.J., Kacew, S. & Singhal, R.L. (1977) Reappraisal of the use of a single dose of
lead for the study of cell proliferation in kidney, liver and lung. *J. Toxicol. environ.*
Health, 2, 1125-1134

Stoner, G.D., Shimkin, M.B., Troxell, M.C., Thompson, T.L. & Terry, L.S. (1976) Test for
carcinogenicity of metallic compounds by the pulmonary tumor response in strain A
mice. *Cancer Res., 36,* 1744-1747

Stowe, H.D. & Goyer, R.A. (1971) The reproductive ability and progeny of F_1 lead-toxic
rats. *Fertil. Steril., 22,* 755-760

Stowe, H.D., Goyer, R.A., Krigman, M.M., Wilson, M. & Cates, M. (1973) Experimental
oral lead toxicity in young dogs. Clinical and morphologic effects. *Arch. Pathol., 95,*
106-116

Stuik, E.J. (1974) Biological response of male and female volunteers to inorganic lead. *Int.*
Arch. Arbeitsmed., 33, 83-97

Sunderman, F.W., Jr (1971) Metal carcinogenesis in experimental animals. *Food Cosmet.*
Toxicol., 9, 105-120

Sunderman, F.W., Jr (1977) *Metal carcinogenesis.* In: Goyer, R.A. & Mehlman, M.A., eds,
Advances in Modern Toxicology, Vol. 2, Washington DC, Hemisphere Publishing Corp.,
pp. 257-295

Teodorescu, F. & Calugaru, A. (1972) Chromosomal changes produced in bone marrow cells of rats following intoxication by lead acetate (Rum.). *St. Si. cerc. biol. seria zoologie T., 24,* 451-457

Tesh, J.M. & Prictchard, A.L. (1977) Lead and the neonate (Abstract). *Teratology, 15,* 23A

Thompson, A.P. (1967) *Lead compounds.* In: Kirk, R.E. & Othmer, D.F., eds, *Encyclopedia of Chemical Technology,* 2nd ed., Vol. 12, New York, NY, John Wiley & Sons, pp. 268-282

van Thoor, J.W., ed. (1968) *Chemical Technology: An Encyclopedic Treatment,* Vol. 1, New York, NY, Barnes & Noble, pp. 559-563

Timperley, M.H. (1977) *The APDC-MIBK Method for the Analysis of Trace Metals in Waters,* Report No. CD 2257, Petone, New Zealand, Department of Scientific & Industrial Research

Torvik, E., Pfitzer, E., Kereiakes, J.G. & Blanchard, R. (1974) Long term effective half-lives for lead-210 and polonium-210 in selected organs of the male rat. *Health Phys., 26,* 81-87

Tsuchiya, K. (1979) *Lead.* In: Friberg, L., Nordberg, G.F. & Vouk, V.B., *Handbook on the Toxicology of Metals,* Amsterdam, Elsevier/North-Holland Biomedical Press, pp. 451-484

Tuna Research Foundation (1974) *Survey of Microconstituents in Canned Seafoods and Development of Protective Procedures,* Report No. NOAA-75013102, for the National Marine Fisheries Service, Springfield, VA, National Technical Information Service

UNEP/WHO (1977) *Lead (Environmental Health Criteria 3),* Geneva, United Nations Environment Programme/World Health Organization, pp. 21-27, 30-41, 44-68, 80-86

US Bureau of the Census (1947) *Facts for Industry, Inorganic Chemicals US Production 1939-1946,* Series M19A Supplement, US Department of Commerce, Washington DC, Industry Division, p. 5

US Bureau of the Census (1978) *US Exports Schedule B Commodity Groupings, Schedule B Commodity by Country,* FT410/December 1977, Washington DC, US Government Printing Office, p. 2-145

US Bureau of the Census (1979) *US Imports of Benzenoid Chemicals and Products: Chemical Elements, Inorganic and Organic Compounds, and Mixtures; and Drugs and Related Products for Consumption, December, 1978,* IM146, Schedule 4, Parts 1-3, US Department of Commerce, Springfield, VA, National Technical Information Service

US Bureau of Mines (1978) *Minerals Yearbook, 1976,* Vol. 1, US Department of the Interior, Washington DC, US Government Printing Office, pp. 727-755

US Bureau of Mines (1980) *Mineral Industry Surveys, Lead Industry in October 1979,* US Department of the Interior, Washington DC, US Government Printing Office, pp. 1-7

US Environmental Protection Agency (1976) *Environmental Protection Agency national interim primary drinking water regulations, 40 CFR 141.* In: *Environment Reporter Reference File,* Washington DC, Bureau of National Affairs, Inc., pp. 132:0101, 132: 0102

US Environmental Protection Agency (1977a) *Environmental Protection Agency effluent guidelines and standards, 40 CFR 421.* In: *Environment Reporter Reference File,* Washington DC, Bureau of National Affairs, Inc., pp. 135:0503-135:0510

US Environmental Protection Agency (1977b) *Environmental Protection Agency effluent guidelines and standards for inorganic chemicals, 40 CFR 415.* In: *Environment Reporter Reference File,* Washington DC, Bureau of National Affairs, Inc., pp. 135: 1301, 135:1322-135:1324

US Environmental Protection Agency (1978) *Environmental Protection Agency regulations on national primary and secondary ambient air quality standards, 40 CFR 50.* In: *Environment Reporter Reference File,* Washington DC, Bureau of National Affairs, Inc., pp. 121:0101-121:0102, 121:0117-121:0122

US International Trade Commission (1978) *Synthetic Organic Chemicals, US Production and Sales, 1977,* ITC Publication 920, Washington DC, US Government Printing Office, pp. 343, 349, 375

US Occupational Safety & Health Administration (1979) *Occupational safety and health standards, subpart Z - toxic and hazardous substances, 29 CFR 1910.* In: *Occupational Safety & Health Reporter Reference File,* Washington DC, Bureau of National Affairs, Inc., pp. 31:8301-31:8304, 31:8421-31:8429

US Tariff Commission (1925) *Census of Dyes and Other Synthetic Organic Chemicals, 1924*, TIS No. 33, Washington DC, US Government Printing Office, pp. 124-125, 130

US Tariff Commission (1946) *Synthetic Organic Chemicals, US Production and Sales, 1944*, Report No. 155, Second Series, Washington DC, US Government Printing Office, pp. 116-117

US Tariff Commission (1949) *Synthetic Organic Chemicals, US Production and Sales, 1947*, Report No. 162, Second Series, Washington DC, US Government Printing Office, p. 140

US Tariff Commission (1961) *Synthetic Organic Chemicals, US Production and Sales, 1960*, TC Publication 34, Washington DC, US Government Printing Office, p. 188

US Tariff Commission (1965) *Synthetic Organic Chemicals, US Production and Sales, 1964*, TC Publication 167, Washington DC, US Government Printing Office, p. 59

Valciukas, J.A., Lilis, R., Fischbein, A., Selikoff, I.J., Eisinger, J. & Blumberg, W.E. (1978) Central nervous system dysfunction due to lead exposure. *Science, 201*, 465-467

Vander, A.J., Taylor, D.L., Kalitis, K., Mouw, D.R. & Victery, W. (1977) Renal handling of lead in dogs: clearance studies. *Am. J. Physiol., 233*, 532-538

Van Esch, G.J. & Kroes, R. (1969) The induction of renal tumours by feeding basic lead acetate to mice and hamsters. *Br. J. Cancer, 23*, 765-771

Van Esch, G.J., Van Genderen, H. & Vink, H.H. (1962) The induction of renal tumours by feeding of basic lead acetate to rats. *Br. J. Cancer, 16*, 289-297

Van Gelder, G.A., Carson, T.L. & Buck, W.B. (1973) Slowed learning in lambs prenatally exposed to lead (Abstract). *Toxicol. appl. Pharmacol., 25*, 466-467

Van Wazer, J.R. (1968) *Phosphoric acids and phosphates.* In: Kirk, R.E. & Othmer, D.F., eds, *Encyclopedia of Chemical Technology*, 2nd ed., Vol. 15, New York, NY, John Wiley & Sons, pp. 275-276

Varma, M.M., Joshi, S.R. & Adeyemi, A.O. (1974) Mutagenicity and infertility following administration of lead sub-acetate to Swiss male mice. *Experientia, 30*, 486-487

Viets, J.G. (1978) Determination of silver, bismuth, cadmium, copper, lead, and zinc in geologic materials by atomic absorption spectrometry with tricaprylylmethyl-ammonium chloride. *Anal. Chem., 50,* 1097-1101

Wallace, G. & Koirtyohann, S.R. (1974) *The analysis of trace metals in sub-milligram quantities of biological material by flameless atomic absorption.* In: Hemphill, D.D., ed., *Trace Substances in Environmental Health,* VIII, Colombia, MO, University of Missouri

Watanabe, T., Iwahana, T. & Ikeda, M. (1977) Comparative study on determination of lead blood by flame and flameless atomic absorption spectrophotometry with and without wet digestion. *Int. Arch. occup. environ. Health, 39,* 121-126

Watkins, D., Corbyons, T., Bradshaw, J. & Winefordner, J. (1976) Determination of lead in confection wrappers by atomic spectrometry. *Anal. chim. Acta, 85,* 403-406

Weast, R.C., (1977) *Handbook of Chemistry and Physics,* 58th ed., Cleveland, OH, The Chemical Rubber Company, pp. B122-B124, C-701

Whitaker, G.C. (1965) *Driers and metallic soaps.* In: Kirk, R.E. & Othmer, D.F., eds, *Encyclopedia of Chemical Technology,* 2nd ed., Vol. 7, New York, NY, John Wiley & Sons, pp. 275-278, 287

White, C. & Patterson, J.W. (1912) Basic lead acetate. *Br. Patent No. 9638,* 23 April [*Chem. Abstr., 7*(19), 3425]

Whitfield, C.L., Ch'ien, L.T. & Whitehead, J.D. (1972) Lead encephalopathy in adults. *Am. J. Med., 52,* 289-298

WHO (1970) *European Standards for Drinking-Water,* 2nd ed., Geneva, World Health Organization, p. 33

WHO (1971) *International Standards for Drinking-Water,* 3rd ed., Geneva, World Health Organization, p. 32

WHO (1977) *Environmental Health Criteria 3: Lead,* Geneva

WHO (1979) *Summary Report of Data Received from Collaborating Centres for Food Contamination Monitoring Stage 1 - 1977 under the Joint FAO/WHO Food and Animal Feed Contamination Monitoring Programme Phase II,* WHO: HCS/FCM/78.2, Geneva

Wibberley, D.G., Khera, A.K., Edwards, J.H. & Rushton, D.I. (1977) Lead levels in human placentae from normal and malformed births. *J. med. Genet., 14,* 339-345

Wide, M. & Nilsson, O. (1977) Differential susceptibility of the embryo to inorganic lead during periimplantation in the mouse. *Teratology, 16,* 273-276

Willes, R.F., Lok, E., Truelove, J.F. & Sundaram, A. (1977) Retention and tissue distribution of ^{210}Pb(NO$_3$)$_2$ administered orally to infant and adult monkeys. *J. Toxicol. environ. Health, 3,* 395-406

Windholz, M., ed. (1976) *The Merck Index,* 9th ed., Rahway, NJ, Merck & Co., pp. 709, 711

Winell, M. (1975) An international comparison of hygienic standards for chemicals in the work environment. *Ambio, 4,* 34-36

Young, D.R., Jan, T.-K. & Moore, M.D. (1977) *Metals in power plant cooling water discharges.* In: *Coastal Water Research Project Annual Report,* El Segundo, CA, Southern Californian Coastal Water Research Project, pp. 25-31

Zawirska, B. & Medras, K. (1968) Tumours and disorders of porphyrin metabolism in rats with chronic lead intoxication (Ger.). *Zbl. allg. Path., 111,* 1-12

Zawirska, B. & Medras, K. (1972) The role of the kidneys in disorders of porphyrin metabolism during carcinogenesis induced with lead acetate. *Arch immunol. ther. exp., 20,* 257-272

Zegarska, Z., Kilkowska, K. & Romankiewicz-Wozniczko, G. (1974) Developmental defects in white rats caused by acute lead poisoning. *Folia Morphol., 33,* 23-28

Zetturlund, B., Winberg, J., Lundren, G. & Johansson, G. (1977) Lead in umbilical cord blood correlated with the blood lead of the mother in areas with low, medium or high atmospheric pollution. *Acta paediatr. scand., 66,* 169-175

Ziegler, E.E., Edwards, B.B., Jensen, R.L., Mahaffey, K.R. & Fomon, S.J. (1978) Absorption and retention of lead by infants. *Pediatr. Res., 12,* 29-34

Zollinger, H.U. (1953) Kidney adenomas and carcinomas in rats following chronic administration of lead and their possible relationship to the corresponding neoplasms in man (Ger.). *Virchows Arch. Pathol. Anat., 326,* 694-710

SUPPLEMENTARY CORRIGENDA TO *IARC MONOGRAPHS* VOLUMES 1-22

Corrigenda covering Volumes 1-6 appeared in Volume 7, others appeared in Volumes 8, 10, 11, 12, 13, 15, 16, 17, 18, 19, 20, 21, 22.

Volume 17

p. 91 (Table 1)	2nd column, last line	*replace* 4 *by* 3
	3rd column, 7th line	*replace* 62 *by* 67
	4th column, 7th line	*replace* 4 *by* 62

Volume 21

p. 63	last line	*add* a,b *after* (Nandi, 1978
p. 78	Nandi, S. (1978	*add* a
	Nandi, S. (1978	*add* b
p. 227	Rüdiger *et al.* (1979)	*replace by* Rüdiger, H.W., Haenisch, F., Metzler, M., Oesch, F. & Glatt, H.R. (1979) Metabolites of diethylstilbestrol induce sister chromatid exchanges in human cultured fibroblasts. *Nature, 281,* 392-394

Supplement 1

p. 23	6. ASBESTOS (Group 1)	*replace first paragraph by* All types of commercial asbestos fibres that have been tested are carcinogenic in mice, rats, hamsters or rabbits, producing lung tumours and/or mesotheliomas after inhalation or after intrapleural or intraperitoneal injection.

CUMULATIVE INDEX TO IARC MONOGRAPHS ON THE EVALUATION

OF THE CARCINOGENIC RISK OF CHEMICALS TO HUMANS

Numbers in bold indicate volume, and numbers in italics indicate page. References to corrigenda are given in parentheses. Compounds marked with an asterisk (*) were considered by the Working Groups, but monographs were not prepared because adequate data on their carcinogenicity were not available.

2-Amino-4-nitrophenol*

2-Amino-5-nitrophenol*

Amitrole   **7,** *31*

Amobarbital sodium*

Anaesthetics, volatile   **11,** *285*

Aniline   **4,** *27*   (corr. **7,***320*)

Anthranilic acid   **16,** *265*

Apholate   **9,** *31*

Aramite®   **5,** *39*

Arsenic and arsenic compounds   **1,** *41*

                                             2, *48*

                                            23, *39*

    Arsanilic acid
    Arsenic pentoxide
    Arsenic sulphide
    Arsenic trioxide
    Arsine
    Calcium arsenate
    Dimethylarsinic acid
    Lead arsenate
    Methanearsonic acid, disodium salt
    Methanearsonic acid, monosodium salt
    Potassium arsenate
    Potassium arsenite
    Sodium arsenate
    Sodium arsenite
    Sodium cacodylate

Asbestos   **2,** *17*   (corr. **7,***319*)

                                            14   (corr. **15,***341*)

                                                             (corr. **17,***351*)

    Actinolite
    Amosite
    Anthophyllite
    Chrysotile
    Crocidolite
    Tremolite

Auramine   **1,** *69*   (corr. **7,***319*)

Aurothioglucose   **13,** *39*

H

Haematite	1,	29
Haematoxylin*		
Heptachlor and its epoxide	5,	173
	20,	129
Hexachlorobenzene	20,	155
Hexachlorobutadiene	20,	179
Hexachlorocyclohexane (α-, β-, δ-, ε-, technical HCH and lindane)	5,	47
	20,	195
Hexachloroethane	20,	467
Hexachlorophene	20,	241
Hexamethylenediamine*		
Hexamethylphosphoramide	15,	211
Hycanthone and its mesylate	13,	91
Hydrazine	4,	127
Hydroquinone	15,	155
4-Hydroxyazobenzene	8,	157
17α-Hydroxyprogesterone caproate	21,	399
8-Hydroxyquinoline	13,	101
Hydroxysenkirkine	10,	265

I

Indeno[1,2,3-cd] pyrene	3,	229	
Iron-dextran complex	2,	161	
Iron-dextrin complex	2,	161	(corr. 7, 319)
Iron oxide	1,	29	
Iron sorbitol-citric acid complex	2,	161	
Isatidine	10,	269	
Isonicotinic acid hydrazide	4,	159	
Isoprene*			
Isopropyl alcohol	15,	223	
Isopropyl oils	15,	223	
Isosafrole	1,	169	
	10,	232	

IARC MONOGRAPHS ON THE EVALUATION
OF THE CARCINOGENIC RISK OF CHEMICALS TO HUMANS

SOME INORGANIC SUBSTANCES, CHLORINATED HYDROCARBONS, AROMATIC AMINES, *N*-NITROSO COMPOUNDS, AND NATURAL PRODUCTS
Volume 1, 1972; 184 pages
US$ 4.20; Sw. fr. 12.—
(OUT OF PRINT)

SOME INORGANIC AND ORGANOMETALLIC COMPOUNDS
Volume 2, 1973; 181 pages
US$ 3.60; Sw. fr. 12.—

CERTAIN POLYCYCLIC AROMATIC HYDROCARBONS AND HETEROCYCLIC COMPOUNDS
Volume 3, 1973; 271 pages
US$ 5.40; Sw. fr. 18.—

SOME AROMATIC AMINES, HYDRAZINE AND RELATED SUBSTANCES, *N*-NITROSO COMPOUNDS AND MISCELLANEOUS ALKYLATING AGENTS
Volume 4, 1974; 286 pages
US$ 7.20; Sw. fr. 18.—

SOME ORGANOCHLORINE PESTICIDES
Volume 5, 1974; 241 pages
US$ 7.20; Sw. fr. 18.—

SEX HORMONES
Volume 6, 1974; 243 pages
US$ 7.20; Sw. fr. 18.—

SOME ANTI-THYROID AND RELATED SUBSTANCES, NITROFURANS AND INDUSTRIAL CHEMICALS
Volume 7, 1974; 326 pages
US$ 12.80; Sw. fr. 32.—

SOME AROMATIC AZO COMPOUNDS
Volume 8, 1975; 357 pages
US$ 14.40; Sw. fr. 36.—

SOME AZIRIDINES, *N*-, *S*- AND *O*-MUSTARDS AND SELENIUM
Volume 9, 1975; 268 pages
US$ 10.80; Sw. fr. 27.—

SOME NATURALLY OCCURRING SUBSTANCES
Volume 10, 1976; 353 pages
US$ 15.00; Sw. fr. 38.—

CADMIUM, NICKEL, SOME EPOXIDES, MISCELLANEOUS INDUSTRIAL CHEMICALS AND GENERAL CONSIDERATIONS ON VOLATILE ANAESTHETICS
Volume 11, 1976; 306 pages
US$ 14.00; Sw. fr. 34.—

SOME CARBAMATES, THIOCARBAMATES AND CARBAZIDES
Volume 12, 1976; 282 pages
US$ 14.00; Sw. fr. 34.—

SOME MISCELLANEOUS PHARMACEUTICAL SUBSTANCES
Volume 13, 1977; 255 pages
US$ 12.00; Sw. fr. 30.—

ASBESTOS
Volume 14, 1977; 106 pages
US$ 6.00; Sw. fr. 14.—

SOME FUMIGANTS, THE HERBICIDES 2,4-D AND 2,4,5-T, CHLORINATED DIBENZODIOXINS AND MISCELLANEOUS INDUSTRIAL CHEMICALS
Volume 15, 1977; 354 pages
US$ 20.00; Sw. fr. 50.—

SOME AROMATIC AMINES AND RELATED NITRO COMPOUNDS—HAIR DYES, COLOURING AGENTS AND MISCELLANEOUS INDUSTRIAL CHEMICALS
Volume 16, 1978; 400 pages
US$ 20.00; Sw. fr. 50.—

SOME *N*-NITROSO COMPOUNDS
Volume 17, 1978; 365 pages
US$ 25.00; Sw. fr. 50.—

POLYCHLORINATED BIPHENYLS AND POLYBROMINATED BIPHENYLS
Volume 18, 1978; 140 pages
US$ 13.00; Sw. fr. 20.—

SOME MONOMERS, PLASTICS AND SYNTHETIC ELASTOMERS, AND ACROLEIN
Volume 19, 1979; 513 pages
US$ 35.00; Sw. fr. 60.—

SOME HALOGENATED HYDROCARBONS
Volume 20, 1979; 609 pages
US$ 35.00; Sw. fr. 60.—

CHEMICALS AND INDUSTRIAL PROCESSES ASSOCIATED WITH CANCER IN HUMANS
IARC MONOGRAPHS SUPPLEMENT 1, 1979; 71 pages
US$ 6.00; Sw. fr. 10.—

SEX HORMONES (II)
Volume 21, 1979; 583 pages
US$ 35.00; Sw. fr. 60.—

SOME NON-NUTRITIVE SWEETENING AGENTS
Volume 22, 1980; 208 pages
US$ 15.00; Sw. fr. 25.—

SOME METALS AND METALLIC COMPOUNDS
Volume 23, 1980; 438 pages
US$ 30.00; Sw. fr. 50.—

IARC Publications continued on inside back cover

IARC SCIENTIFIC PUBLICATIONS

WHO/IARC publications may be obtained, direct or through booksellers, from:

ALGERIA: Société Nationale d'Edition et de Diffusion, 3 bd Zirout Youcef, ALGIERS

ARGENTINA: Carlos Hirsch SRL, Florida 165, Galerías Güemes, Escritorio 453/465, BUENOS AIRES

AUSTRALIA: *Mail Order Sales:* Australian Government Publishing Service, P.O. Box 84, CANBERRA A.C.T. 2600; *or over the counter from* Australian Government Publishing Service Bookshops *at:* 70 Alinga Street, CANBERRA CITY A.C.T. 2600; 294 Adelaide Street, BRISBANE, Queensland 4000; 347 Swanston Street, MELBOURNE, VIC 3000; 309 Pitt Street, SYDNEY, N.S.W. 2000; Mt Newman House, 200 St. George's Terrace, PERTH, WA 6000; Industry House, 12 Pirie Street, ADELAIDE, SA 5000; 156–162 Macquarie Street, HOBART, TAS 7000 — Hunter Publications, 58A Gipps Street, COLLINGWOOD, VIC 3066 — R. Hill & Son Ltd, 608 St. Kilda Road, MELBOURNE, VIC 3004; Lawson House, 10–12 Clark Street, CROW'S NEST, NSW 2065

AUSTRIA: Gerold & Co., Graben 31, 1011 VIENNA I

BANGLADESH: The WHO Programme Coordinator, G.P.O. Box 250, DACCA 5 — The Association of Voluntary Agencies, P.O. Box 5045, DACCA 5

BELGIUM: Office international de Librairie, 30 avenue Marnix, 1050 BRUSSELS — *Subscriptions to World Health only:* Jean de Lannoy, 202 avenue du Roi, 1060 BRUSSELS

BRAZIL: Biblioteca Regional de Medicina OMS/OPS, Unidade de Venda de Publicações, Caixa Postal 20.381, Vila Clementino, 04023 SÃO PAULO, S.P.

BURMA: *see* India, WHO Regional Office

CANADA: *Single and bulk copies of individual publications (not subscriptions):* Canadian Public Health Association, 1335 Carling Avenue, Suite 210, OTTAWA, Ont. K1Z 8N8. *Subscriptions: Subscription orders, accompanied by cheque made out to the* Royal Bank of Canada, OTTAWA, Account World Health Organization, *should be sent to the* World Health Organization, P.O. Box 1800, Postal Station B, OTTAWA, Ont. K1P 5R5. *Correspondence concerning subscriptions should be addressed to the* World Health Organization, Distribution and Sales, 1211 GENEVA 27, Switzerland

CHINA: China National Publications Import Corporation, P.O. Box 88, BEIJING (PEKING)

COLOMBIA: Distrilibros Ltda, Pío Alfonso García, Carrera 4a, Nos 36–119, CARTAGENA

CYPRUS: Publishers' Distributors Cyprus, 30 Democratias Ave Ayios Dhometious, P.O. Box 4165, NICOSIA

CZECHOSLOVAKIA: Artia, Ve Smeckach 30, 111 27 PRAGUE 1

DENMARK: Munksgaard Ltd, Nørregade 6, 1165 COPENHAGEN K

ECUADOR: Librería Científica S.A., P.O. Box 362, Luque 223, GUAYAQUIL

EGYPT: Nabaa El Fikr Bookshop, 55 Saad Zaghloul Street, ALEXANDRIA

EL SALVADOR: Librería Estudiantil, Edificio Comercial B No 3, Avenida Libertad, SAN SALVADOR

FIJI: The WHO Programme Coordinator, P.O. Box 113, SUVA

FINLAND: Akateeminen Kirjakauppa, Keskuskatu 2, 00101 HELSINKI 10

FRANCE: Librairie Arnette, 2 rue Casimir-Delavigne, 75006 PARIS

GERMAN DEMOCRATIC REPUBLIC: Buchhaus Leipzig, Postfach 140, 701 LEIPZIG

GERMANY, FEDERAL REPUBLIC OF: Govi-Verlag GmbH, Ginnheimerstrasse 20, Postfach 5360, 6236 ESCHBORN — W. E. Saarbach, Postfach 101610, Follerstrasse 2, 5000 KÖLN 1 — Alex. Horn, Spiegelgasse 9, Postfach 3340, 6200 WIESBADEN

GHANA: Fides Enterprises, P.O. Box 1628, ACCRA

GREECE: G. C. Eleftheroudakis S.A., Librairie internationale, rue Nikis 4, ATHENS (T. 126)

HAITI: Max Bouchereau, Librairie "A la Caravelle", Boîte postale 111-B, PORT-AU-PRINCE

HONG KONG: Hong Kong Government Information Services, Beaconsfield House, 6th Floor, Queen's Road, Central, VICTORIA

HUNGARY: Kultura, P.O.B. 149, BUDAPEST 62 — Akadémiai Könyvesbolt, Váci utca 22, BUDAPEST V

ICELAND: Snaebjørn Jonsson & Co., P.O. Box 1131, Hafnarstraeti 9, REYKJAVIK

INDIA: WHO Regional Office for South-East Asia, World Health House, Indraprastha Estate, Ring Road, NEW DELHI 110002 — Oxford Book & Stationery Co., Scindia House, NEW DELHI 110001; 17 Park Street, CALCUTTA 700016 (*Sub-agent*)

INDONESIA: M/s Kalaman Book Service Ltd, Kwitang Raya No. 11, P.O. Box 3105/Jkt., JAKARTA

IRAN: Iranian Amalgamated Distribution Agency, 151 Khiaban Soraya, TEHERAN

IRAQ: Ministry of Information, National House for Publishing, Distributing and Advertising, BAGHDAD

IRELAND: The Stationery Office, DUBLIN 4

ISRAEL: Heiliger & Co., 3 Nathan Strauss Street, JERUSALEM

ITALY: Edizioni Minerva Medica, Corso Bramante 83–85, 10126 TURIN; Via Lamarmora 3, 20100 MILAN

JAPAN: Maruzen Co. Ltd, P.O. Box 5050, TOKYO International, 100-31

KOREA, REPUBLIC OF: The WHO Programme Coordinator, Central P.O. Box 540, SEOUL

KUWAIT: The Kuwait Bookshops Co. Ltd, Thunayan Al-Ghanem Bldg, P.O. Box 2942, KUWAIT

LAO PEOPLE'S DEMOCRATIC REPUBLIC: The WHO Programme Coordinator, P.O. Box 343, VIENTIANE

LEBANON: The Levant Distributors Co. S.A.R.L., Box 1181, Makdassi Street, Hanna Bldg, BEIRUT

LUXEMBOURG: Librairie du Centre, 49 bd Royal, LUXEMBOURG

MALAWI: Malawi Book Service, P.O. Box 30044, Chichiti, BLANTYRE 3

MALAYSIA: The WHO Programme Coordinator, Room 1004, Fitzpatrick Building, Jalan Raja Chulan, KUALA LUMPUR 05-02 — Jubilee (Book) Store Ltd, 97 Jalan Tuanku Abdul Rahman, P.O. Box 629, KUALA LUMPUR 01-08 — Parry's Book Center, K. L. Hilton Hotel, Jln. Treacher, P.O. Box 960, KUALA LUMPUR

MEXICO: La Prensa Médica Mexicana, Ediciones Científicas, Paseo de las Facultades 26, Apt. Postal 20–413, MEXICO CITY 20, D.F.

MONGOLIA: *see* India, WHO Regional Office

MOROCCO: Editions La Porte, 281 avenue Mohammed V, RABAT

MOZAMBIQUE: INLD, Caixa Postal 4030, MAPUTO

NEPAL: *see* India, WHO Regional Office

NETHERLANDS: Medical Books Europe BV, Noorderwal 38, 7241 BL LOCHEM

NEW ZEALAND: Government Printing Office, Mulgrave Street, Private Bag, WELLINGTON 1. *Government Bookshops at:* Rutland Street, P.O. 5344, AUCKLAND; 130 Oxford Terrace, P.O. Box 1721, CHRISTCHURCH; Alma Street, P.O. Box 857, HAMILTON; Princes Street, P.O. Box 1104, DUNEDIN — R. Hill & Son Ltd, Ideal House, Cnr Gillies Avenue & Eden St., Newmarket, AUCKLAND 1

NIGERIA: University Bookshop Nigeria Ltd, University of Ibadan, IBADAN — G. O. Odatuwa Publishers & Booksellers Co., 9 Benin Road, Okirigwe Junction, SAPELE, BENDEL STATE

NORWAY: J. G. Tanum A/S, P.O. Box 1177 Sentrum, OSLO 1

PAKISTAN: Mirza Book Agency, 65 Shahrah-E-Quaid-E-Azam, P.O. Box 729, LAHORE 3

PAPUA NEW GUINEA: The WHO Programme Coordinator, P.O. Box 5896, BOROKO

PHILIPPINES: World Health Organization, Regional Office for the Western Pacific, P.O. Box 2932, MANILA — The Modern Book Company Inc., P.O. Box 632, 926 Rizal Avenue, MANILA

POLAND: Składnica Księgarska, ul Mazowiecka 9, 00052 WARSAW (*except periodicals*) — BKWZ Ruch, ul Wronia 23, 00840 WARSAW (*periodicals only*)

PORTUGAL: Livraria Rodrigues, 186 Rua do Ouro, LISBON 2

SIERRA LEONE: Njala University College Bookshop (University of Sierra Leone), Private Mail Bag, FREETOWN

SINGAPORE: The WHO Programme Coordinator, 144 Moulmein Road, G.P.O. Box 3457, SINGAPORE 1 — Select Books (Pte) Ltd, 215 Tanglin Shopping Centre, 2/F, 19 Tanglin Road, SINGAPORE 10

SOUTH AFRICA: Van Schaik's Bookstore (Pty) Ltd, P.O. Box 724, 268 Church Street, PRETORIA 0001

SPAIN: Comercial Atheneum S.A., Consejo de Ciento 130–136, BARCELONA 15; General Moscardó 29, MADRID 20 — Librería Díaz de Santos, Lagasca 95 y Maldonado 6, MADRID 6; Balmes 417 y 419, BARCELONA 22

SRI LANKA: *see* India, WHO Regional Office

SWEDEN: Aktiebolaget C.E. Fritzes Kungl. Hovbokhandel, Regeringsgatan 12, 10327 STOCKHOLM

SWITZERLAND: Medizinischer Verlag Hans Huber, Länggass Strasse 76, 3012 BERN 9

SYRIAN ARAB REPUBLIC: M. Farras Kekhia, P.O. Box No. 5221, ALEPPO

THAILAND: *see* India, WHO Regional Office

TUNISIA: Société Tunisienne de Diffusion, 5 avenue de Carthage, TUNIS

TURKEY: Haset Kitapevi, 469 Istiklal Caddesi, Beyoglu, ISTANBUL

UNITED KINGDOM: H.M. Stationery Office: 49 High Holborn, LONDON WC1V 6HB; 13a Castle Street, EDINBURGH EH2 3AR; 41 The Hayes, CARDIFF CF1 1JW; 80 Chichester Street, BELFAST BT1 4JY; Brazennose Street, MANCHESTER M60 8AS; 258 Broad Street, BIRMINGHAM B1 2HE; Southey House, Wine Street, BRISTOL BS1 2BQ. *All mail orders should be sent to* P.O. Box 569, LONDON SE1 9NH

UNITED STATES OF AMERICA: *Single and bulk copies of individual publications (not subscriptions):* WHO Publications Centre USA, 49 Sheridan Avenue, ALBANY, N.Y. 12210. *Subscriptions: Subscription orders, accompanied by check made out to the* Chemical Bank, New York, Account World Health Organization, *should be sent to the* World Health Organization, P.O. Box 5284, Church Street Station, NEW YORK, N.Y. 10249. *Correspondence concerning subscriptions should be addressed to the* World Health Organization, Distribution and Sales, 1211 GENEVA 27, Switzerland. *Publications are also available from the* United Nations Bookshop, NEW YORK, N.Y. 10017 (*retail only*), *and single and bulk copies of individual* International Agency for Research on Cancer *publications (not subscriptions) may also be ordered from the* Franklin Institute Press, Benjamin Franklin Parkway, Philadelphia, PA 19103

USSR: *For readers in the USSR requiring Russian editions:* Komsomolskij prospekt 18, Medicinskaja Kniga, MOSCOW — *For readers outside the USSR requiring Russian editions:* Kuzneckij most 18, Meždunarodnaja Kniga, MOSCOW G-200

VENEZUELA: Editorial Interamericana de Venezuela C.A., Apartado 50.785, CARACAS 105 — Librería del Este, Apartado 60.337, CARACAS 106 — Librería Médica Paris, Apartado 60.681, CARACAS 106

YUGOSLAVIA: Jugoslovenska Knjiga, Terazije 27/II, 11000 BELGRADE

ZAIRE: Librairie universitaire, avenue de la Paix Nº 167, B.P. 1682, KINSHASA I

Special terms for developing countries are obtainable on application to the WHO Programme Coordinators or WHO Regional Offices listed above or to the World Health Organization, Distribution and Sales Service, 1211 Geneva 27, Switzerland. Orders from countries where sales agents have not yet been appointed may also be sent to the Geneva address, but must be paid for in pounds sterling, US dollars, or Swiss francs.

Price: Sw. fr. 50.— US$ 30.00 Prices are subject to change without notice.

IARC/2/80